Advances in Organic Synthesis in Pharmaceuticals, Agrochemicals and Materials

Advances in Organic Synthesis in Pharmaceuticals, Agrochemicals and Materials

Guest Editors

Zhao-Yang Wang
Jiuzhong Huang

MDPI

Basel • Beijing • Wuhan • Barcelona • Belgrade • Novi Sad • Cluj • Manchester

Guest Editors

Zhao-Yang Wang
School of Chemistry
South China Normal University
Guangzhou
China

Jiuzhong Huang
School of Pharmacy
Gannan Medical University
Ganzhou
China

Editorial Office
MDPI AG
Grosspeteranlage 5
4052 Basel, Switzerland

This is a reprint of the Special Issue, published open access by the journal *Molecules* (ISSN 1420-3049), freely accessible at: https://www.mdpi.com/journal/molecules/special_issues/KEN2ILRU4H.

For citation purposes, cite each article independently as indicated on the article page online and as indicated below:

Lastname, A.A.; Lastname, B.B. Article Title. *Journal Name* **Year**, *Volume Number*, Page Range.

ISBN 978-3-7258-5861-3 (Hbk)
ISBN 978-3-7258-5862-0 (PDF)
https://doi.org/10.3390/books978-3-7258-5862-0

Contents

About the Editors

Zhao-Yang Wang

Zhao-Yang Wang is a professor at School of Chemistry, South China Normal University since 2005 and a provincial-level talent of "Guangdong Thousand Hundred and Ten Project" since 2010. With the support of scientific funds received from institutions such as National Natural Science Foundation of China, as a corresponding author or editor-in-chief, he has published more than 200 papers in SCI-cited journals, e.g., *Angew. Chem. Int. Ed.*, *Green Chem.*, *Org. Lett.*, and a series of chemistry textbooks, such as *Organic Chemistry*, *Green Chemistry General Textbook*, *Chemical History Humanities Textbook*, *Higher Organic Chemistry*, etc. As testament to his scientific research achievements in green chemistry, organic synthesis, functional molecules, polymeric materials, and fine chemicals, including over 30 authorized patents, he won the first-class prize of "Guangdong Provincial Science and Technology Award" in 2011, and the "China Patent Excellence Award" in 2022.

Jiuzhong Huang

Jiuzhong Huang is an associate professor in the School of Pharmacy at Gannan Medical University, China. His career bridges academic research and industrial application, positioning him at the forefront of pharmaceutical innovation. He earned his Ph.D. from the South China University of Technology, a foundation that equipped him with a strong background in advanced chemical research. Meanwhile, Dr. Huang spent nearly a decade from 2011 to 2020 in the pharmaceutical industry, working at HEC Pharm Group. During this period, he focused his research and development efforts on innovative drugs, gaining invaluable experience in the practical and applied aspects of drug discovery. His research interests are multifaceted, primarily centering on drug discovery and transition-metal catalysis. This dual focus allows him to explore novel synthetic methodologies and apply them directly to the development of new therapeutic agents.

molecules

MDPI

Editorial

Editorial on the Advances in Organic Synthesis in Pharmaceuticals, Agrochemicals and Materials

Jiuzhong Huang [1] and Zhao-Yang Wang [2,*]

[1] Jiangxi Province Key Laboratory of Pharmacology of Traditional Chinese Medicine, School of Pharmacy, Gannan Medical University, Ganzhou 341000, China; huangjz@gmu.edu.cn
[2] School of Chemistry, South China Normal University, Guangzhou 510006, China
* Correspondence: wangzy@scnu.edu.cn

This Special Issue, entitled "Advances in Organic Synthesis in Pharmaceuticals, Agrochemicals and Materials", offers a comprehensive overview of the latest progress and multifaceted applications in organic synthesis. It showcases the intricate science and artistry involved in molecular construction and highlights the field's profound impact across multiple disciplines.

A central theme of this collection is the development of novel synthetic methodologies that enable precise and controlled assembly of complex molecular architectures. These advances not only improve reactivity and selectivity but also open new pathways for producing pharmaceuticals, agrochemicals, and functional materials [1–6]. The eight selected contributions exemplify this evolution, presenting innovative approaches—including synthetic methodology, element organic chemistry, natural product total synthesis, and biological activity of small molecules—that enrich the synthetic toolkit while offering mechanistic insights and potential applications in catalysis, medicinal chemistry, and materials science [7–10].

Firstly, Ye et al. (2024) report a molybdenum-catalyzed anti-Markovnikov hydrosilylation of alkynes with high (E)-selectivity [11]. Using a commercially available $Mo(CO)_6$/dppb catalyst system under mild conditions, the method exhibits excellent functional group tolerance and regioselectivity. This work offers a cost-effective and sustainable alternative to noble-metal catalysts, with a proposed mechanism involving oxidative addition, migratory insertion, and reductive elimination supported by control experiments. The next contribution, by Ashirov et al. (2025), describes the synthesis and characterization of hydrogen-bonded di(hydroperoxy)alkane adducts with tricyclohexylphosphine oxide (Cy_3PO) [12]. These shelf-stable, crystalline compounds display high solubility in organic solvents and act as efficient oxidants, as shown in the rapid oxidation of triphenylphosphine. Structural and spectroscopic analyses have confirmed that hydrogen bonding weakens the P=O bond. This weakening enhances the compound's oxidative reactivity. Consequently, the solid peroxides now have new and promising possibilities for use in synthesis. In the third paper, Xu et al. (2025) investigate the dual role of N, N-dimethylformamide (DMF) in copper-catalyzed domino reactions toward Se-phenyl dimethylcarbamoselenoates [13]. Starting from aryl halides and selenium powder, the reaction proceeds under mild conditions with a broad substrate scope. Deuterium labeling and mass spectrometry studies indicate oxidative addition as the rate-determining step, offering an economical route to valuable organoselenium compounds. Liu et al. (2025), in the fourth paper, present a one-pot Heck/dehydration strategy for the total synthesis of trans-dehydroosthol and citrubuntin—key meroterpenoid intermediates [14]. By employing less reactive bromocoumarins and optimized base/solvent systems, the authors achieved high yields and stereoselectivity without protecting groups. This redox-neutral and atom-economical approach streamlines access to complex natural product frameworks.

The fifth contribution revisits the bioactivity of shikonin, previously identified as a strong SARS-CoV-2 Mpro inhibitor [15]. Cross-validation studies, however, revealed that inhibition occurred only in the absence of reducing agents such as DTT, suggesting shikonin acts as a non-specific cysteine protease inhibitor with associated cytotoxicity. Reactive oxygen species generation and bioreductive alkylation were implicated in its off-target toxicity. These findings highlight the need to modify the naphthazarin scaffold to develop specific Mpro inhibitors with improved safety profiles. In the sixth study, twenty novel 5-(1-amino-4-phenoxybutylidene)barbituric acid derivatives bearing an enamino diketone motif were synthesized and evaluated for herbicidal activity [16]. One compound, BA-1, demonstrated promising efficacy, a broad herbicidal spectrum, and good crop safety. Structure-activity relationship (SAR) studies indicated that steric, electronic, and lipophilic properties significantly influence activity. Molecular docking suggested that BA-1 binds effectively to NtPPO, indicating potential as a novel PPO inhibitor and a candidate for further optimization.

The seventh paper highlights disubstituted Meldrum's acid as a new carbon-based scaffold with sulfur(VI) fluoride exchange (SuFEx)-like reactivity [17]. Phenols proved optimal nucleophiles, while thiols and thiophenols—often problematic in classical SuFEx—exhibited comparable reactivity. Alcohols and amines required elevated temperatures, and sterically hindered nucleophiles remain challenging, motivating ongoing catalyst development. Lastly, Guest Editor Prof. Wang and Dr. Huang developed a nickel-catalyzed [2 + 2 + 2] cycloaddition of alkynes, nitriles, and allyl boronates [18]. This concise catalytic system allows efficient, regioselective synthesis of fused pyridine derivatives from readily available materials. Mechanistic studies underscored the essential role of the terminal double bond and the Bpin group.

As of 13 October 2025, these eight articles have collectively attracted 8303 views, averaging 1038 views per publication. Together, these studies underscore the critical roles of catalyst design, solvent participation, and reaction engineering in modern synthetic chemistry. They also reflect a shift toward sustainability—employing earth-abundant metals, stable oxidants, and domino processes to reduce waste and synthetic steps [19–21]. By bridging organic, inorganic, and materials chemistry, this Issue embodies the collaborative and interdisciplinary spirit driving innovation in the field.

We commend the authors for their contributions and encourage continued exploration into the mechanisms and applications of these promising methodologies.

Funding: The authors thanks to the National Natural Science Foundation of China (22361003), the Jiangxi Provincial Natural Science Foundation (20242BAB25591).

Conflicts of Interest: The authors declare no conflicts of interest.

References

1. Campbell, M.G.; Tobias Ritter, T. Late-Stage Fluorination: From Fundamentals to Application. *Org. Process Res. Dev.* **2014**, *18*, 474. [CrossRef]
2. Zhang, N.; Samanta, S.R.; Rosen, B.M.; Virgil Percec, V. Single Electron Transfer in Radical Ion and Radical-Mediated Organic, Materials and Polymer Synthesis. *Chem. Rev.* **2014**, *114*, 5848. [CrossRef]
3. Devendar, P.; Qu, R.-Y.; Kang, W.-M.; He, B.; Yang, G.-F. Palladium-Catalyzed Cross-Coupling Reactions: A Powerful Tool for the Synthesis of Agrochemicals. *J. Agric. Food Chem.* **2018**, *66*, 8914. [CrossRef]
4. Yang, X.; Jiang, S.; Jin, Z.; Li, T. Application of Asymmetric Catalysis in Chiral Pesticide Active Molecule Synthesis. *J. Agric. Food Chem.* **2024**, *72*, 17153. [CrossRef]
5. Yang, H.; Yu, H.; Stolarzewicz, I.A.; Tang, W. Enantioselective Transformations in the Synthesis of Therapeutic Agents. *Chem. Rev.* **2023**, *123*, 9397. [CrossRef] [PubMed]

6. Wang, Y.; Dana, S.; Long, H.; Xu, Y.; Li, Y.; Kaplaneris, N.; Ackermann, L. Electrochemical Late-Stage Functionalization. *Chem. Rev.* **2023**, *123*, 11269. [CrossRef]
7. Eftekhari-Sis, B.; Zirak, M.; Akbari, A. Arylglyoxals in Synthesis of Heterocyclic Compounds. *Chem. Rev.* **2013**, *113*, 2958. [CrossRef]
8. Liu, J.; Ren, H.; Tang, T.; Wang, J.; Fang, J.; Huang, C.; Zheng, Z.; Qin, B. The Biocatalysis in Cancer Therapy. *ACS Catal.* **2023**, *13*, 7730. [CrossRef]
9. Magano, J.; Dunetz, J.R. Large-Scale Applications of Transition Metal-Catalyzed Couplings for the Synthesis of Pharmaceuticals. *Chem. Rev.* **2011**, *111*, 2177. [CrossRef]
10. Brovetto, M.; Gamenara, D.; Méndez, P.S.; Seoane, G.A. C−C Bond-Forming Lyases in Organic Synthesis. *Chem. Rev.* **2011**, *111*, 4346. [CrossRef] [PubMed]
11. Ye, F.; Huang, Z.; Li, J.; Wang, Q.; Wu, L.; Li, X. Molybdenum-Catalyzed (E)-Selective Anti-Markovnikov Hydrosilylation of Alkynes. *Molecules* **2024**, *29*, 5952. [CrossRef] [PubMed]
12. Ashirov, R.; Todorovic, M.; Bhuvanesh, N.; Blümel, J. HydrogenBonded Di(hydroperoxy)alkane Adducts of the Type $Cy_3P{=}O{\cdot}(HOO)_2CHR$ (R = Alkyl). *Molecules* **2025**, *30*, 329. [CrossRef] [PubMed]
13. Xu, R.; Hu, S.; Wu, L.; Ning, Y.; Xu, J. N, N-Dimethylformamide's Participation in Domino Reactions for the Synthesis of Se-Phenyl Dimethylcarbamoselenoate Derivatives. *Molecules* **2025**, *30*, 747. [CrossRef]
14. Liu, Z.; Ge, B.; Gong, X.; Wang, F.; Lei, T.; Jiang, S. Novel One-Step Total Synthesis of trans-Dehydroosthol and Citrubuntin. *Molecules* **2025**, *30*, 1067. [CrossRef] [PubMed]
15. Cui, J.; Xiang, S.; Zhang, Q.; Xiao, S.; Yuan, G.; Liu, C.; Li, S. Design, Synthesis, and Biological Evaluation of 5,8-Dimethyl Shikonin Oximes as SARS-CoV-2 Mpro Inhibitors. *Molecules* **2025**, *30*, 1321. [CrossRef]
16. Chen, K.; Wang, S.; Fu, S.; Zhang, Y.; Gao, W.; Liu, J.; Liu, R.; Lei, K. Design, Synthesis and Herbicidal Activity of 5-(1-Amino-4-phenoxybutylidene)barbituric Acid Derivatives Containing an Enamino Diketone Motif. *Molecules* **2025**, *30*, 3445. [CrossRef]
17. Chen, B.; Wang, Z.; Peng, X.; Xie, J.; Sun, Z.; Li, L. Disubstituted Meldrum's Acid: Another Scaffold with SuFEx-like Reactivity. *Molecules* **2025**, *30*, 3534. [CrossRef]
18. Du, K.; Zhu, T.; Li, G.; Shi, T.; Li, C.; Hu, S.; Gao, R.; Wang, Z.-Y.; Huang, J. Ni-Catalyzed [2 + 2 + 2] Cycloaddition via the Capture of Azametallacyclopentadienes with Allyl Boronate: Facile Access to Fused Pyridine Derivatives. *Molecules* **2025**, *30*, 3629. [CrossRef]
19. Tang, C.; Qiu, X.; Cheng, Z.; Jiao, N. Molecular oxygen-mediated oxygenation reactions involving radicals. *Chem. Soc. Rev.* **2021**, *50*, 8067. [CrossRef]
20. Wang, X.; He, J.; Wang, Y.-N.; Zhao, Z.; Jiang, K.; Yang, W.; Zhang, T.; Jia, S.; Zhong, K.; Niu, L.; et al. Strategies and Mechanisms of First-Row Transition Metal-Regulated Radical C−H Functionalization. *Chem. Rev.* **2024**, *124*, 10192. [CrossRef]
21. Jia, H.; Tan, Z.; Zhang, M. Reductive Functionalization of Pyridine-Fused N-Heteroarene. *Acc. Chem. Res.* **2024**, *57*, 795. [CrossRef] [PubMed]

molecules

MDPI

Communication

Molybdenum-Catalyzed (*E*)-Selective Anti-Markovnikov Hydrosilylation of Alkynes

Feihua Ye, Zhaoyang Huang, Jiahao Li, Qiumin Wang, Lihuan Wu * and Xiang Li *

School of Environmental and Chemical Engineering, Zhaoqing University, Zhaoqing 526061, China; yefeihua@zqu.edu.cn (F.Y.); 18359851060@163.com (Z.H.); 13726079874@163.com (J.L.); 18129625361@163.com (Q.W.)

* Correspondence: zqwlh@126.com (L.W.); lix@zqu.edu.cn (X.L.)

Abstract: Herein, we report the first example of molybdenum-catalyzed (*E*)-Selective anti-Markovnikov hydrosilylation of alkynes. The reaction operates effectively with the utilization of minute amounts of the inexpensive, bench-stable pre-catalyst and ligand under mild conditions. Moreover, this molybdenum-catalyzed hydrosilylation process features the advantages of simple operation, excellent selectivity, and broad functional groups tolerance.

Keywords: (*E*)-vinysilanes; hydrosilylation; alkynes; molybdenum catalyst; synthetic method

1. Introduction

Silicon-containing molecules have been widely served as versatile building blocks towards modern organic synthesis and pharmaceutical chemistry [1–3]. Among these synthons, vinylsilanes possess the advantages of incomparable reactivity, low toxicity, high stability, and simple operations, and offer ample opportunities for post-synthesis manipulations in synthetic chemistry [4,5]. Therefore, the preparation of these molecules has been thoroughly investigated in recent years [6]. The most straightforward and atom-economic approach for accessing multifunctional vinylsilanes was the transition metal catalyzed hydrosilylation of alkynes [7]. However, the addition products of alkynes with silanes could be Markovnikov type α-vinylsilane isomers, anti-Markovnikov addition type β-(*E*), or β-(*Z*) vinylsilane isomers. Hence, the most challenging issue of these methods was the precise controlling of both regioselectivity and stereoselectivity of the desired addition products. Over the past few decades, noble metal catalysts (such as platinum [8,9], rhodium [10–12], palladium [13], iridium [14,15], ruthenium [16,17], and gold [18,19]) have been well established to tackle these selectivity challenges. For example, Jiménez's group reported the complete β-(*Z*) selectivity synthesis of vinylsilane via the cyclometalated rhodium(III)-triazolylidene homogeneous and heterogeneous terminal alkyne hydrosilylation catalysts [11]. Despite the ubiquitous utilization of these noble metal catalysts, restrictions like elevated and fluctuating catalyst expenses, prevalent side reactions, expensive and complex ligands have limited their applications. On the other hand, concerning the sustainable development of green chemistry, the combination of chemical, economic, and environmental concerns has stimulated the expedition of inexpensive, low-toxic base-metal catalysts, such as cobalt [20–28], iron [29–32], manganese [33], copper [34,35], and nickel catalysts [36].

In the past decades, cobalt catalysts have exhibited exceptional catalytic performance in the precise preparation of the desired isomers. As shown in Scheme 1, Deng and coworkers realized the Markovnikov hydrosilylation of alkynes by dicobalt carbonyl N-heterocyclic carbene catalyst with excellent α/β selectivity and functional group compatibility [26]. In addition, highly Z-selective Co-catalyzed hydrosilylation of alkynes has also been achieved by Ge' group, and both primary and secondary hydrosilanes were well-tolerated in this transformation [21]. Compared with β-(Z) products, the β-(E) isomers were thermodynamically more stable. As a consequence, effective catalytic systems for the highly regio- and stereoselective construction of β-(E) isomers have been investigated thoroughly in the past decades. Thomas reported a complex of the $MesBIPCoCl_2$ for stereoselective hydrosilylation of for electronically unbiased alkyl alkynes and primary hydrosilanes to synthesize the (E)-β-vinylsilanes with moderate (E)-selectivity [37]. In 2018, Ge and coworkers employed a combination of bench-stable $Co(acac)_2$ and bisphoshpine ligands for the regioselective and stereoselective hydrosilylation of terminal alkynes [38]. This catalytic system was activated by the reaction with hydrosilanes rather than air-sensitive activators, such as Grignard reagents or $NaBHEt_3$. The reaction conditions were extremely mild and practical, providing an effective method for the construction of (E)-β-vinylsilanes. Except for the cobalt catalyst, Zhan reported that iron catalyst also served as an alternative choice for the regio- and stereoselective (E)-β-vinylsilanes synthesis [29]. In 2024, Zhao and coworkers demonstrated significant progress in Cu-catalyzed asymmetric hydrosilylation to construct Si-seterogenic alkenyl silanes [35]. The simple Cu/(S)-Tol-BINAP catalytic system enabled the excellent regio-, stereo-, and enantioselectivities in the reaction. Despite the significant achievements that have been made in this field, considering the environmental and economic aspects, the exploration of new types of non-noble metal catalysts for highly selective hydrosilylation of alkynes remains appealing and desirable.

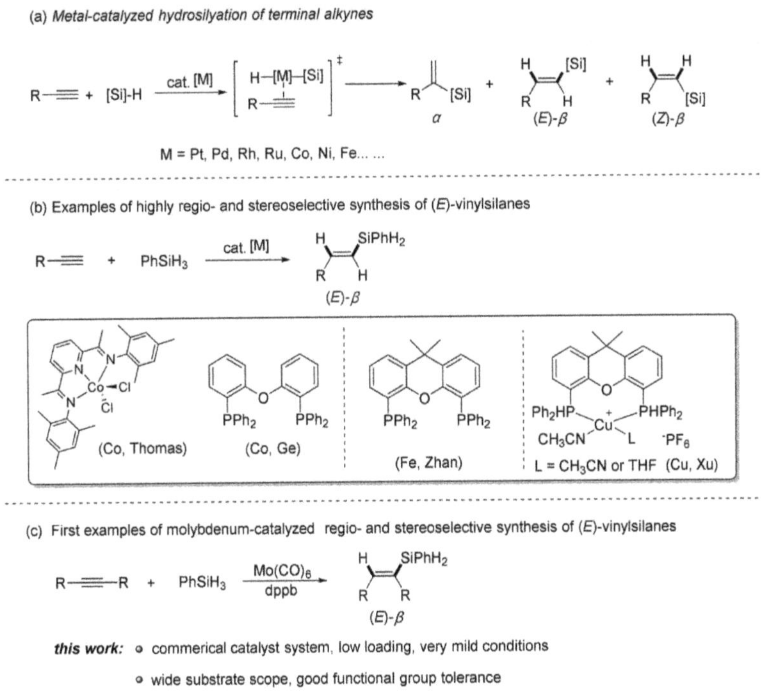

Scheme 1. Transition-Metal-Catalyzed Hydrosilylation of Terminal Alkynes.

Our group is committed to developing effective and practical organic reactions with excellent regio- and stereoselectivity [39–41]. Consequently, we disclose the first example of molybdenum-catalyzed regiodivergent and stereoselective synthesis of (E)-vinylsilanes with both aromatic and aliphatic alkynes after tremendous efforts.

2. Results and Discussion

Initially, our studies commenced with the hydrosilylation of phenylacetylene (**1a**) and $PhSiH_3$ (**2a**) as representative substrates to evaluate the optimal reaction conditions. Based on our previous work, we chose non-noble tungsten catalysis, such as W(CO)6, $W(CH_3CN)_3(CO)_3$, and $Mo(CO)_6$ as catalyst, t-BuOK as additive, PPh_3 as ligand, and MeCN as solvent. To our delight, the addition of product **3a** was indeed generated as expected with the combination of $Mo(CO)_6$ and PPh_3 (entries 1). However, the regioselectivity and stereoselectivity were not satisfied. The Markovnikov addition side product was generated in comparable yields (entries 1). For the purpose of increasing the efficiency and selectivity of this reaction, several commercial phosphine ligands (such as tri-tert-butylphosphine, dppb, dppe, dppbz, xantphos) were screened under identical conditions. These experiments revealed that the bidentate phosphine ligands demonstrated better selectivity than the monodentate phosphine ligands. Among these ligands, dppb displayed optimal regioselectivity and stereoselectivity (entries 3–9). Further investigation was concentrated on different types of solvents, such as THF, Et_2O, Toluene, EtOH, and H_2O. Fortunately, the implementation of THF was the better solvent both with respect to the reaction yield and the selectivity (entries 10–14). Subsequently, when adjusting the temperature from room temperature to 80 °C, neither the yield nor the selectivity of the reaction was enhanced (entries 15–16). Finally, controlled experiments indicated that the molybdenum catalysis and ligand were essential for this reaction (entries 17–18). Up to this point, the optimal reaction conditions were determined as follows: 1 mol% $Mo(CO)_6$, 1.2 mol% dppb, 5 mol% t-BuOK in 2 mL anhydrous THF at room temperature for 4 h.

Under the identified optimal conditions (entry 10 in Table 1), we turned to study the scope of aromatic terminal alkynes that underwent this molybdenum-catalyzed *E*-selective hydrosilylation reaction, and the results were presented in Scheme 2. Generally, a diverse array of terminal alkynes with various electronic substituents on the phenyl ring could participate very well to construct the (*E*)-vinylsilane products in high yield and selectivity. The electronic characteristics of aryl substituents in aromatic alkynes had no significant influence on the regioselectivity of this hydrosilylation process. Diverse substitution patterns (including methyl-, phenyl, trifluoromethyl- and halogen-) were all compatible in this reaction (**3a**–**3o**). These halogen substituents (F, Br and Cl) allowed further structural modification of these (*E*)-vinylsilanes. Moreover, the position of the substituents did not affect the generation of the expected products (**3k**–**3p**). Considering the synthetic interests, the fused-ring substrate was examined, the corresponding product obtained only in a slight decrease in the reaction yield (**3o**).

Table 1. Optimization of the reaction conditions [a].

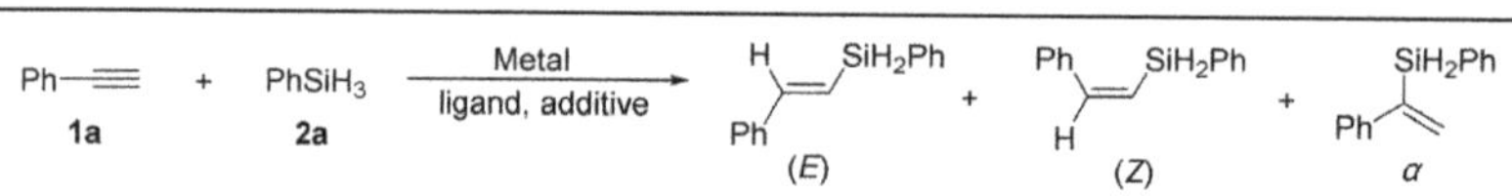

Entry	Catalyst	Ligand	Solvent	Yield (%) [b]	*E*/*Z*/α [b]
1	$W(CO)_6$	PPh_3	MeCN	n.d.	-
2	$W(CO)_3(CH_3CN)_3$	PPh_3	MeCN	n.d.	-
3	$Mo(CO)_6$	PPh_3	MeCN	80	75/0/25
4	$Mo(CO)_6$	$P(p\text{-Tol})_3$	MeCN	78	70/0/30
5	$Mo(CO)_6$	$P(^tBu)_3$	MeCN	n.d.	trace

Table 1. *Cont.*

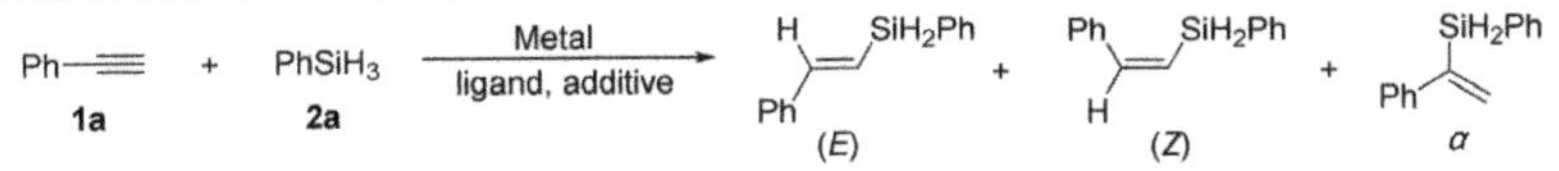

Entry	Catalyst	Ligand	Solvent	Yield (%) [b]	E/Z/α [b]
6	$Mo(CO)_6$	dppb	MeCN	85	98/0/2
7	$Mo(CO)_6$	dppe	MeCN	82	97/0/3
8	$Mo(CO)_6$	dppbz	MeCN	65	80/7/13
9	$Mo(CO)_6$	xantphos	MeCN	79	85/5/10
10	$Mo(CO)_6$	dppb	THF	90	98/0/2
11	$Mo(CO)_6$	dppb	Et_2O	78	95/0/5
12	$Mo(CO)_6$	dppb	Toluene	54	91/0/9
13	$Mo(CO)_6$	dppb	EtOH	trace	-
14	$Mo(CO)_6$	dppb	H_2O	n.d.	-
15 [c]	$Mo(CO)_6$	dppb	THF	86	95/0/5
16 [d]	$Mo(CO)_6$	dppb	THF	80	90/0/10
17	-	dppb	THF	n.d.	-
18	$Mo(CO)_6$	-	THF	43	54/12/34

[a] phenylacetylene **1a** (0.5 mmol), $PhSiH_3$ **2a** (0.75 mmol), ^{t}BuOK (5 mol%), catalyst (1 mol%), ligand (1.2 mol%), solvent (2 mL), room temperature, 4 h; dppb = 1,4-bis(diphenylphosphino)butane; dppe = 1,2-bis(diphenylphosphino)ethane; dppbz = 1,2-bis(diphenylphosphanyl)benzene; xantphos = 4,5-bis(diphenylphosphino)-9,9-dimethylxanthene; n.d. = not detected. [b] calculated by GC with decane as internal standard; [c] the reaction temperature was 40 °C; [d] the reaction temperature was 80 °C.

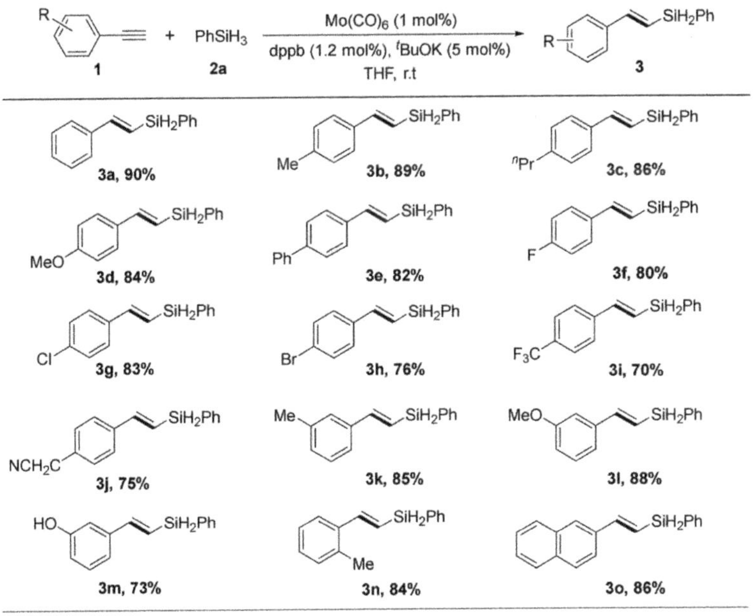

Scheme 2. Scope of terminal alkynes for the Mo/dppb catalyzed anti-Markovnikov hydrosilylation with $PhSiH_3$. Alkynes **1** (0.5 mmol), $PhSiH_3$ **2a** (0.75 mmol), $Mo(CO)_6$ (1 mol%), dppb (1.2 mol%), t-BuOK (5 mol %), anhydrous THF (2 mL), r. t., 4 h. Yields of isolated products. The selectivity for product (*β*-*E*-vinylsilane product: *α*-isomers) was ≥20:1, unless otherwise noted, determined by ^{1}H NMR spectroscopy.

The catalytic efficiency of the $Mo(CO)_6$/dppb system was further explored by using a variety of electronically unbiased alkyl alkynes. Pleasingly, all substrates transformed into the corresponding (*E*)-vinylsilane in good yields and excellent selectivity (both high stereoselectivity and regioselectivity) (Scheme 3). The halogen-substituted alkyl alkyne substrates were well-tolerated in this reaction with no dehalogenation observing. These halogen substituents undoubtedly allowed further structural modification of the vinylsilane. Except for the terminal alkynes, the internal substrates hex-3-yne (**2s**) could proceed this anti-Markovnikov hydrosilylation with lower yields and comparable selectivity. Unfortunately, secondary hydrosilane (Ph_2SiH_2) and tertiary hydrosilanes ($(EtO)_3SiH$) turned out to be inactive in this reaction.

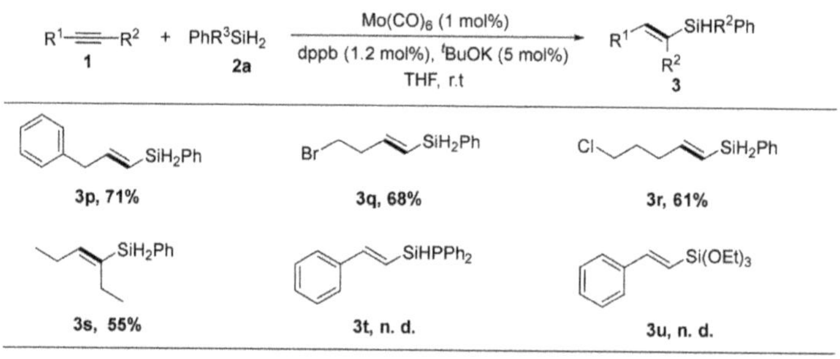

Scheme 3. Scope of alkynes for the Mo/dppb catalyzed anti-Markovnikov hydrosilylation with silanes. Alkynes **1** (0.5 mmol), $PhSiH_3$ **2a** (0.75 mmol), $Mo(CO)_6$ (1 mol%), dppb (1.2 mol%), *t*-BuOK (5 mol %), anhydrous THF (2 mL), r. t., 4 h, n.d. = not detected. Yields of isolated products. The selectivity for product (β-*E*-vinylsilane product: α-isomers) was $\geq$20:1, unless otherwise noted, determined by ^{1}H NMR spectroscopy.

To emphasize the usefulness of this practical procedure for the construction of (*E*)-vinylsilane, phenylacetylene (**1a**) and $PhSiH_3$ (**3a**), in the presence of $Mo(CO)_6$ and dppb, could be reacted to yield 87% at room temperature in 4 h on a 10 mmol scale. In addition, we also conducted further conversion of vinylsilanes via the Hiyama–Denmark coupling reaction to synthesize internal (*E*)-vinylarenes in 80% yield (Scheme 4).

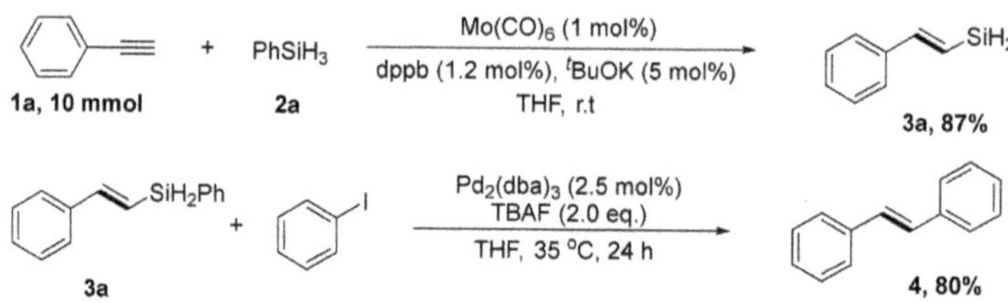

Scheme 4. Gram-Scale Synthesis and further transformations.

Based on mechanical experiments and prior studies [29,31,38], the plausible mechanism accounting for the syhthesis of (*E*)-vinylsilane was discussed in Scheme 5. Firstly, in the presence of dppb ligand and the base additive ^{t}BuOK, the molybdenum catalysis could react with $PhSiH_3$ to form the monohydrido species $L_nMo(H)(SiH_2Ph)$ (B) through the oxidative addition process. Subsequently, the key intermediate (C) was generated after the coordination of the alkyne and migratory insertion into the Mo-H bond. Finally, the expected product, (*E*)-vinylsilane, was afforded via the reductive elimination procedure.

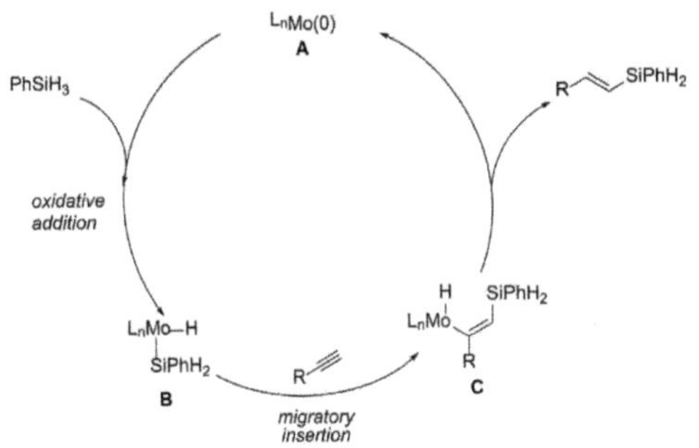

Scheme 5. Plausible Mechanistic Pathway.

3. Materials and Methods

3.1. Materials

All the reagents were obtained from commercial sources and used directly without further purification, unless otherwise noted. ^1H NMR and ^{13}C NMR spectra were recorded on a Bruker AVANCE III 400 MHz. ^1H NMR and ^{13}C NMR chemical shifts were determined relative to the internal standard TMS at δ 0.0. Chemical shifts (δ) are reported in ppm, and coupling constants (J) are reported in Hertz (Hz).

3.2. General Methods for the Preparation of (E)-Vinylsilanes

A 25 mL Schlenk tube was charged with $Mo(CO)_6$ (1 mol%) and was mixed with anhydrous THF (2 mL) in a glass vial equipped with a magnetic stirring bar. Then, dppb (1.2 mol%), ^{t}BuOK (5 mol%), phenylacetylene (**1a**; 0.5 mmol), and $PhSiH_3$ (**2a**, 0.75 mmol) were added. The mixture was stirred vigorously at room temperature for 4–6 h. After completing the reaction, then cooling to room temperature, the reaction mixture was washed with 10 mL H_2O, then diluted with EtOAc (10 mL). The organic phase was dried over $MgSO_4$ and concentrated in vacuo. The residue was purified by flash chromatography on silica gel using petroleum ether/ethyl acetate as the eluent to give the desired product (*E*)-phenyl(styryl)silane (**3a**).

4. Conclusions

In summary, a convenient and efficient molybdenum-catalyzed (*E*)-selective anti-Markovnikov hydrosilylation of alkynes and $PhSiH_3$ is disclosed. Compared with the reported works, we cannot claim that we possess the discernible superior advantages over the selectivity, scope, and efficiency. But considering the importance of the (*E*)-vinylsilanes, our reaction could provide alternatives for the construction of these compounds. This catalytic system relies on the natural abundance of molybdenum and the commercial, inexpensive dppb ligand. Furthermore, the advantages of readily available reagents, mild reaction conditions (room temperature, short reaction time and low catalyst and ligand loading), and good functional-group tolerance make this protocol practical for (*E*)-selective vinylsilane synthesis.

Supplementary Materials: The following supporting information can be downloaded at: https://www.mdpi.com/article/10.3390/molecules29245952/s1, the NMR data and spectra of the catalytic products.

Author Contributions: Writing—review and editing, F.Y.; investigation and methodology, Z.H., Q.W. and J.L.; data curation, Z.H. and L.W.; funding acquisition, F.Y. and X.L.; conceptualization, L.W. All authors have read and agreed to the published version of the manuscript.

Funding: This research was funded by the Zhaoqing University Science Fund (ZD202413), College Students' innovation and entrepreneurship training program (S202410580062, S202410580066), Zhaoqing University High-Level Project Training Programme Project (GCCZK202406), Zhaoqing

University Innovation Research Team Project (TD202413), Guangdong Provincial Key Laboratory of Eco-environmental Studies and Low-carbon Agriculture in Peri-urban Areas (2020B121201014).

Institutional Review Board Statement: Not applicable.

Informed Consent Statement: Not applicable.

Data Availability Statement: Data are contained within the article and Supplementary Materials.

Conflicts of Interest: The authors declare no conflicts of interest.

References

1. Langkopf, E.; Schinzer, D. Uses of Silicon-Containing Compounds in the Synthesis of Natural Products. *Chem. Rev.* **1995**, *95*, 1375–1408. [CrossRef]
2. Bracegirdle, S.; Anderson, E.A. Recent advances in the use of temporary silicon tethers in metal-mediated reactions. *Chem. Soc. Rev.* **2010**, *39*, 4114–4129. [CrossRef] [PubMed]
3. Rémond, E.; Martin, C.; Martinez, J.; Cavelier, F. Siliconcontaining amino acids: Synthetic aspects, conformational studies, and applications to bioactive peptides. *Chem. Rev.* **2016**, *116*, 11654–11684. [CrossRef] [PubMed]
4. Blumenkopf, T.A.; Overman, L.E. Vinylsilane- and Alkynylsilane-Terminated Cyclization Reactions. *Chem. Rev.* **1986**, *86*, 857. [CrossRef]
5. Komiyama, T.; Minami, Y.; Hiyama, T. Recent Advances in Transition-Metal-Catalyzed Synthetic Transformations of Organosilicon Reagents. *ACS Catal.* **2017**, *7*, 631–651. [CrossRef]
6. Roy, A.K. A review of recent progress in catalyzed homogeneous hydrosilation (hydrosilylation). *Adv. Organomet. Chem.* **2007**, *55*, 1–59.
7. Anderson, E.; Lim, D. Synthesis of Vinylsilanes. *Synthesis* **2012**, *44*, 983–1010. [CrossRef]
8. Shvydkiy, N.V.; Rimskiy, K.V.; Perekalin, D.S. Cyclobutadiene platinum complex as a new type of precatalyst for hydrosilylation of alkenes and alkynes. *Appl. Organomet. Chem.* **2023**, *33*, e7008. [CrossRef]
9. Ibáñez-Ibáñez, K.; Lázaro, A.; Mejuto, C.; Crespo, M.; Vicent, C.; Rodríguez, L.; Mata, J.A. Visible light harvesting alkyne hydrosilylation mediated by pincer platinum complexes. *J. Catal.* **2023**, *428*, 115155. [CrossRef]
10. Puerta-Oteo, R.; Munarriz, J.; Polo, V.; Jiménez, M.V.; Pérez-Torrente, J.J. Carboxylate-Assisted β-(Z) Stereoselective Hydrosilylation of Terminal Alkynes Catalyzed by a Zwitterionic Bis-NHC Rhodium(III) Complex. *ACS Catal.* **2020**, *10*, 7367–7380. [CrossRef]
11. Sánchez-Page, B.; Munarriz, J.; Jiménez, M.V.; Pérez-Torrente, J.J.; Blasco, J.; Subias, G.; Passarelli, V.; Álvarez, P. *β*-(Z) Selectivity Control by Cyclometalated Rhodium(III)-Triazolylidene Homogeneous and Heterogeneous Terminal Alkyne Hydrosilylation Catalysts. *ACS Catal.* **2020**, *10*, 13334–13351. [CrossRef]
12. Zhang, Z.; Yang, L.; Yi, M.; Wu, X.; Lu, Y. Dirhodium(II)/XantPhos Catalyzed Synthesis of β-(E)-Vinylsilanes via Hydrosilylation and Isomerization from Alkynes. *Chem. Eur. J.* **2024**, *30*, e202402406.
13. Ren, S.; Ye, B.; Li, S.; Pang, L.; Pan, Y.; Tang, H. Well-defined coordination environment breaks the bottleneck of organic synthesis: Single-atom palladium catalyzed hydrosilylation of internal alkynes. *Nano Res.* **2022**, *15*, 1500–1508. [CrossRef]
14. Roemer, M.; Gonçales, V.R.; Keaveney, S.T.; Pernik, I.; Lian, J.; Downes, J.; Gooding, J.J.; Messerle, B.A. Carbon supported hybrid catalysts for controlled product selectivity in the hydrosilylation of alkynes. *Catal. Sci. Technol.* **2021**, *11*, 1888–1898. [CrossRef]
15. Li, Q.; Gu, D.; Yu, D.; Liu, Y. Caged Iridium Catalyst for Hydrosilylation of Alkynes with High Site Selectivity. *ChemCatChem* **2022**, *14*, e202101727. [CrossRef]
16. Dai, W.; Wu, X.; Li, C.; Zhang, R.; Wang, J.; Liu, H. Regio-selective and stereo-selective hydrosilylation of internal alkynes catalyzed by ruthenium complexes. *RSC Adv.* **2018**, *8*, 28261–28265. [CrossRef]
17. Kanno, K.; Noguchi, S.; Ono, Y.; Egawa, S.; Otsuka, N.; Mita, M.; Kyushin, S. Ruthenium-catalyzed hydrosilylation of alkynes with preservation of the Si–Si bond of hydrooligosilanes: Regio- and stereoselective synthesis of (Z)-alkenyloligosilanes and carbonyl-functionalized alkenyldisilanes. *J. Organomet. Chem.* **2022**, *961*, 122234. [CrossRef]
18. Saridakis, I.; Kidonakis, M.; Stratakis, M. Unique Reactivity of Dihydrosilanes under Catalysis by Supported Gold Nanoparticles: *cis*-1,2-Dehydrogenative Disilylation of Alkynes. *ChemCatChem* **2018**, *10*, 980–983. [CrossRef]
19. Feng, X.; Guo, J.; Wang, S.; Wu, Q.; Chen, Z. Atomically dispersed gold anchored on carbon nitride nanosheets as effective catalyst for regioselective hydrosilylation of alkynes. *J. Mater. Chem. A* **2021**, *9*, 17885–17892. [CrossRef]
20. Lu, Z.; Guo, J. Highly Chemo-, Regio-, and Stereoselective Cobalt-Catalyzed Markovnikov Hydrosilylation of Alkynes. *Angew. Chem. Int. Ed.* **2016**, *55*, 10835–10838.
21. Teo, W.; Wang, C.; Tan, Y.; Ge, S. Cobalt-Catalyzed Z-Selective Hydrosilylation of Terminal Alkynes. *Angew. Chem. Int. Ed.* **2017**, *56*, 4328–4332. [CrossRef] [PubMed]
22. Du, X.; Hou, W.; Zhang, Y.; Huang, Z. Pincer cobalt complex-catalyzed Z-selective hydrosilylation of terminal alkyne. *Org. Chem. Front.* **2017**, *4*, 1517–1521. [CrossRef]
23. Wu, G.; Chakraborty, U.; Wangelin, A.J. Regiocontrol in the cobalt-catalyzed hydrosilylation of alkynes. *Chem. Commun.* **2018**, *54*, 12322–12325. [CrossRef] [PubMed]

24. Li, R.-H.; An, X.-M.; Yang, M.; Li, D.-C.; Hu, Z.-L.; Zhan, Z.-P. Highly Regio- and Stereoselective Heterogeneous Hydrosilylation of Terminal Alkynes over Cobalt-Metalated Porous Organic Polymer. *Org. Lett.* **2018**, *20*, 5023–5026. [CrossRef]
25. Skrodzki, M.; Patroniak, V.; Pawluć, P. Schiff Base Cobalt(II) Complex-Catalyzed Highly Markovnikov-Selective Hydrosilylation of Alkynes. *Org. Lett.* **2021**, *23*, 663–667. [CrossRef]
26. Wang, D.; Lai, Y.; Wang, P.; Leng, X.; Xiao, J.; Deng, L. Markovnikov Hydrosilylation of Alkynes with Tertiary Silanes Catalyzed by Dinuclear Cobalt Carbonyl Complexes with NHC Ligation. *J. Am. Chem. Soc.* **2021**, *143*, 12847–12856. [CrossRef]
27. Park, J.-W. Cobalt-catalyzed alkyne hydrosilylation as a new frontier to selectively access silyl-hydrocarbons. *Chem. Commun.* **2022**, *58*, 491–504. [CrossRef]
28. Stachowiak-Dłużyńska, H.; Kuciński, K.; Wyrzykiewicz, B.; Kempe, R.; Hreczycho, G. Co-catalyzed Selective syn-Hydrosilylation of Internal Alkynes. *ChemCatChem* **2023**, *15*, e202300592. [CrossRef]
29. Liu, Z.-K.; Zhang, G.-L.; Li, D.-C.; Yang, Y.; Chen, L.; Zhan, Z.-P. Iron-Catalyzed Synthesis of (E)-β-Vinylsilanes via a Regio- and Stereoselective Hydrosilylation from Terminal Alkynes. *Synlett* **2019**, *30*, 235–239.
30. Guo, Z.; Wen, H.; Liu, G.; Huang, Z. Iron-Catalyzed Regio- and Stereoselective Hydrosilylation of 1,3-Enynes To Access 1,3-Dienylsilanes. *Org. Lett.* **2021**, *23*, 2375–2379. [CrossRef]
31. Hu, W.-Y.; He, P.; Qiao, T.-Z.; Sun, W.; Li, W.-T.; Lian, J.; Li, J.-H.; Zhu, S.-F. Iron-Catalyzed Regiodivergent Alkyne Hydrosilylation. *J. Am. Chem. Soc.* **2020**, *142*, 16894–16902. [CrossRef] [PubMed]
32. Sen, A.; Sen, T.; Kumar, R.; Kumar, C.P.; Kumar, H.; Kumar, K.; Kumar, S.H. Iron-catalyzed (*E*)-selective hydrosilylation of alkynes: Scope and mechanistic insights. *Catal. Sci. Technol.* **2024**, *14*, 2752–2760. [CrossRef]
33. Behera, R.R.; Saha, R.; Kumar, A.A.; Sethi, S.; Jana, N.C.; Bagh, B. Hydrosilylation of Terminal Alkynes Catalyzed by an Air-Stable Manganese-NHC Complex. *J. Org. Chem.* **2023**, *88*, 8133–8149. [CrossRef] [PubMed]
34. Wang, Z.-L.; Zhang, F.-L.; Xu, J.-L.; Shan, C.-C.; Zhao, M.; Xu, Y.-H. Copper-Catalyzed Anti-Markovnikov Hydrosilylation of Terminal Alkynes. *Org. Lett.* **2020**, *22*, 7735–7742. [CrossRef]
35. Xu, J.-L.; Wang, Z.-L.; Zhao, J.-B.; Xu, Y.-H. Enantioselective construction of Si-stereogenic linear alkenylhydrosilanes via copper-catalyzed hydrosilylation of alkynes. *Chem Catal.* **2024**, *4*, 100887. [CrossRef]
36. Bai, D.; Cheng, R.; Yang, J.; Xu, W.; Chen, X.; Chang, J. Regiodivergent hydrosilylation in the nickel(0)-catalyzed cyclization of 1,6-enynes. *Org. Chem. Front.* **2022**, *9*, 5285–5291. [CrossRef]
37. Docherty, J.H.; Peng, J.; Dominey, A.P.; Thomas, S.P. Activation and discovery of earth-abundant metal catalysts using sodium tert-butoxide. *Nat. Chem.* **2017**, *9*, 595–600. [CrossRef]
38. Wu, C.; Teo, W.; Ge, S. Cobalt-Catalyzed (E)-Selective anti-Markovnikov Hydrosilylation of Terminal Alkynes. *ACS Catal.* **2018**, *8*, 5896–5900. [CrossRef]
39. Li, C.; Li, J.; Tan, C.; Wu, W.; Jiang, H. DDQ-mediated regioselective C-S bond formation: Efficient access to allylic sulfides. *Org. Chem. Front.* **2018**, *5*, 3158–3162. [CrossRef]
40. Li, C.; Li, M.; Zhong, W.; Jin, Y.; Li, J.; Wu, W.; Jiang, H. Palladium-Catalyzed Oxidative Allylation of Sulfoxonium Ylides: Regioselective Synthesis of Conjugated Dienones. *Org. Lett.* **2019**, *21*, 872–875. [CrossRef]
41. Li, C.; Liao, M.; He, Z.; Chen, Y.; Mai, J.; Dong, R.; Chen, J.; Chen, L. Metal-Free Oxidative Cross-Dehydrogenative Coupling of Alkenes with Thiophenols. *ChemistrySelect* **2023**, *8*, e202300845. [CrossRef]

molecules

MDPI

Article

Hydrogen-Bonded Di(hydroperoxy)alkane Adducts of the Type $Cy_3P{=}O{\cdot}(HOO)_2CHR$ (R = Alkyl)

Rahym Ashirov, Maya Todorovic, Nattamai Bhuvanesh and Janet Blümel *

Department of Chemistry, Texas A&M University, College Station, TX 77842-3012, USA; rahymashirov@tamu.edu (R.A.); maya.todorovic@tamu.edu (M.T.); nbhuv@chem.tamu.edu (N.B.)
* Correspondence: bluemel@tamu.edu

Abstract: Five representatives of a novel type of di(hydroperoxy)alkane adducts of phosphine oxides have been synthesized and fully characterized, including their solubility in organic solvents. The phosphine oxide Cy_3PO (**1**) has been used in combination with the corresponding aldehydes to create the adducts $Cy_3PO{\cdot}(HOO)_2CHCH_3$ (**2**), $Cy_3PO{\cdot}(HOO)_2CHCH_2CH_3$ (**3**), $Cy_3PO{\cdot}(HOO)_2CH(CH_2)_2CH_3$ (**4**), $Cy_3PO{\cdot}(HOO)_2CH(CH_2)_3CH_3$ (**5**), and $Cy_3PO{\cdot}(HOO)_2CH(CH_2)_7CH_3$ (**6**). All adducts crystallize easily and contain the peroxide and phosphine oxide hydrogen-bonded in 1:1 ratios. The single crystal X-ray structures of **2–6** and their unique features are discussed. The ^{31}P NMR spectra of the adducts **2–6** show downfield-shifted signals as compared to Cy_3PO. In the IR spectra, the ν(P=O) wavenumbers of the adducts have smaller values than the neat phosphine oxide. All spectroscopic results of **2–6** show that the P=O bond is weakened by hydrogen-bonding to the di(hydroperoxy)alkane moieties. Adduct **6** selectively oxidizes PPh_3 to $OPPh_3$ within minutes, and nonanal is reformed in the process. The easy synthesis, handling, and administration of these stable, solid, and soluble peroxides with well-defined composition will have a positive impact on synthetic chemistry.

Keywords: phosphine oxides; di(hydroperoxy)alkanes; X-ray structures; multinuclear NMR; IR data

1. Introduction

General Introduction

Hydrogen peroxide (H_2O_2) is an important and versatile oxidant used for diverse applications in industrial and academic settings [1–3]. However, H_2O_2 is commercially available only as dilute aqueous solution. Therefore, biphasic reactions are needed when reactants and products are only soluble in organic solvents that are not miscible with water. The latter may lead to secondary reactions and side-products. Aqueous H_2O_2 also decays at unpredictable rates and needs to be titrated prior to use [4]. Other types of peroxides have been applied, for example, urea hydrogen peroxide adducts [5–7], organic peroxocarbonates [8–10], peroxoborates [10], and organic peroxides [11]. However, these peroxides are not soluble in organic solvents, their composition is not stoichiometric, and, in the case of organic peroxides, there is a safety issue. Adducts of H_2O_2 with organic solvents are known, but they also pose safety risks, and are not shelf-stable, and have to be prepared immediately before being applied as oxidizers [12–15].

Superior, alternative solid adducts of peroxides have been sought. Phosphine oxides can act as electron pair donors for diverse HO groups and form strong hydrogen bonds [16–20]. Indeed, phosphine oxides could successfully be used to stabilize H_2O_2

and di(hydroperoxy)alkanes, and they facilitate crystallization [21–29]. While phosphines are ubiquitous as ligands and play crucial roles in catalysis [30–34], phosphine oxides are less prominent. However, they are important for characterizing surfaces [35–39] and as synthetic targets [40–44]. Phosphine oxides have been used previously for Mitsunobu reactions [45,46] and recently in redox-free Mitsunobu organocatalysis [47].

All of the phosphine oxide adducts of the type $R_3PO{\cdot}(HOO)_2CR'R''$ (R = alkyl, aryl) are shelf-stable over months, their composition is well-defined, they have high melting points, and they are soluble in organic solvents. These adducts have been successfully employed in diverse reactions, e.g., selective phosphine oxidation, sulfide to sulfoxide oxidation, the direct oxidative esterification of aldehydes, and Baeyer–Villiger oxidations [21–29].

In this contribution, we describe a hitherto unrealized type of peroxide adduct of phosphine oxides in order to probe and expand the range of possible adducts. From a practical point of view, we sought to reduce the "dead weight" of the adducts to render them more competitive with commercial aqueous H_2O_2 while retaining their oxidative power. Therefore, the new adducts $Cy_3PO{\cdot}(HOO)_2CHR$ (R = alkyl) are derived from aldehydes, and, instead of two, there is only one hydrogen atom and one alkyl substituent bound to the $(HOO)_2C$ moiety. It is noteworthy that aldehyde-based unsupported di(hydroperoxy)alkanes are unstable oils that are hard to purify and handle because they decompose swiftly and form mixtures with the ensuing hydroxy(hydroperoxy)alkanes [12]. Therefore, another goal was to probe whether phosphine oxides could also stabilize the aldehyde-derived di(hydroperoxy)alkanes and render the adducts $Cy_3PO{\cdot}(HOO)_2CHR$ crystalline and easy to handle.

In the following sections, it is demonstrated that in spite of reducing the size and weight of the peroxides substantially, the new di(hydroperoxy)alkane adducts of tricyclohexylphosphine oxide can easily be synthesized, crystallized, and characterized. Their interesting structural features are discussed along with their NMR and IR characteristics, and their superb solubility in common organic solvents is quantified.

2. Results and Discussion

2.1. Synthesis and Characterization

The syntheses of the di(hydroperoxy)alkane adducts of tricyclohexylphosphine oxide **2–6** (Figure 1) were straightforward and followed one standard procedure. Combining DCM solutions of the clean phosphine oxide **1** [22] with the di(hydroperoxy)alkanes [12] in a 1:1 ratio, the adducts **2–6** formed instantly and could be obtained in crystalline form by the slow evaporation of the solvent at ambient temperature under the atmosphere. All adducts **2–6** have been obtained with a stoichiometrically precise 1:1 composition of peroxide and phosphine oxide.

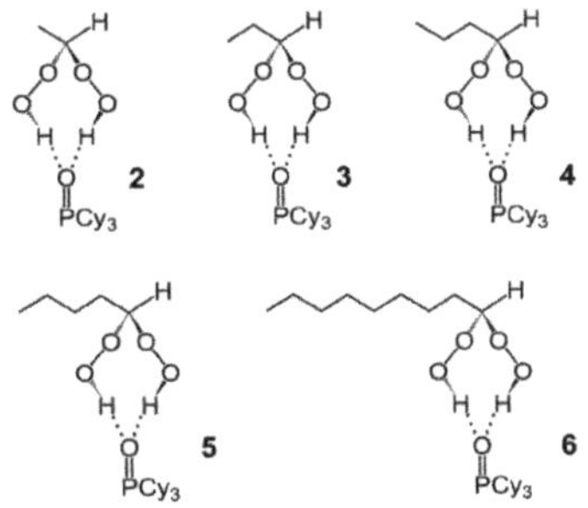

Figure 1. Di(hydroperoxy)alkane adducts **2–6** of Cy_3PO (**1**).

The colorless adducts **2–6** (Figure 1) are stable at ambient temperature and only start to decompose during melting at temperatures higher than 84 °C. Besides the melting characteristics, the single crystal X-ray structures [48], the IR spectra [49], and the ^{1}H, ^{13}C, and ^{31}P NMR spectroscopic data are reported for the adducts. Furthermore, selected solubilities in representative organic solvents have been quantified.

2.2. X-Ray Crystallography of the Adducts $Cy_3PO{\cdot}(HOO)_2CHR$

The adducts $Cy_3PO{\cdot}(HOO)_2CHR$ **2–6** (Figure 1) crystallize readily in large colorless specimens of single crystal X-ray quality. The ease of crystallization is most probably due to the Cy_3PO carrier that is favorable for packing the adducts in crystal lattices. More recently, we reported that various R_3POs also enable the crystallization of hydrogen-bonded H_2O_2 and ketone-derived di(hydroperoxy)alkanes [21–29]. The single crystal X-ray structures of the adduct assemblies $Cy_3PO{\cdot}(HOO)_2CHR$ (**2–6**) are displayed in Figures 2 and 3 (**2**), Figure 4 and Figure S1 (**3**), Figure 5 and Figure S2 (**4**), Figures 6 and 7 (**5**), and Figure 8 (**6**) [48]. Relevant structural data are summarized in Tables 1 and 2 and Tables S1 and S2 in the Supplementary Materials. The single crystal X-ray structures of all adducts **2–6** confirm the stoichiometrically precise 1:1 composition of the phosphine oxide and the di(hydroperoxy)alkane.

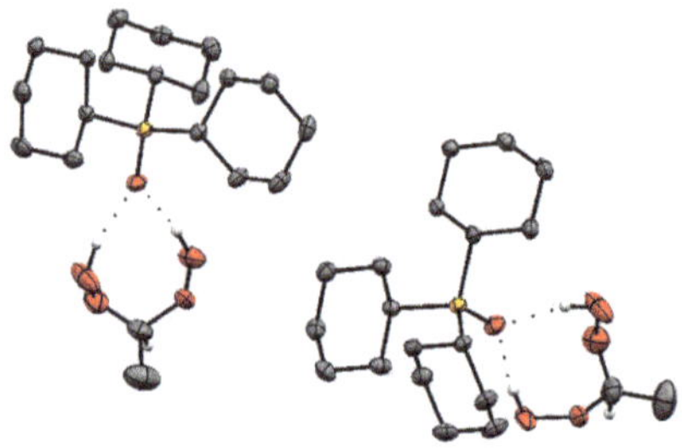

Figure 2. Two adduct assemblies of $Cy_3PO{\cdot}(HOO)_2CHCH_3$ (**2**). Hydrogen atoms except those in the $CH(OOH)_2$ moieties are omitted for clarity.

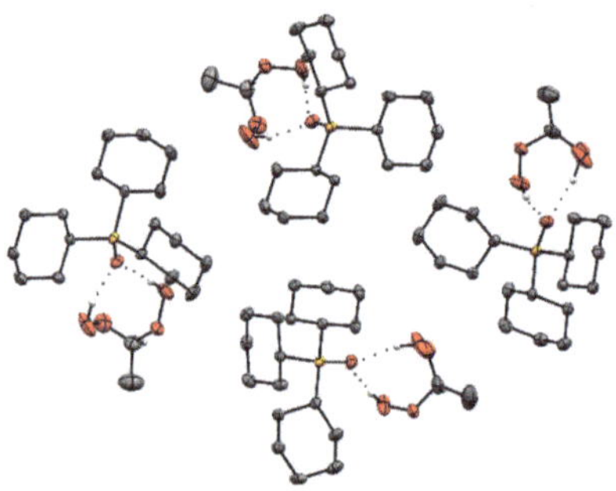

Figure 3. Stacking pattern of four adduct assemblies of $Cy_3PO{\cdot}(HOO)_2CHCH_3$ (**2**). Hydrogen atoms except those in the $CH(OOH)_2$ moieties are omitted for clarity.

Interestingly, crystalline **2** (Figure 2) does not follow the arrangement of adduct assemblies observed with all adducts of the type $R_3PO{\cdot}(HOO)_2CR'R''$ (R, R′, R″ = alkyl, aryl) [21–29]. The latter adducts, without exception, feature two adducts with the P=O groups being aligned and pointing in opposite directions. This conventional arrangement is observed also for **3** (Figure 4 and Figure S1). In **2**, the P=O groups are nearly perpendicular, and the overall stacking pattern is unprecedented and resembles a molecular roundabout (Figure 3). We assume that the unusual stacking of **2** is due to the small steric demand of the di(hydroperoxy)ethane moiety that is unable to fill the void created by the large Cy_3PO of the adjacent assembly.

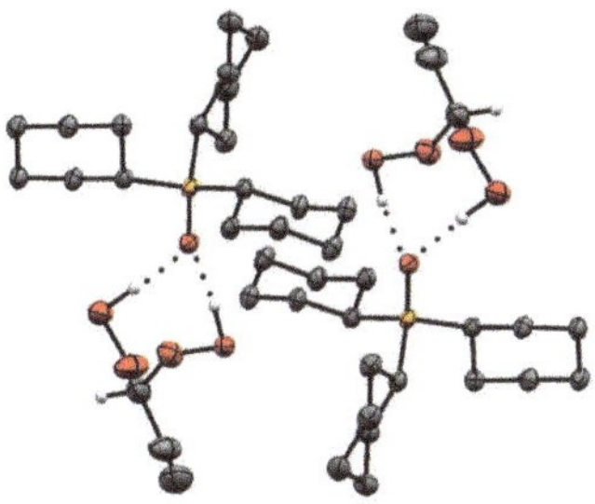

Figure 4. Stacking pattern of two adduct assemblies of $Cy_3PO{\cdot}(HOO)_2CHCH_2CH_3$ (**3**). Hydrogen atoms except those in $CH(OOH)_2$ moieties are omitted for clarity.

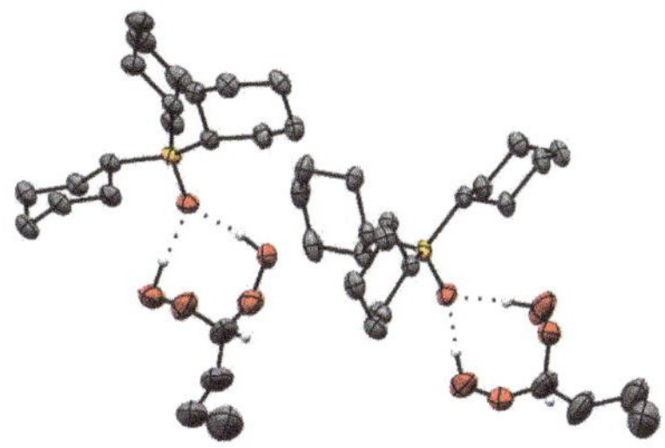

Figure 5. Stacking pattern of two adduct assemblies of $Cy_3PO{\cdot}(HOO)_2CH(CH_2)_2CH_3$ (**4**). Hydrogen atoms except those in $CH(OOH)_2$ moieties are omitted for clarity.

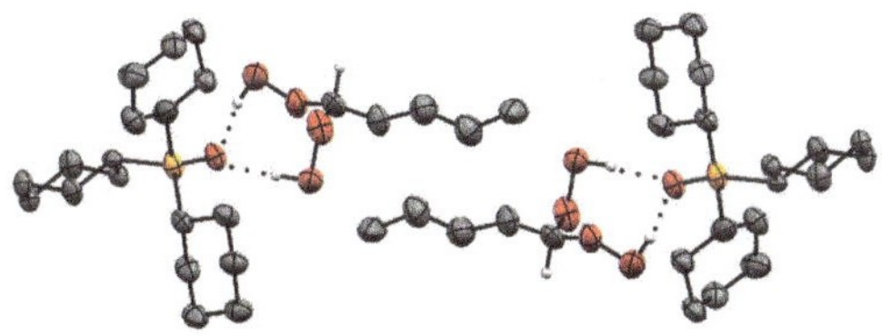

Figure 6. Stacking pattern of two adduct assemblies of $Cy_3PO{\cdot}(HOO)_2CH(CH_2)_3CH_3$ (**5**). Hydrogen atoms except those in $CH(OOH)_2$ moieties are omitted for clarity.

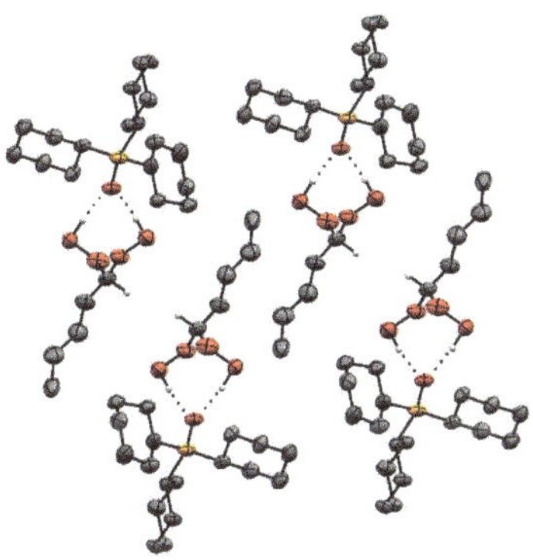

Figure 7. Stacking pattern of four adduct assemblies of $Cy_3PO{\cdot}(HOO)_2CH(CH_2)_3CH_3$ (**5**). Hydrogen atoms except those in $CH(OOH)_2$ moieties are omitted for clarity.

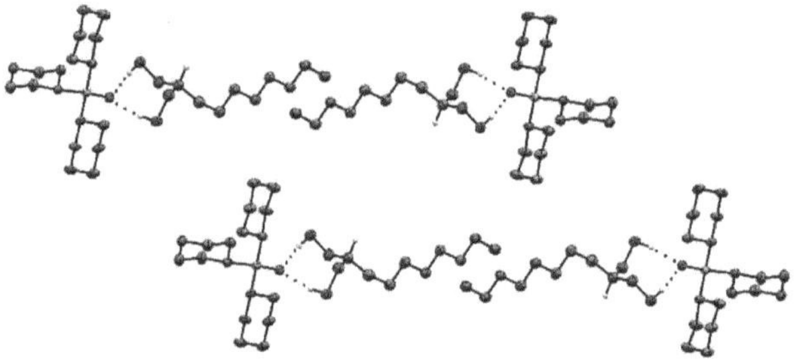

Figure 8. Stacking pattern of two adduct assemblies of $Cy_3PO{\cdot}(HOO)_2CH(CH_2)_7CH_3$ (**6**). Hydrogen atoms except those in $CH(OOH)_2$ moieties are omitted for clarity.

The larger propyl groups in the assemblies of adduct **3**, on the other hand, allow for the conventional, antiparallel stacking with the P=O groups pointing in opposite directions (Figures 4 and S1). The minor space requirement of the hydrogen atom in the $(HOO)_2CH$ group as compared to adducts with all alkyl substituents described previously [21–29] does not impact the structure of **3**, and the usual stacking motif is realized.

Differing from the scenario of **2**, **3**, and structures reported previously [21–29], the adduct assemblies of **4** show another different packing motif (Figures 5 and S2). In this case, the P=O groups of two adjacent adducts are nearly parallel and oriented in the same direction. This unprecedented packing motif produces a crowded scenario in the stacking pattern (Figure S2) and a noticeable kink at the terminal end of the butyl group.

The adduct assemblies of **5** follow the usual stacking motif with the P=O groups being aligned and pointing in opposite directions (Figures 6 and 7). The pentyl chains perfectly align parallel to each other and create a well-organized pattern with optimal space filling. The adduct assemblies of **6** also align in the classic manner of two assemblies each oriented antiparallel to each other (Figure 8). Regarding **6**, it is remarkable that the methylene chains are fully extended. A similar scenario has been described for diphosphine dioxides with long alkyl chains previously [38]. Interestingly, the long methylene chains are not aligned over their full length like in **5** but only over the three terminal carbon atoms. Overall, the structure of **6** resembles a tenside with hydrophobic and hydrophilic sections.

The P=O bond lengths in **2**–**6** (Table 1) are in the same range as those observed for the doubly hydrogen-bonded peroxide adducts of diverse trialkyl- and triarylphosphine oxides of the types $(R_3PO{\cdot}H_2O_2)_2$ (bond length range 1.4882 to 1.5046 Å) [18–20] and $R_3PO{\cdot}(HOO)_2CR'R''$ (1.4992 to 1.5047 Å) [24–29]. Due to the strong hydrogen bonding of the di(hydroperoxy)alkanes to the oxygen atom in the P=O bonds, the latter are elongated in the adducts **2**–**6** as compared to the neat phosphine oxide **1** (Table 1). The bond length differences Δ(P=O) range between 0.0169 Å and 0.0253 Å.

Therewith, the P=O bonds in **2**–**6** are lengthened to about the same extent as observed for ketone-derived adducts [24–29]. The weakening of the P=O bonds due to adduct formation is confirmed by ^{31}P NMR and IR spectroscopy (see below). The differences in the Δ(P=O) values of the diverse adducts **2**–**6** do not follow a trend (Table 1). Therefore, it can be assumed that the methylene chain length does not play a role, and the slight differences in the Δ(P=O) values between the adducts **2**–**6** are due to crystal packing effects.

Another criterion for the strength of the hydrogen bonds in the adducts **2**–**6** is the distance between the oxygen atoms in the O–H···O bridges. Distances between 2.75 and 2.85 Å are regarded as typical for these oxygen–oxygen distances [50,51]. Nearly all of the distances found for the adducts **2**–**6** are even shorter, with values ranging from 2.689 Å to 2.751 Å (Table 1). Therefore, it can be concluded that the phosphine oxide forms two strong hydrogen bonds with the di(hydroperoxy)alkanes. Again, there is no obvious trend that would link the oxygen–oxygen distance in the O–H···O assembly with the length of the alkyl chains.

Table 1. Distances O–H···O and P=O bond lengths in **2–6** (Å) and differences Δ(P=O) between the P=O bond lengths of the adducts $Cy_3PO·(HOO)_2CHR$ (**2–6**) and the corresponding phosphine oxide Cy_3PO (**1**) (1.490(2) Å).

Adduct	O–H···O (Å)	P=O (Å)	Δ(P=O) (Å)
2	2.689/2.751	1.5071 (17)	0.0169 (17)
3	2.719/2.741	1.5110 (9)	0.0208 (9)
4	2.711/2.719	1.5082 (14)	0.0180 (14)
5	2.701/2.702	1.5074 (11)	0.0172 (11)
6	2.712/2.737	1.5155 (10)	0.0253 (10)

Finally, we considered the bond angles at the CH carbon atoms of the di(hydroperoxy) alkane moieties in **2–6** (Table 2). These angles should indicate whether the formation of the two nearly linear hydrogen bonds to the phosphine oxide leads to a distortion of the tetrahedral geometry in order to accommodate the packing in the single crystals. All O–C–O angles of **2–6** fall within the narrow range of 112.5° and 114.5° and, therewith, are substantially larger than the tetrahedral angle 109.5°. The values are even larger than those of comparable adducts incorporating cyclic alkanes [28]. For example, the O–C–O angle in the adduct $Cy_3PO·(HOO)_2C(CH_2)_4$ where the quaternary carbon is part of a cyclopentyl ring amounts to only 111.8° [28]. Regarding the O–C–C angles of **2–6** (Table 2), the values scatter between 103.8° and 121.2°. Both extreme values are found in adduct **2**, which also shows a very different packing of the adduct assemblies in the unit cell (Figure 3). Overall, the bond angles around the di(hydroperoxy)alkane CH carbon in **2–6** reflect the accommodation of the individual structures to the packing motif of the adducts.

Table 2. Bond angles at the CH carbon atom of the di(hydroperoxy)alkane moieties in the adducts **2–6**.

$Cy_3PO·(HOO)_2CHR$	O–C–O (°)	O1–C–C/O2–C–C (°)
2	114.5 (2)	103.8 (3)/121.2 (3)
3	112.5 (3)	113.7 (3)/106.5 (3)
4	113.6 (3)	114.3 (5)/119.0 (5)
5	113.66 (17)	114.0 (2)/114.44 (19)
6	113.05 (12)	105.40 (12)/115.43 (12)

2.3. NMR Spectroscopy of the Adducts of $Cy_3PO·(HOO)_2CHR$

All NMR spectra of **2–6** are displayed in the Supplementary Materials (Figures S3–S13). ^{1}H and ^{13}C NMR spectroscopies prove the successful transformation of the starting aldehydes into the di(hydroperoxy)alkanes. The most diagnostic resonance stems from the aldehyde proton C*H*O that is located between 9.4 to 9.8 ppm for all alkyl aldehydes used in this study. This signal vanishes during the formation of the adducts **2–6,** and a new signal in the range from 5.01 ppm to 5.24 ppm appears, corresponding to the protons in the $(HOO)_2CH$ moieties (Figures S4–S8). The ^{3}J(H-H) coupling to the adjacent CH_3 protons for **2** and CH_2 protons for **3–6** splits these signals into a characteristic quartet and triplets, respectively. In ^{13}C NMR, the transitions from the aldehydes to the di(hydroperoxy)alkanes manifest in the CHO resonance of the alkyl aldehydes in the range from 200 ppm to 203 ppm [52] disappearing and new signals between 110.94 ppm and 106.26 ppm emerging for the $(HOO)_2CH$ moieties (Figures S9–S13). All ^{13}C NMR signals could be assigned by comparison with different adducts described previously [22–29] and by using chemical shift tables (Figures S9–S13) [52]. Furthermore, the $^{n}J(^{31}P\text{-}^{13}C)$ couplings that were only visible for the cyclohexyl carbon signals and were not propagated beyond the hydrogen bonds were utilized. Where needed, HMBC and HSQC spectra were recorded.

While ^{1}H and ^{13}C NMR spectroscopies clearly indicate the transformation of the aldehydes to the corresponding di(hydroperoxy)alkanes, the proof of adduct formation is based on ^{31}P NMR. Compared to the chemical shift of Cy_3PO (49.91 ppm), the ^{31}P NMR signals of the adducts **2–6** are substantially downfield-shifted by more than 7 ppm (Table 3, Figure S3). The hydrogen bonding of the P=O group to the two hydroperoxy groups in the adducts reduces the electron density at the phosphorus nucleus. As a result, the signal of the deshielded ^{31}P nucleus is shifted downfield. Similar changes in the ^{31}P NMR chemical shifts have been described for other di(hydroperoxy)alkane adducts of phosphine oxides previously, with the largest chemical shift changes being observed for adducts of Cy_3PO [28].

Table 3. ^{31}P NMR chemical shifts. The chemical shift differences $\Delta\delta$ (ppm) refer to the chemical shift of the phosphine oxide Cy_3PO (49.91 ppm). The solvent was $CDCl_3$ for all samples.

$Cy_3PO\cdot(HOO)_2CHR$	$\delta(^{31}P)$ (ppm)	$\Delta\delta(^{31}P)$ (ppm)
2	57.35	7.44
3	57.05	7.14
4	56.96	7.05
5	57.20	7.29
6	57.43	7.52

2.4. IR Spectroscopy of the Adducts of $Cy_3PO\cdot(HOO)_2CHR$

The IR stretching frequencies [49,53] for the O–H and P=O groups of the adducts **2–6** are summarized in Table 4. The IR data complement the results from the single crystal X-ray diffraction and ^{31}P NMR measurements. The strong hydrogen bonds in the adducts manifest in a weakening of the P=O bond and correspondingly lower wavenumbers in **2–6** as compared to the neat phosphine oxide **1**. This effect is rather pronounced, and the differences amount to 25 to 30 cm^{-1}. These differences $\Delta\nu$(P=O) are in the same order of magnitude as those obtained for di(hydroperoxy)alkanes of the type $R_3PO\cdot(HOO)_2CR'R''$ hydrogen-bonded to the electron-rich Cy_3PO reported previously [24–29].

Table 4. IR wavenumbers for the stretching vibrations of the O–H and P=O groups (cm^{-1}) of the adducts **2–6**. The wavenumber differences $\Delta\nu$(P=O) (cm^{-1}) refer to the ν(P=O) of the phosphine oxide Cy_3PO (1157 cm^{-1}) [22].

$Cy_3PO\cdot(HOO)_2CHR$	ν(O–H) (cm^{-1})	ν(P=O) (cm^{-1})	Δν(P=O) (cm^{-1})
2	3195	1129	28
3	3193	1127	30
4	3198	1131	26
5	3200	1131	26
6	3196	1132	25

Another consequence of the adduct formation is that the O–H bond is weakened in **2–6** by the strong hydrogen bonds with the P=O group of the phosphine oxide carrier.

In nonpolar solvents, dilute substances containing OH groups exhibit sharp absorption peaks between 3650 cm^{-1} and 3590 cm^{-1} [49]. However, the O–H stretching bands for **2–6** are found at much lower wavenumbers and within the narrow range from 3193 cm^{-1} to 3200 cm^{-1} (Table 4). This result confirms that in the solid adducts, the P=O groups are firmly hydrogen-bonded to the di(hydroperoxy)alkane moieties.

2.5. Solubilities of the Adducts in Organic Solvents

Aqueous H_2O_2 is a very potent oxidizer and used extensively in academia and industry [1–3]. However, besides its lack of shelf stability, high cost, and safety issues, the crucial drawback is that most oxidations have to be performed in biphasic mixtures. Since the actual reaction only occurs at the interface between the aqueous and organic solvent layers, longer reaction times are required. Furthermore, the work-up necessitates additional phase separation and product-drying steps. Water-sensitive educts or products are not amenable to treatment with aqueous H_2O_2. Recently, we succeeded in immobilizing a phosphine oxide carrier on a silica surface that stabilized H_2O_2 and di(hydroperoxy)alkanes by strong hydrogen bonds [21]. This material allowed the use of diverse protic and nonprotic solvents in oxidation reactions because the peroxide was exposed to the substrate in a monolayer on the mesoporous high-surface area silica [21]. However, this method requires an immobilization step and support material.

Earlier, favorable phosphine oxides have been utilized to render H_2O_2 and di(hydroperoxy)alkanes soluble in organic solvents [22–29]. The phosphine oxide Cy_3PO should be uniquely suited for increasing the solubilities of the peroxide moieties in the adducts **2–6**. In fact, the quantified solubilities of the adducts that incorporate the shortest and longest alkyl chains, $Cy_3PO{\cdot}(HOO)_2CHCH_3$ (**2**) and $Cy_3PO{\cdot}(HOO)_2CH(CH_2)_7CH_3$ (**6**), in representative organic solvents are very high (Figure 9). In most solvents, the adducts **2** and **6** are even more soluble than the carrier Cy_3PO (**1**). The only exception is the protic solvent methanol, which might lead to the dissociation of the adduct hydrogen bonds in solution. The higher solubilities of the smaller fragments of **2,** as compared to those of **6** with the hydrophobic octyl substituent at the $(HOO)_2CH$ group, support the assumption of dissociation in methanol. The solubilities of **2** and **6** are remarkably high in the aromatic solvent benzene and the chlorinated solvents DCM and chloroform. In DCM, for example, more than 1.2 g of **6** are soluble per mL of DCM, and nearly 1.1 g per mL of **2** can be dissolved (Figure 9). The polar, non-protic solvent acetonitrile is the least favorable solvent for all species, **1**, **2**, and **6**.

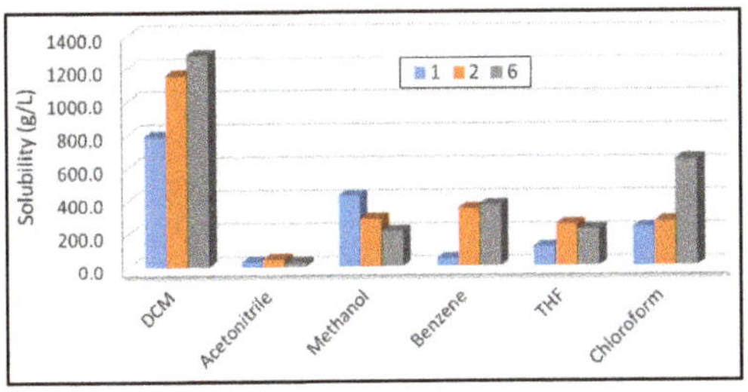

Figure 9. Solubilities of the adducts $Cy_3PO{\cdot}(HOO)_2CHCH_3$ (**2**) and $Cy_3PO{\cdot}(HOO)_2CH(CH_2)_7CH_3$ (**6**) in representative organic solvents, compared to Cy_3PO (**1**).

In summary, the adducts of $Cy_3PO{\cdot}(HOO)_2CHR$ are highly soluble in many organic solvents without the decomposition of the peroxide moiety. Therefore, in contrast to aqueous hydrogen peroxide or insoluble inorganic peroxides, they can be applied for oxidation reactions in one homogeneous organic phase. The solubilities of the new adducts in non-protic and chlorinated solvents allow a broader range of applications for oxidation reactions. Biphasic liquid/liquid and liquid/solid reaction mixtures that prolong the reaction times, complicate the work-up, and diminish the product yields and selectivities can be avoided by choosing any of the adducts **2–6**.

2.6. Application for the Selective Oxidation of PPh_3

Finally, we sought to demonstrate that the new adducts of the type $Cy_3PO{\cdot}(HOO)_2CHR$ (R = alkyl) are able to selectively oxidize phosphines in analogy to the ketone-derived adducts described previously [21–29]. We chose adduct **6** in combination with PPh_3 as the substrate because triarylphosphines are not oxidized in air, even in solution and at high temperatures [22]. The outcome of the oxidation reaction can be determined by ^{31}P NMR spectroscopy. The original resonance at about –6 ppm vanishes, while the signal for $OPPh_3$ appears at 29.10 ppm [22]. Another question about the new adducts can be answered unequivocally with this experiment. After the active oxygen atoms of the adduct are spent, the aldehyde is obtained again. This is clearly visible in the ^{1}H and ^{13}C NMR spectra (Figures S14 and S15). The aldehyde proton signal at about 9.5 ppm reappears in the ^{1}H NMR spectrum after the reaction, matching the corresponding peak in the spectrum of nonanal. Analogously, the ^{13}C NMR spectrum of the reaction mixture displays the aldehyde carbon signal at about 203 ppm, while the resonance of the adduct **6** that stems from the carbon atom attached to the two hydroperoxy groups at ca. 110 ppm has vanished. In summary, this reaction shows that the new adduct is a powerful oxidant that led to the full and selective oxidation of a triarylphosphine within minutes and that the reaction product besides the oxidized species and the supporting phosphine oxide Cy_3PO is the corresponding aldehyde.

3. Experimental Section

General Considerations. All reactions were carried out under the atmosphere unless mentioned otherwise. Cy_3PO was synthesized water-free from the phosphine using air oxygen after adsorption on activated carbon (AC) as described earlier [54]. The absence of water was checked by IR spectroscopy. The solvents, hydrogen peroxide (30% aqueous solution), and aldehydes were used as obtained from the supplier. All di(hydroperoxy)alkanes and their Cy_3PO adducts **2–6** were synthesized in analogy to the representative procedure outlined for **2** below. The ^{31}P (Figure S3), ^{1}H (Figures S4–S8), and ^{13}C NMR spectra (Figures S9–S13) were recorded at ambient temperature on a Bruker 400 MHz NMR instrument at 161.82, 399.76, and 100.53 MHz, respectively. The ^{31}P and ^{13}C NMR spectra were proton-decoupled. For referencing the ^{31}P NMR spectra, neat Ph_2PCl ($\delta(^{31}P) = +81.92$ ppm), placed in a capillary that was centered in the 5 mm NMR tube, was used. The ^{1}H and ^{13}C NMR spectra were referenced using the signals of the solvent $CDCl_3$ (residual protons: $\delta(^{1}H) = 7.26$ ppm; $\delta(^{13}C) = 77.16$ ppm). The IR spectra of the neat powders of the adducts **2–6** were obtained with a Shimadzu IRAffinity-1 FTIR spectrometer equipped with a Pike Technologies MIRacle ATR plate.

Representative Synthesis of $Cy_3PO{\cdot}(HOO)_2CHCH_3$ (2). Syntheses of $(HOO)_2CHCH_3$: acetaldehyde (120.0 mg, 2.727 mmol, 1.000 eq.), phosphomolybdic acid (83.3 mg, 0.0456 mmol, 0.0167 eq.), and $MgSO_4$ (448.7 mg, 3.728 mmol, 1.367 eq.) were added to 14 mL of 3-fold concentrated ethereal H_2O_2 solution [12] in a reaction vial and stirred for 24 h at ambient temperature. The solids were filtered off through Celite and washed with 10 mL of EtOAc. EtOAc (10 mL) and H_2O (10 mL) were added to the combined filtrate and washing solutions. Then, the organic and aqueous phases were separated with a separatory funnel. The aqueous layer was extracted two times with 20 mL portions of EtOAc, and all organic phases were combined. They were washed with 15 mL of H_2O and 15 mL of a brine solution. Finally, the organic phase was dried over anhydrous Na_2SO_4. The Na_2SO_4 was filtered off, and the organic phase was stripped of the solvent by rotary evaporation. The resulting oily residue was subjected to oil pump vacuum, and the di(hydroperoxy)ethane was obtained as slightly yellow oil (196.8 mg, 2.094 mmol, and 76.77% yield with respect to acetaldehyde). All other di(hydroperoxy)alkanes were synthesized according to this representative procedure and were obtained as colorless oils with 52–64% yields with respect to their corresponding aldehydes.

Adduct synthesis: tricyclohexylphosphine oxide (**1**, 96.8 mg, 0.327 mmol, 1.00 eq.) and di(hydroperoxy)ethane (39.4 mg, 0.419 mmol, 1.28 eq.) were dissolved in 1 mL of DCM, and the reaction mixture was homogenized by treatment with a Pasteur pipette for 1 min. The solution was placed on a watch glass, and the solvent was allowed to evaporate overnight under ambient conditions. The resulting solid was scraped off and dried further under vacuum. The adduct $Cy_3PO{\cdot}(HOO)_2CHCH_3$ (**2**) was obtained as a white powder (109.8 mg, 0.2812 mmol, 86.1% isolated yield with respect to **1**). All of the other adducts (**3**–**6**) were synthesized following the same procedure, except for one additional step. After drying **3**–**6** overnight on a watch glass, the adducts were washed five times with 1 mL portions of hexanes to obtain the pure products. After further drying under ambient conditions overnight, the adducts **3**–**6** were obtained as white powders with 29–54% isolated, not-optimized yields with respect to **1**. For obtaining single crystals of X-ray quality, see Supplementary Materials.

NMR data of **2** (δ, $CDCl_3$). $^{31}P\{^1H\}$ 57.35 (s); ^1H 11.98 (O*H*), 5.24 (q, $^3J(^1H–^1H)$ = 5.6 Hz, 1H, OC*H*), 1.87 (br d, 6H, $^2J(^1H–^1H)$ = 11.3 Hz, PCHC*H*eq), 1.84–1.75 (m, 9H, $PCH_{ax}CH_2CH_{eq}$), 1.75–1.61 (m, 3H, $PCH(CH_2)_2CH_{eq}$), 1.50–1.30 (m, 6H, $PCHCH_{ax}$), 1.33 (d, $^3J(^1H–^1H)$ = 5.6 Hz, 3H, CH_3), 1.30–1.12 (m, 9H, $PCHCH_2CH_{ax}CH_{ax}$). $^{13}C\{^1H\}$ 106.26 (s, OC), 34.89 (d, $^1J(^{31}P–^{13}C)$ = 60.6 Hz, PC), 26.81 (d, $^3J(^{31}P–^{13}C)$ = 11.9 Hz, PC_2C), 26.08 (d, $^2J(^{31}P–^{13}C)$ = 2.8 Hz, PCC), 26.01 (s, PC_3C), 15.10 (s, CH_3).

NMR data of **3**. (δ, $CDCl_3$). $^{31}P\{^1H\}$ 57.05 (s); ^1H 11.99 (O*H*), 5.01 (t, $^3J(^1H–^1H)$ = 5.8 Hz, 1H, OC*H*), 1.90 (br d, 6H, $^2J(^1H–^1H)$ = 11.0 Hz, $PCHCH_{eq}$), 1.86–1.78 (m, 9H, $PCH_{ax}CH_2CH_{eq}$), 1.78–1.63 (m, 3H, $PCH(CH_2)_2CH_{eq}$), 1.72 (quint, $^3J(^1H–^1H)$ = 5.8 Hz, 2H, $OCHCH_2$), 1.53–1.33 (m, 6H, $PCHCH_{ax}$), 1.33–1.13 (m, 9H, $PCHCH_2CH_{ax}CH_{ax}$), 0.99 (t, $^3J(^1H–^1H)$ = 7.4 Hz, 3H, CH_3). $^{13}C\{^1H\}$ 110.94 (s, OC), 34.91 (d, $^1J(^{31}P–^{13}C)$ = 60.8 Hz, PC), 26.86 (d, $^3J(^{31}P–^{13}C)$ = 11.7 Hz, PC_2C), 26.14 (s, PCC), 26.05 (s, PC_3C), 22.29 (s, OCC), 9.40 (s, CH_3).

NMR data of **4**. (δ, $CDCl_3$). $^{31}P\{^1H\}$ 56.96 (s); ^1H 11.96 (O*H*), 5.09 (t, $^3J(^1H–^1H)$ = 6.0 Hz, 1H, OC*H*), 1.90 (dd, 6H, $^2J(^1H–^1H)$ = 2.4 Hz, $^2J(^1H–^1H)$ = 10.9 Hz, $PCHCH_{eq}$), 1.87–1.77 (m, 9H, $PCH_{ax}CH_2CH_{eq}$), 1.77–1.61 (m, 3H, $PCH(CH_2)_2CH_{eq}$), 1.67 (dt, $^3J(^1H–^1H)$ = 6.4 Hz, $^3J(^1H–^1H)$ = 9.0 Hz, 2H, $OCHCH_2$), 1.55–1.32 (m, 6H, $PCHCH_{ax}$), 1.46 (sextet, $^3J(^1H–^1H)$ = 7.7 Hz, 2H, $OCHCH_2CH_2$), 1.33–1.12 (m, 9H, $PCHCH_2CH_{ax}CH_{ax}$), 0.92 (t, $^3J(^1H–^1H)$ = 7.4 Hz, 3H, CH_3); $^{13}C\{^1H\}$ 109.69 (s, OC), 34.88 (d, $^1J(^{31}P–^{13}C)$ = 60.5 Hz, PC), 30.92 (s, OCC), 26.85 (d, $^3J(^{31}P–^{13}C)$ =11.9 Hz, PC_2C), 26.12 (d, $^2J(^{31}P–^{13}C)$ = 2.9 Hz, PCC), 26.04 (s, PC_3C), 18.35 (s, OC_2C), 13.99 (s, CH_3).

NMR data of **5**. (δ, $CDCl_3$). $^{31}P\{^1H\}$ 57.20 (s); ^1H 12.01 (O*H*), 5.08 (t, $^3J(^1H–^1H)$ = 6.0 Hz, 1H, OC*H*), 1.90 (dd, 6H, $^2J(^1H–^1H)$ = 2.5 Hz, $^2J(^1H–^1H)$ = 11.1 Hz, $PCHCH_{eq}$), 1.86–1.78 (m, 9H, $PCH_{ax}CH_2CH_{eq}$), 1.78–1.63 (m, 3H, $PCH(CH_2)_2CH_{eq}$), 1.70 (dt, $^3J(^1H–^1H)$ = 6.5 Hz, $^3J(^1H–^1H)$ = 9.0 Hz, 2H, $OCHCH_2$), 1.56–1.32 (m, 6H, $PCHCH_{ax}$), 1.56–1.39 (quintet, 2H, $OCHCH_2CH_2$), 1.33 (sextet, $^3J(^1H–^1H)$ = 7.5 Hz, 2H, $OCHCH_2CH_2CH_2$), 1.32–1.14 (m, 9H, $PCHCH_2CH_{ax}CH_{ax}$), 0.89 (t, $^3J(^1H–^1H)$ = 7.2 Hz, 3H, CH_3); $^{13}C\{^1H\}$ 109.89 (s, OC), 34.99 (d, $^1J(^{31}P–^{13}C)$ = 60.6 Hz, PC), 28.67 (s, OCC), 27.17 (s, OC_2C), 26.90 (d, $^3J(^{31}P–^{13}C)$ = 11.9 Hz, PC_2C), 26.20 (d, $^2J(^{31}P–^{13}C)$ = 2.9 Hz, PCC), 26.10 (s, PC_3C), 22.60 (s, OC_3C), 14.05 (s, CH_3).

NMR data of **6**. (δ, $CDCl_3$). $^{31}P\{^1H\}$ 57.43 (s); ^1H 11.96 (O*H*), 5.07 (t, $^3J(^1H–^1H)$ = 6.0 Hz, 1H, OC*H*), 1.89 (dd, 6H, $^2J(^1H–^1H)$ = 2.6 Hz, $^2J(^1H–^1H)$ = 10.9 Hz, $PCHCH_{eq}$), 1.86–1.77

(m, 9H, PCH_{ax}CH$_2$CH_{eq}), 1.77–1.61 (m, 3H, PCH(CH$_2$)$_2$CH_{eq}), 1.68 (dt, $^3J(^1H–^1H)$ = 6.2 Hz, $^3J(^1H–^1H)$ = 9.3 Hz, 2H, OCHCH_2), 1.56–1.33 (m, 6H, PCHCH_{ax}), 1.56–1.15 (m, 12H, OCHCH$_2$(CH_2)$_6$CH$_3$), 1.33–1.15 (m, 9H, PCHCH$_2$CH_{ax}CH_{ax}), 0.85 (t, $^3J(^1H–^1H)$ = 7.0 Hz, 3H, CH_3); $^{13}C\{^1H\}$ 109.91 (s, OC), 34.87 (d, $^1J(^{31}P–^{13}C)$ = 60.6 Hz, PC), 31.96 (s, OC$_6$C), 29.52 (s, OC$_3$C)*, 29.49 (s, OC$_5$C)*, 29.30 (s, OC$_4$C)*, 28.95 (s, OCC), 26.85 (d, $^3J(^{31}P–^{13}C)$ = 11.9 Hz, PC$_2$C), 26.11 (d, $^2J(^{31}P–^{13}C)$ = 2.8 Hz, PCC), 26.03 (s, PC$_3$C), 25.01 (s, OC$_2$C), 22.76 (s, OC$_7$C), 14.20 (s, CH$_3$). * Assignments interchangeable.

Melting ranges. The melting ranges of the adducts **2–6** (Table 5) were obtained using sealed capillaries and a conventional melting point apparatus (Optimelt). All melting ranges were lower than the melting point of neat Cy_3PO (155–157 °C). The adducts **2–6** started melting at the given lower values and reached the clear points at the high values. The reason why the adducts have no single melting points is because they start to decompose at the temperatures required for melting.

Table 5. Melting ranges of the adducts **2-6**.

$Cy_3PO{\cdot}(HOO)_2CHR$	mp (°C)
2	87–99
3	84–90
4	100–105
5	84–90
6	89–92

Solubilities of **1**, **2**, and **6**. The corresponding phosphine oxide or adduct (10–16 mg) was weighed in a 20 mL vial. The selected solvent was added in dropsized portions to the vial while manually shaking it. The temperature was maintained at 20 °C. Once all solid was dissolved, the weight of the added solvent was recorded, and the solvent volume was calculated.

Oxidation of PPh_3. Adduct **6** (22.0 mg, 0.0451 mmol, 1 equiv.) was added to PPh_3 (20.0 mg, 0.0762 mmol, 1.69 equiv.), dissolved in 0.5 mL $CDCl_3$. The reaction mixture was stirred for 5 min at RT and subsequently analyzed with ^1H, ^{13}C, and ^{31}P NMR spectroscopies.

IR Spectroscopy. The IR spectra of the polycrystalline materials were recorded using a Shimadzu IRAffinity-1 FTIR spectrometer equipped with a Pike Technologies MIRacle ATR plate.

X-Ray Diffraction. See Supplementary Materials and references [55–59].

4. Conclusions

Five representative hydrogen-bonded peroxide adducts of the novel type $Cy_3PO{\cdot}(HOO)_2CHR$ (R = alkyl) (**2–6**) have been synthesized and fully characterized. Single crystal X-ray diffraction studies confirmed that all adducts feature a precise 1:1 composition of di(hydroperoxy)alkane moiety and the hydrogen-bonded phosphine oxide. The arrangements of the adduct assemblies in the solid state follow the classic pattern for **3**, **5**, and **6**, but different new packing motifs are found for **2** and **4**. In accordance with the elongation of the P=O bonds detected by X-ray diffraction, the ^{31}P NMR spectra display downfield-shifted signals, and the IR wavenumbers ν(P=O) of all adducts are smaller as compared to the values of neat Cy_3PO. The solubilities of the adducts are high in common organic solvents and have been quantified for **1**, for comparison, and **2** and **6**.

In summary, the described new adducts, derived from aldehydes, represent a hitherto missing link of di(hydroperoxy)alkane adducts of phosphine oxides. It has been demonstrated that this new type of adduct is stable, crystallizes easily, and is amenable to full spectroscopic characterization. The strong hydrogen bonds between the peroxide and phosphine oxide result in shelf-stable, crystalline material with high solubility in organic solvents, allowing for oxidation reactions in one phase. As one preliminary application, a phosphine has been oxidized selectively to the phosphine oxide. The easy synthesis, handling, and dosing of these solid peroxides will make a positive impact on synthetic chemistry.

Supplementary Materials: The following supporting information for X-ray diffraction [55–59] and NMR spectroscopy can be downloaded at https://www.mdpi.com/article/10.3390/molecules30020329/s1. Table S1: Crystallographic data for **2**, **3**, and **4**; Table S2: Crystallographic data for **5** and **6**; Figure S1: Stacking pattern of two adduct assemblies of $Cy_3PO{\cdot}(HOO)_2CHCH_2CH_3$ (**3**). Hydrogen atoms except those in $CH(OOH)_2$ moieties are omitted for clarity; Figure S2: Stacking pattern of four adduct assemblies of $Cy_3PO{\cdot}(HOO)_2CH(CH_2)_2CH_3$ (**4**). Hydrogen atoms except those in $CH(OOH)_2$ moieties are omitted for clarity; Figure S3: ^{31}P NMR spectra of the adducts **2–6** in $CDCl_3$. All signals are downfield-shifted as compared to the resonance of Cy_3PO ($\delta(^{31}P)$ = 49.91 ppm); Figure S4: ^{1}H NMR spectrum of the adduct $Cy_3PO{\cdot}(HOO)_2CHCH_3$ (**2**); Figure S5: ^{1}H NMR spectrum of the adduct $Cy_3PO{\cdot}(HOO)_2CHCH_2CH_3$ (**3**); Figure S6: ^{1}H NMR spectrum of the adduct $Cy_3PO{\cdot}(HOO)_2CH(CH_2)_2CH_3$ (**4**); Figure S7: ^{1}H NMR spectrum of the adduct $Cy_3PO{\cdot}(HOO)_2CH(CH_2)_3CH_3$ (**5**); Figure S8: ^{1}H NMR spectrum of the adduct $Cy_3PO{\cdot}(HOO)_2CH(CH_2)_7CH_3$ (**6**); Figure S9: ^{13}C NMR spectrum of the adduct $Cy_3PO{\cdot}(HOO)_2CHCH_3$ (**2**); Figure S10: ^{13}C NMR spectrum of the adduct $Cy_3PO{\cdot}(HOO)_2CHCH_2CH_3$ (**3**); Figure S11: ^{13}C NMR spectrum of the adduct $Cy_3PO{\cdot}(HOO)_2CH(CH_2)_2CH_3$ (**4**); Figure S12: ^{13}C NMR spectrum of the adduct $Cy_3PO{\cdot}(HOO)_2CH(CH_2)_3CH_3$ (**5**); Figure S13: ^{13}C NMR spectrum of the adduct $Cy_3PO{\cdot}(HOO)_2CH(CH_2)_7CH_3$ (**6**). Assignments for C4, C5, and C6 are interchangeable; Figure S14: ^{1}H NMR spectra of nonanal (top) and the reaction mixture after combining adduct **6** with 2 equivalents of PPh_3 (bottom); Figure S15: ^{13}C NMR spectra of nonanal (top), the adduct $Cy_3PO{\cdot}(HOO)_2CH(CH_2)_7CH_3$ (**6**) (middle), and the reaction mixture after combining adduct **6** with 2 equivalents of PPh_3 (bottom). The supporting information is available free of charge. Detailed description of materials and methods used for X-ray crystallography. Crystallographic information for **2–5** with selected data in tables. ^{31}P, ^{13}C, and ^{1}H NMR spectra.

Author Contributions: Conceptualization, J.B.; Methodology, R.A., N.B. and J.B.; Software, N.B.; Validation, N.B. and J.B.; Formal analysis, R.A., M.T., N.B. and J.B.; Investigation, R.A., M.T. and J.B.; Resources, J.B.; Data curation, R.A. and N.B.; Writing—original draft, J.B.; Writing—review & editing, R.A. and N.B.; Visualization, R.A. and N.B.; Supervision, J.B.; Project administration, J.B.; Funding acquisition, J.B. All authors have read and agreed to the published version of the manuscript.

Funding: This work was supported by the National Science Foundation (CHE-1900100).

Institutional Review Board Statement: Not applicable.

Informed Consent Statement: Not applicable.

Data Availability Statement: CCDC 2404335 (**2**), 2404336 (**3**), 2404337 (**4**), 2404338 (**5**), and 2404339 (**6**) contain the crystallographic data for this paper. These data can be obtained free of charge via www.ccdc.cam.ac.uk/data_request/cif (accessed on 19 December 2024), or by emailing data_request@ccdc.cam.ac.uk, or by contacting the Cambridge Crystallographic Data Centre, 12 Union Road, Cambridge CB2 1EZ, UK; fax: +44-1223-336033.

Conflicts of Interest: There are no conflicts of interest to declare.

References

1. Duprey, D.; Cavani, F. *Handbook of Advanced Methods and Processes in Oxidation Catalysis*; Imperial College Press: London, UK, 2014.
2. Cavani, F.; Teles, J.H. Sustainability in Catalytic Oxidation: An Alternative Approach or a Structural Evolution? *ChemSusChem* **2009**, *2*, 508–534. [CrossRef]
3. Comyns, A.E. Peroxides and Peroxide Compounds. In *Van Nostrand's Encyclopedia of Chemistry*; John Wiley & Sons, Inc.: Hoboken, NJ, USA, 2005.
4. Klassen, N.V.; Marchington, D.; McGowan, H.C.E. H_2O_2 Determination by the I_3^- Method and by $KMnO_4$ Titration. *Anal. Chem.* **1994**, *66*, 2921–2925. [CrossRef]
5. Azizi, M.; Maleki, A.; Hakimpoor, F. Solvent, Metal- and Halogen-Free Synthesis of Sulfoxides by Using a Recoverable Heterogeneous Urea-Hydrogen Peroxide Silica-Based Oxidative Catalytic System. *Catal. Commun.* **2017**, *100*, 62–65. [CrossRef]
6. Taliansky, S. Urea-Hydrogen Peroxide Complex. *Synlett* **2005**, *12*, 1962–1963. [CrossRef]
7. Ji, L.; Wang, Y.-N.; Qian, C.; Chen, X.-Z. Nitrile-Promoted Alkene Epoxidation with Urea-Hydrogen Peroxide (UHP). *Synth. Commun.* **2013**, *43*, 2256–2264. [CrossRef]
8. Koukabi, N. Sodium Percarbonate: A Versatile Oxidizing Reagent. *Synlett* **2010**, *19*, 2969–2970. [CrossRef]
9. McKillop, A.; Sanderson, W.R. Sodium Perborate and Sodium Percarbonate: Further Applications in Organic Synthesis. *J. Chem. Soc. Perkin Trans.* **2000**, *1*, 471–476. [CrossRef]
10. Habibi, D.; Zolfigol, M.A.; Safaiee, M.; Shamsian, A.; Ghorbani-Choghamarani, A. Catalytic Oxidation of Sulfides to Sulfoxides using Sodium Perborate and/or Sodium Percarbonate and Silica Sulfuric Acid in the Presence of KBr. *Catal. Commun.* **2009**, *10*, 1257–1260. [CrossRef]
11. Arzumanyan, A.V.; Novikov, R.A.; Terent'ev, A.O.; Platonov, M.M.; Lakhtin, V.G.; Arkhipov, D.E.; Korlyukov, A.A.; Chernyshev, V.V.; Fitch, A.N.; Zdvizhkov, A.T.; et al. Nature Chooses Rings: Synthesis of Silicon-Containing Macrocyclic Peroxides. *Organometallics* **2014**, *33*, 2230–2246. [CrossRef]
12. Zha, Q.; Wu, Y. Synthesis of Primary *gem*-Dihydroperoxides and Their Peroxycarbenium [3 + 2] Cycloaddition Reactions with Alkenes. *J. Org. Chem.* **2020**, *85*, 14121–14138. [CrossRef] [PubMed]
13. Dove, J.E.; Riddick, J. Concerning the preparation of anhydrous hydrogen peroxide. *Can. J. Chem.* **1968**, *46*, 330–332. [CrossRef]
14. Wolanov, Y.; Lev, O.; Churakov, A.V.; Medvedev, A.G.; Novotortsev, V.M.; Prikhodchenko, P.V. Preparation of pure hydrogen peroxide and anhydrous peroxide solutions from crystalline serine perhydrate. *Tetrahedron* **2010**, *66*, 5130–5133. [CrossRef]
15. Cofré, P.; Sawyer, D.T. Redox Chemistry of Hydrogen Peroxide in Anhydrous Acetonitrile. *Inorg. Chem.* **1986**, *25*, 2089–2092. [CrossRef]
16. Kharel, S.; Bhuvanesh, N.; Gladysz, J.A.; Blümel, J. New Hydrogen Bonding Motifs of Phosphine Oxides with a Silanediol, a Phenol, and Chloroform. *Inorg. Chim. Acta* **2019**, *490*, 215–219. [CrossRef]
17. Tupikina, E.Y.; Bodensteiner, M.; Tolstoy, P.M.; Denisov, G.S.; Shenderovich, I.G. P=O Moiety as an Ambidextrous Hydrogen Bond Acceptor. *J. Phys. Chem. C* **2018**, *122*, 1711–1720. [CrossRef]
18. Begimova, G.; Tupikina, E.Y.; Yu, V.K.; Denisov, G.S.; Bodensteiner, M.; Shenderovich, I.G. Effect of Hydrogen Bonding to Water on the ^{31}P Chemical Shift Tensor of Phenyl- and Trialkylphosphine Oxides and α-Amino Phosphonates. *J. Phys. Chem. C* **2016**, *120*, 8717–8729. [CrossRef]
19. Cuypers, R.; Sudhölter, E.J.R.; Zuilhof, H. Hydrogen Bonding in Phosphine Oxide/Phosphate–Phenol Complexes. *ChemPhysChem* **2010**, *11*, 2230–2240. [CrossRef] [PubMed]
20. Bewick, N.A.; Arendt, A.; Li, Y.; Szafert, S.; Lis, T.; Wheeler, K.A.; Young, J.; Dembinski, R. Synthesis and Solid-State Structure of (4-Hydroxy-3,5-diiodophenyl)phosphine Oxides. Dimeric Motifs with the Assistance of O-H···O=P Hydrogen Bonds. *Curr. Org. Chem.* **2015**, *19*, 469–474. [CrossRef]
21. Hoefler, J.C.; Vu, A.; Perez, A.J.; Blümel, J. Immobilized Di(hydroperoxy)propane Adducts of Phosphine Oxides as Traceless and Recyclable Oxidizing Agents. *Appl. Surf. Sci.* **2023**, *629*, 157333. [CrossRef]
22. Hilliard, C.R.; Bhuvanesh, N.; Gladysz, J.A.; Blümel, J. Synthesis, Purification, and Characterization of Phosphine Oxides and Their Hydrogen Peroxide Adducts. *Dalton Trans.* **2012**, *41*, 1742–1754. [CrossRef]
23. Arp, F.F.; Bhuvanesh, N.; Blümel, J. Hydrogen Peroxide Adducts of Triarylphosphine Oxides. *Dalton Trans.* **2019**, *48*, 14312–14325. [CrossRef] [PubMed]
24. Ahn, S.H.; Cluff, K.J.; Bhuvanesh, N.; Blümel, J. Hydrogen Peroxide and Di(hydroperoxy)propane Adducts of Phosphine Oxides as Stoichiometric and Soluble Oxidizing Agents. *Angew. Chem. Int. Ed.* **2015**, *54*, 13341–13345. [CrossRef] [PubMed]
25. Arp, F.F.; Bhuvanesh, N.; Blümel, J. Di(hydroperoxy)cycloalkane Adducts of Triarylphosphine Oxides: A Comprehensive Study Including Solid-State Structures and Association in Solution. *Inorg. Chem.* **2020**, *59*, 13719–13732. [CrossRef] [PubMed]
26. Arp, F.F.; Ahn, S.H.; Bhuvanesh, N.; Blümel, J. Selective Synthesis and Stabilization of Peroxides via Phosphine Oxides. *New J. Chem.* **2019**, *43*, 17174–17181. [CrossRef]

27. Ahn, S.H.; Bhuvanesh, N.; Blümel, J. Di(hydroperoxy)alkane Adducts of Phosphine Oxides: Safe, Solid, Stoichiometric, and Soluble Oxidizing Agents. *Chem. Eur. J.* **2017**, *23*, 16998–17009. [CrossRef] [PubMed]
28. Ahn, S.H.; Lindhardt, D.; Bhuvanesh, N.; Blümel, J. Di(hydroperoxy)cycloalkanes Stabilized via Hydrogen Bonding by Phosphine Oxides: Safe and Efficient Baeyer-Villiger Oxidants. *ACS Sustain. Chem. Eng.* **2018**, *6*, 6829–6840. [CrossRef]
29. Arp, F.F.; Ashirov, R.; Bhuvanesh, N.; Blümel, J. Di(hydroperoxy)adamantane Adducts: Synthesis, Characterization and Application as Oxidizers for the Direct Esterification of Aldehydes. *Dalton Trans.* **2021**, *50*, 15296–15309. [CrossRef] [PubMed]
30. Blümel, J. Linkers and Catalysts Immobilized on Oxide Supports: New Insights by Solid-State NMR Spectroscopy. *Coord. Chem. Rev.* **2008**, *252*, 2410–2423. [CrossRef]
31. Guenther, J.; Reibenspies, J.; Blümel, J. Synthesis and Characterization of Tridentate Phosphine Ligands Incorporating Long Methylene Chains and Ethoxysilane Groups for Immobilizing Molecular Rhodium Catalysts. *Mol. Catal.* **2019**, *479*, 110629–110642. [CrossRef]
32. Pope, J.C.; Posset, T.; Bhuvanesh, N.; Blümel, J. The Palladium Component of an Immobilized Sonogashira Catalyst System: New Insights by Multinuclear HRMAS NMR Spectroscopy. *Organometallics* **2014**, *33*, 6750–6753. [CrossRef]
33. Shakeri, E.; Blümel, J. Creating Well-Defined Monolayers of Phosphine Linkers Incorporating Ethoxysilyl Groups on Silica Surfaces for Superior Immobilized Catalysts. *Appl. Surf. Sci.* **2023**, *615*, 156380–156387. [CrossRef]
34. Posset, T.; Guenther, J.; Pope, J.; Oeser, T.; Blümel, J. Immobilized Sonogashira Catalyst Systems: New Insights by Multinuclear HRMAS NMR Studies. *Chem. Commun.* **2011**, *47*, 2059–2061. [CrossRef]
35. Hayashi, S.; Jimura, K.; Kojima, N. Adsorption of Trimethylphosphine Oxide on Silicalite Studied by Solid-State NMR. *Bull. Chem. Soc. Jpn.* **2014**, *87*, 69–75. [CrossRef]
36. Machida, S.; Sohmiya, M.; Ide, Y.; Sugahara, Y. Solid-State ^{31}P Nuclear Magnetic Resonance Study of Interlayer Hydroxide Surfaces of Kaolinite Probed with an Interlayer Triethylphosphine Oxide Monolayer. *Langmuir* **2018**, *34*, 12694–12701. [CrossRef] [PubMed]
37. Hubbard, P.J.; Benzie, J.W.; Bakhmutov, V.I.; Blümel, J. Disentangling Different Modes of Mobility of Triphenylphosphine Oxide Adsorbed on Alumina. *J. Chem. Phys.* **2020**, *152*, 054718-1–054718-8. [CrossRef] [PubMed]
38. Kharel, S.; Cluff, K.J.; Bhuvanesh, N.; Gladysz, J.A.; Blümel, J. Structures and Dynamics of Secondary and Tertiary Alkylphosphine Oxides Adsorbed on Silica. *Chem. Asian J.* **2019**, *14*, 2704–2711. [CrossRef] [PubMed]
39. Hilliard, C.R.; Kharel, S.; Cluff, K.J.; Bhuvanesh, N.; Gladysz, J.A.; Blümel, J. Structures and Unexpected Dynamic Properties of Phosphine Oxides Adsorbed on Silica Surfaces. *Chem. Eur. J.* **2014**, *20*, 17292–17295. [CrossRef] [PubMed]
40. Ashirov, R.; Kimball, M.R.; O'Brien, M.; Bhuvanesh, N.; Blümel, J. Aluminum Trichloride Adducts of Phosphine Oxides: A Single Crystal X-Ray and Solid-State NMR Study. *Inorg. Chim. Acta* **2024**, *564*, 121952. [CrossRef]
41. Chrzanowski, J.; Krasowska, D.; Drabowicz, J. Synthesis of Optically Active Tertiary Phosphine Oxides: A Historical Overview and the Latest Advances. *Heteroat. Chem.* **2018**, *29*, e21476. [CrossRef]
42. Kharel, S.; Jia, T.; Bhuvanesh, N.; Reibenspies, J.H.; Blümel, J.; Gladysz, J.A. A Non-templated Route to Macrocyclic Dibridgehead Diphosphorus Compounds: Crystallographic Characterization of a "Crossed-Chain" Variant of *in/out* Stereoisomers. *Chem. Asian J.* **2018**, *13*, 2632–2640. [CrossRef]
43. Fletcher, M.D. *Organophosphorus Reagents, a Practical Approach in Chemistry*; Murphy, P.J., Ed.; Oxford University Press: London, UK, 2004; pp. 171–214. ISBN 9780198502623.
44. Adams, H.; Collins, R.C.; Jones, S.; Warner, C.J.A. Enantioselective Preparation of P-Chiral Phosphine Oxides. *Org. Lett.* **2011**, *13*, 6576–6579. [CrossRef]
45. Swamy, K.C.K.; Kumar, N.N.B.; Balaraman, E.; Kumar, K.V.P.P. Mitsunobu and Related Reactions: Advances and Applications. *Chem. Rev.* **2009**, *109*, 2551–2651.
46. Dembinski, R. Recent Advances in the Mitsunobu Reaction: Modified Reagents and the Quest for Chromatography-Free Separation. *Eur. J. Org. Chem.* **2004**, *2004*, 2763–2772. [CrossRef]
47. Beddoe, R.H.; Andrews, K.G.; Magne, V.; Cuthbertson, J.D.; Saska, J.; Shannon-Little, A.L.; Shanahan, S.E.; Sneddon, H.F.; Denton, R.M. Redox-Neutral Organocatalytic Misunobu Reactions. *Science* **2020**, *365*, 910–914. [CrossRef] [PubMed]
48. The Following CCDC Reference Numbers Contain the Supplementary Crystallographic Data for the Corresponding Compounds **2–6** for This Paper: 2404335 (**2**), 2404336 (**3**), 2404337 (**4**), 2404338 (**5**), and 2404339 (**6**). These Data Can Be Obtained Free of Charge from the Cambridge Crystallographic Data Centre. Available online: www.ccdc.cam.ac.uk/data_request/cif (accessed on 19 December 2024).
49. Günzler, H.; Gremlich, H.-U. *IR Spektroskopie*, 4th ed.; Wiley-VCH: Weinheim, Germany, 2003.
50. Jeffrey, G.A. *An Introduction to Hydrogen Bonding*; Oxford University Press: Oxford, UK, 1997.
51. Baker, E.N.; Hubbard, R.E. Hydrogen Bonding in Globular Proteins. *Prog. Biophys. Mol. Bio.* **1984**, *44*, 97–179. [CrossRef]
52. Kalinowski, H.-O.; Berger, S.; Braun, S. *^{13}C-NMR-Spektroskopie*; Georg Thieme Verlag Stuttgart: New York, NY, USA, 1984.
53. Hesse, M.; Meier, H.; Zeeh, B. *Spektroskopische Methoden in der Organischen Chemie*; Georg Thieme Verlag Stuttgart: New York, NY, USA, 1984.

54. Hoefler, J.C.; Jackson, D.; Blümel, J. Surface-Assisted Selective Air Oxidation of Phosphines Adsorbed on Activated Carbon. *Inorg. Chem.* **2024**, *63*, 9275–9287. [CrossRef]
55. CrysAlisPro Software System, Rigaku Oxford Diffraction 2003. Available online: https://rigaku.com/products/crystallography/x-ray-diffraction/crysalispro (accessed on 19 December 2024).
56. Sheldrick, G.M. A short history of SHELX. *Acta Cryst.* **2008**, *A64*, 112–122. [CrossRef]
57. Sheldrick, G.M. Crystal structure solution with ShelXT. *Acta Cryst.* **2015**, *A71*, 3–8.
58. Dolomanov, O.V.; Bourhis, L.J.; Gildea, R.J.; Howard, J.A.K.; Puschmann, H.J. OLEX2. *Appl. Cryst.* **2009**, *42*, 339–341. [CrossRef]
59. Taylor, R.; Macrae, C.F. Mercury. *Acta Cryst.* **2001**, *B57*, 815–827. [CrossRef] [PubMed]

molecules

MDPI

Article

N,N-Dimethylformamide's Participation in Domino Reactions for the Synthesis of Se-Phenyl Dimethylcarbamoselenoate Derivatives

Runsheng Xu *, Shenhuanran Hu, Luhui Wu, Yifan Ning and Jin Xu *

College of Life and Health, Huzhou College, Huzhou 211300, China; com1241613607@163.com (S.H.); wuluhui141@gmail.com (L.W.); fansxmy@outlook.com (Y.N.)
* Correspondence: xurunsheng@zjhzu.edu.cn (R.X.); xujin@zjhzu.edu.cn (J.X.)

Abstract: *N,N*-dimethylformamide's (DMF) participation in domino reactions has been developed. Starting from substituted halogenobenzenes and selenium powder, versatile biologically active Se-phenyl dimethylcarbamoselenoate derivatives were efficiently synthesized under mild reaction conditions. The reaction mechanism was studied using control experiments. These protocols involve a wider substrate scope and provide an economical approach toward C–selenium bond formation.

Keywords: dual role; DMF; domino reaction; C–selenium bond formation; copper catalyst

1. Introduction

Selenium compounds are widely used in various fields, such as synthetic chemistry, pharmaceutical pesticides, and functional materials [1,2]. Furthermore, selenium is one of the most important markers in the human body and has a variety of important functions for human health. First, selenium can enhance the ability of the immune system to identify pathogens in the body. Selenium also helps to maintain the sensitivity of the nervous system [3,4]. Secondly, selenium is an effective antioxidant that can eliminate free radicals in the body, reducing oxidative damage to cells and thereby preventing and reducing the severity of certain chronic diseases. Selenium can reduce cholesterol levels in the blood, prevent the occurrence of arteriosclerosis, inhibit platelet agglomeration, and preserve cardiovascular health [5–7]. Selenium also has a positive impact on male reproductive health, improving sperm quality and enhancing fertility. In terms of the digestive system, selenium can improve and enhance the absorption function of the digestive system, accelerate gastrointestinal motility, promote the decomposition and absorption of gastrointestinal content, and help to reduce the symptoms of indigestion [8–11]. Taninia reported a click reaction of selenols with isocyanates (Scheme 1) [12]. In this method, selenols react with isocyanates under mild catalyst-free conditions to generate selenocarbamates in good yield and with high selectivity over potentially competing nucleophilic additions. The methodology enables the incorporation of a wide variety of functional groups, providing access to a broad array of densely functionalized selenocarbamates. Therefore, the synthesis of organic selenium compounds with a variety of functions is of great significance.

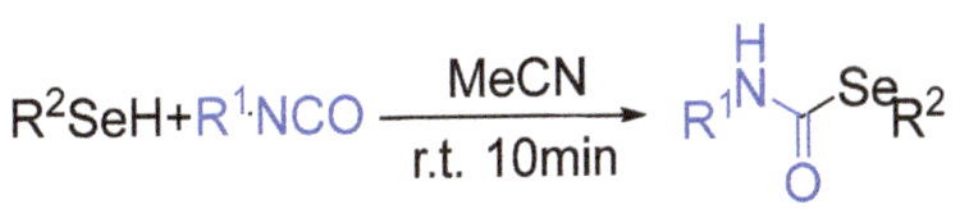

Scheme 1. Click reaction of selenols with isocyanates.

Being a favorable solvent, *N,N*-dimethylformamide (DMF) is also an important synthetic structure [13–15]. It can be used as a parental reagent, a nuclear test agent, and in free radical reactions. It can participate in multiple chemical reactions in organic synthesis. For example, DMF plays an important role in methyl-based reactions. Through the Vilsmeier reagent, the metacimal part of DMF is transferred to the double bond to realize alfalized compounds, heterogenic circular compounds, and pitro-enriched reactions of the e-electronic olefin. DMF can also react with metal reagents to produce aldehydes [16]. When bromine aromatics or iodine-aged aromatics respond to metal halogen with organic lithium reagents or grid reagents, the generated aromatherapy reagent reacts with DMF to efficiently prepare a series of aromatic Aldo [17]. DMF also plays an important role in a vital method for reducing the amino reactor aldosone to amine. For example, a Lewis acid catalyzes the DMF triangle to participate in restorative amino reactions [18]. The reaction substrate is very broad, and the functional group is also very inclusive. In cyanide reactions, DMF can also be used as a C-H functionalized reagent [19–21].

In addition to the above reactions, DMF can be used as a ligand that participates in metal catalytic reactions to achieve amino-based reactions of halogen aromatics. Furthermore, DMF can be used as an important source of dihylaminel, and it can be utilized to realize bigramine-based reactions of various marinated hydrocarbons. Moreover, DMF can participate in the reaction of a cord additional [2+2] bonus to a cyclolar bonus. In summary, DMF plays multiple roles in organic synthesis and can participate in multiple chemical reactions. Its unique structure and properties make DMF a very useful tool in synthesis, providing new means and methods for organic synthesis.

Our interest focuses on traditional metal-catalyzed C-H bond functionalization. Over the past decade, many reactions involving S-C and Se-C bond formation have been developed by our group [22–24]. Herein, a dual role of DMF's participation in domino reactions has been developed. Starting from substituted halogenobenzenes and selenium powder, versatile biologically active Se-phenyl dimethylcarbamoselenoate derivatives were efficiently synthesized under mild reaction conditions. The reaction mechanism was studied by means of deuterium isotope experiments. These protocols involve a wider substrate scope and provide an economical approach toward C–selenium bond formation.

2. Results and Discussion

At the beginning of our experiments, we investigated the model reaction of iodobenzene **1a** and selenium powder **2** to study the reaction conditions, including the optimization of catalysts, bases, and solvents. As shown in Table 1, at the outset, copper salts were used as the catalyst (entries 1–6), and no desired product was gained when the reaction was conducted in the presence of CuO as the catalyst in DMSO (entry 1). These results show that using the proper solvent is critical for this reaction as, when the reactions were conducted in an apolar solvent, the DMF product was detected in a moderate yield. $CuBr_2$ was proven to be the most efficient catalyst species in this reaction (entry 5). Gratifyingly, the yield of product **4a** was obtained at 75% when the catalyst was changed to $Cu(OAc)_2$ (entry 6). By screening different bases for the reaction, Cs_2CO_3 was demonstrated to be a more suitable base than others such as NaOH, Na_2CO_3, Na_2SO_4, NaOEt, K_2CO_3, and K_2PO_3 (entries 6–12). A reduced yield was obtained in the reactions operated at 100 °C (72% yield, entry 13) and 120 °C (77% yield, entry 13). We also found that the yields of the product decreased when the amount of copper catalyst used was higher or lower than 10 mol% equivalent (entries 17 and 18). Finally, we determined that the optimal reaction conditions were as follows: $Cu(OAc)_2$ used as the catalyst, Cs_2CO_3 used as the base, a ratio of **1a**:**2** of 1:1.5:1, a N_2 atmosphere, 110 °C, and preparation for 24 h.

Table 1. Optimization of the reaction conditions [a].

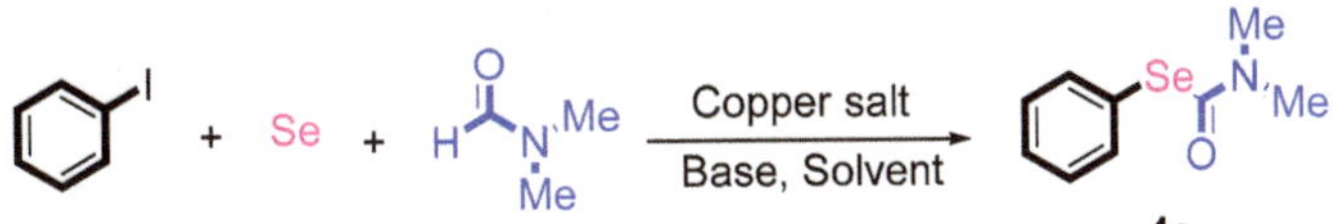

1a **2** **3** **4a**

Entry	Copper Salt	Base	Solvent	1a:2	Yield (%) [b]
1	CuO	Na_2CO_3	DMSO	1:1	0
2	$CuSO_4$	Na_2CO_3	DMF	1:1	18
3	CuI	Na_2CO_3	DMF	1:1	29
4	$CuCl_2$	Na_2CO_3	DMF	1:1	34
5	$CuBr_2$	Na_2CO_3	DMF	1:1	60
6	$Cu(OAc)_2$	Na_2CO_3	DMF	1:1	75
7	$Cu(OAc)_2$	Cs_2CO_3	DMF	1:1	86
8	$Cu(OAc)_2$	NaOH	DMF	1:1	56
9	$Cu(OAc)_2$	Na_2SO_4	DMF	1:1	49
10	$Cu(OAc)_2$	NaOEt	DMF	1:1	65
11	$Cu(OAc)_2$	K_2CO_3	DMF	1:1	55
12	$Cu(OAc)_2$	K_2PO_3	DMF	1:1	57
13	$Cu(OAc)_2$	Cs_2CO_3	DMF	1:1	5
14	$Cu(OAc)_2$	Cs_2CO_3	DMF	1:1	48
15	$Cu(OAc)_2$	Cs_2CO_3	DMF	1:1.5	72 [c]
16	$Cu(OAc)_2$	Cs_2CO_3	DMF	1:1.5	77 [d]
17	$Cu(OAc)_2$	Cs_2CO_3	DMF	1:1.5	64 [e]
18	$Cu(OAc)_2$	Cs_2CO_3	DMF	1:1.5	69 [f]

[a] Unless otherwise noted, reactions conditions were **1a** (10 mmol), **2** (10 mmol), copper catalyst (10 mol%), base (2 equivalent, under N_2 atmosphere), solvent (10 mL), and 110 °C for 24 h. [b] Isolated yield. [c] 100 °C. [d] 120 °C. [e] $Cu(OAc)_2$ (15 mol%). [f] $Cu(OAc)_2$ (5 mol%).

Next, the substrate scope was examined under the optimal conditions, and the results are shown in Table 2. Aryl iodides **1**, selenium powder **2**, and DMF **3** were subjected to this reaction and the products were produced in good to excellent yields (79–92%). A variety of functional groups, including methyl, methoxy, halogen, and naphthyl groups, were compatible with aryl iodides **1**. It was found that both the electron-donating and electron-withdrawing aryl iodides **1** reacted smoothly with selenium powder **2** and DMF **3**. Aryl iodides **1** bearing electron-withdrawing groups showed better activity than those bearing electron-donating groups. This suggests that the conjugated structure could strongly coordinate with the copper catalyst, providing good yields (**4g**, 92% yield; **4h**, 88% yield). Despite the strong electron-donating effect of the trimethyl group, the corresponding product **4f** was still obtained at a 79% yield.

Table 2. *N*,*N*-dimethylformamide's participation in domino reactions [a].

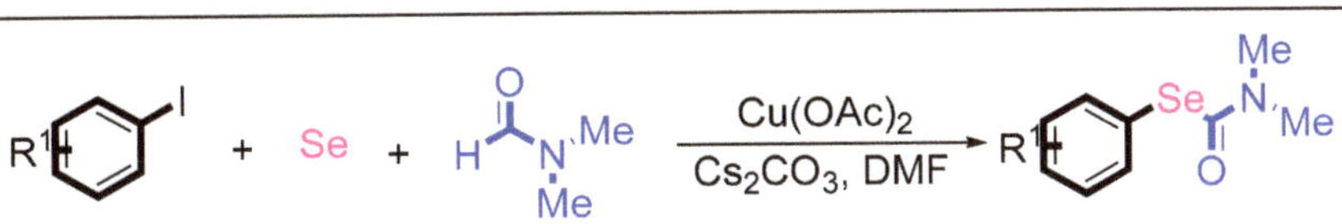

1 **2** **3** **4**

Entry	1	Product	Yield (%) [b]
1	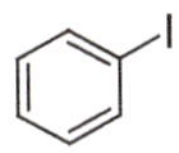	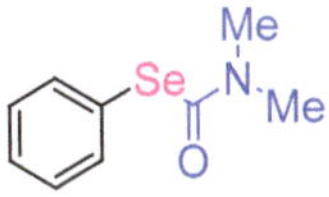 **4a**	86

Table 2. *Cont.*

Entry	1	Product	Yield (%) [b]
2	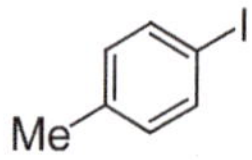	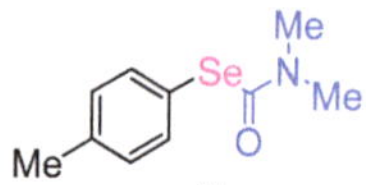 **4b**	84
3	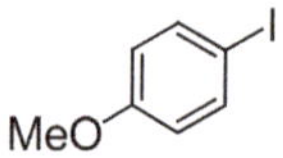	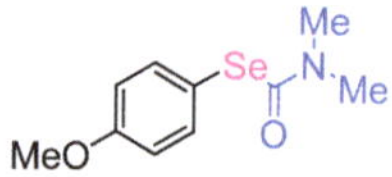 **4c**	81
4	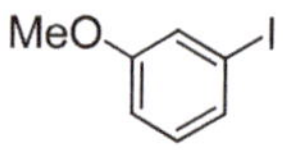	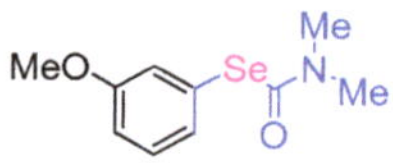 **4d**	83
5	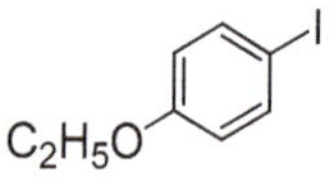	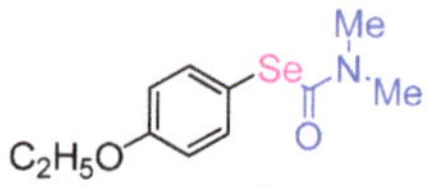 **4e**	80
6	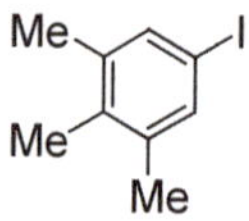	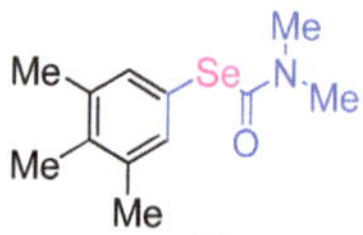 **4f**	79
7	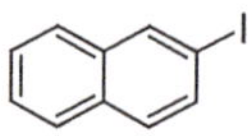	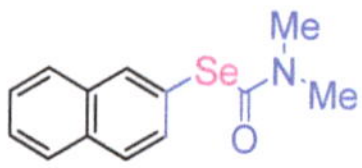 **4g**	92
8	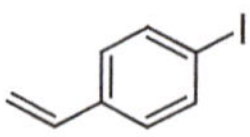	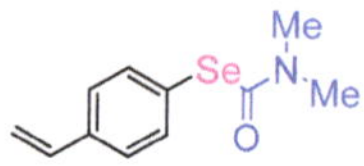 **4h**	90
9	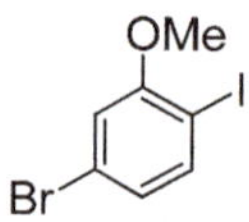	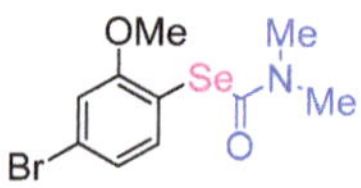 **4i**	88
10	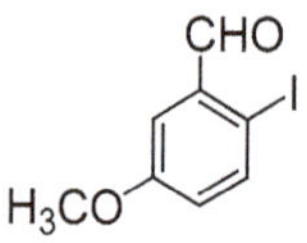	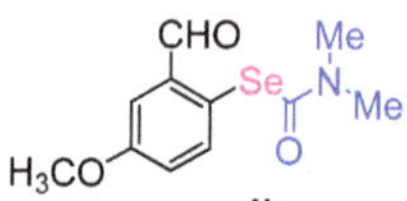 **4j**	89

[a] Unless otherwise noted, the reaction conditions were as follows: **1** (10 mmol), **2** (15 mmol), $Cu(OAc)_2$ (10 mol%), Cs_2CO_3 (2 equivalent), a N_2 atmosphere, DMF (10 mL), and 110 °C for 24 h. [b] Isolated yield.

After the group tolerance of aryl iodides **1** was demonstrated, the diversity of bromine-substituted benzene derivative **5** partners was further investigated under the optimized reaction conditions. A wide array of bromine-substituted benzene derivatives **5** were subjected to this reaction and the products were produced in moderate to good yields (70–86%). A variety of functional groups, including methyl, methoxy, halogen, and biphenyl groups, were compatible. The results are shown in Table 3. We also attempted to use strong electron-withdrawing groups such as trifluoromethyl and nitro under the current reaction conditions; however, this only led to the decomposition of the starting material without the expected product.

To gain a better understanding of this side reaction, tandem mass spectrometry (MS/MS) confirmed the position of the kinetic deuterium isotope effects, as shown in Scheme 2. In the mass spectrometry analysis, the fragment peak of m/z 219.88 ($C_6H_5SeCu^+$) was absent. This demonstrates that oxidative addition is the rate-determining step for C-Se coupling in this reaction. Furthermore, the absence of the fragment peak of m/z 72.04 in the mass spectrometry analysis demonstrates that $C_3H_6NO^+$ may be a key intermediate.

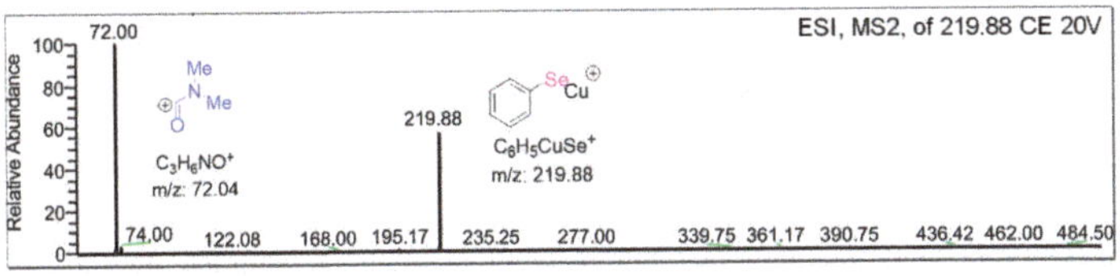

Scheme 2. MS–MS analysis of the isolated product reaction mixture.

To gain more insights into the reaction mechanism, some selective and control experiments were performed (Scheme 3). We examined the chemical competence of PhSeCu under optimal conditions in the presence of benzothiazole under a N_2 atmosphere, and the desired product **4a** was obtained in an 82% isolated yield (Scheme 3, eq1). These data for stoichiometric reactions of PhSeCu suggest that elemental selenium plays a key role in the process of C-Se formation, as shown in Scheme 3, eq2. This is consistent with our hypothesis that PhSeH may be a chemically competent intermediate, primarily through Ullman-type selenation between aryl iodides and selenium in situ during the catalytic cycle. Finally, through the addition of dimethylamine under the optimized reaction conditions (Scheme 3, eq3), the desired transformation was achieved.

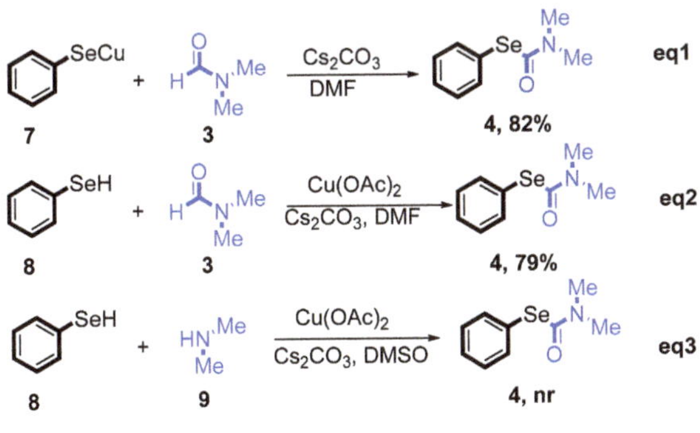

Scheme 3. Preliminary mechanism investigation.

Based on the above results, a possible reaction mechanism is proposed (Scheme 4) [25–28]. At the beginning, the coordination process of Cu^{II} and substituted halogenobenzenes **1** generated a Cu^{IV} intermediate **10**. Then, the substituted halogenobenzenes **1** were converted to intermediate **11c** by reacting with the selenium powder. Finally, the desired products **4** and **6** were obtained via C–Se bond cross coupling from intermediate **11** with DMF. Then, the Cu^{II} species was generated, which re-entered the catalytic cycle.

Table 3. *N*,*N*-dimethylformamide' participation in domino reactions [a].

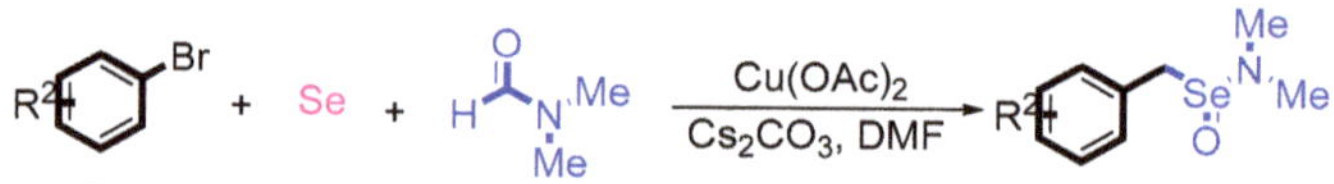

5 2 3 6

Entry	5	Product	Yield (%) [b]
1	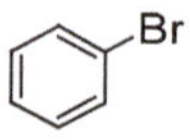	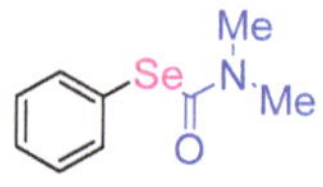 **6a**	81
2	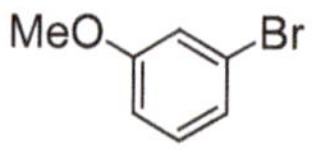	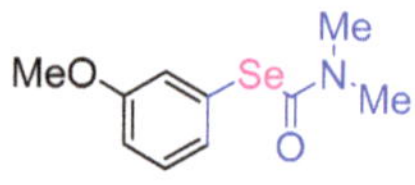 **6b**	78
3	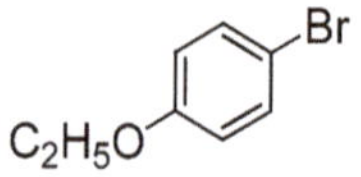	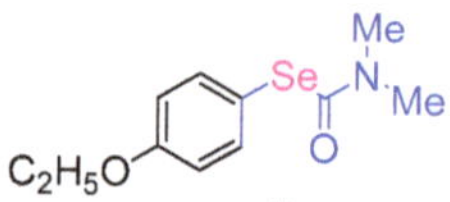 **6c**	76
4	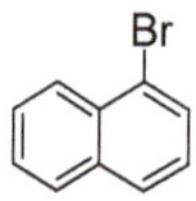	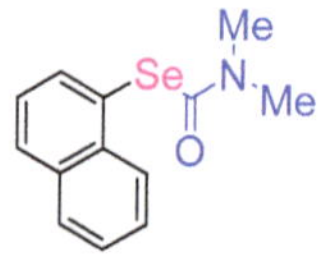 **6d**	85
6	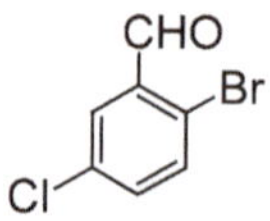	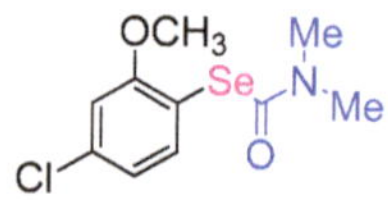 **6e**	86
5	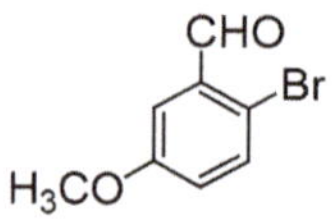	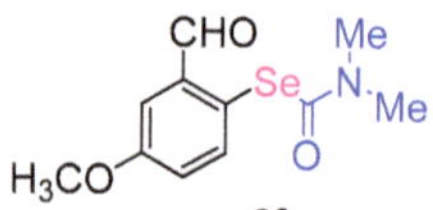 **6f**	83
7	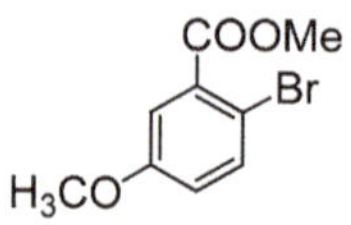	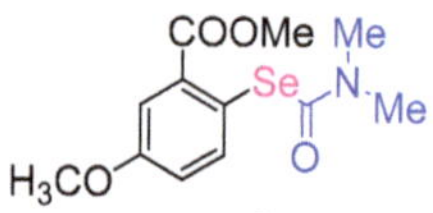 **6g**	72
8	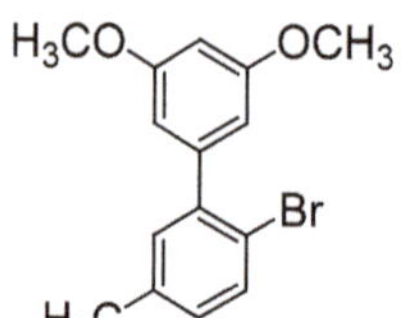	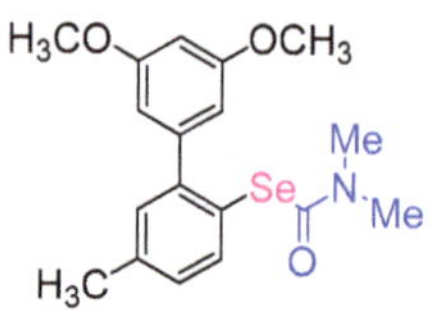 **6h**	70

[a] Unless otherwise noted, the reaction conditions were as follows: **5** (10 mmol), **2** (15 mmol), $Cu(OAc)_2$ (10 mol%), Cs_2CO_3 (2 equivalent), a N_2 atmosphere, DMF (10 mL), and 110 °C for 12 h. [b] Isolated yield.

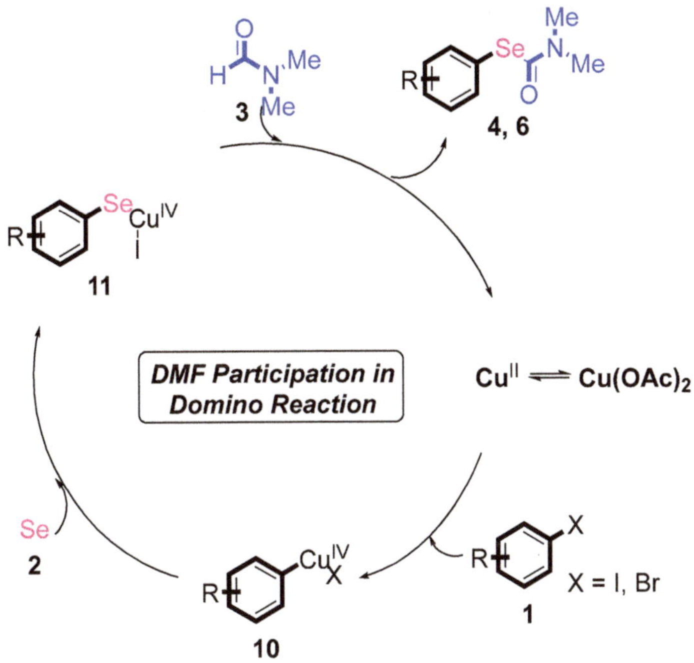

Scheme 4. Proposed mechanism for N, N-dimethylformamide's participation in domino reactions.

3. Materials and Methods

All reagents used in experiment were obtained from commercial sources and used without further purification. Solvents for chromatography were technical grade and distilled prior for using. Solvent mixtures were understood as volume/volume. Chemical yields refer to pure isolated substances. Catalysts were purchased for analytical reagent. Thin layer chromatography employed glass 0.25 mm silica gel plates with F_{254} indicator, visualized by irradiation with UV light. Reactions were carried out under argon in flame-dried or oven-dried glassware unless otherwise specified. Dichloroethane, dichloromethane, acetonitrile, toluene (after distilling from sodium), dimethyl sulfoxide, and tetrahydrofuran (after distilling from sodium) were dried from 4Å molecular sieves. Synthesis-grade solvents were used after as purchased. Chromatographic purification of products was accomplished using silica gel (300–400 mesh). For thin layer chromatography (TLC) analysis, Merck pre-coated TLC plates (silica gel 60 GF_{254}, 0.25 mm) were employed, using UV light as the visualizing agent. The compounds were isolated using Biotage flash column chromatography.

A mixture of iodobenzene **1a** (2.04 g, 10 mmol) and selenium powder **2** (0.79 g, 15 mmol), $Cu(OAc)_2$ (182 mg, 10 mol%), Cs_2CO_3 (6.52 g, 2 equiv), DMF (10 mL). The tube was evacuated and refilled with N_2 three times. The reaction is carried out under nitrogen protection. The reaction mixture was stirred at 110 °C for 12 h. After it was cooled, the reaction mixture was diluted with 20 mL of ethyl ether for 3 times. The filtrate was washed with water (3 × 15 mL). The organic phase was dried over Na_2SO_4, filtered, and concentrated under reduced pressure. and filtered through a pad of silica gel, followed by washing the pad of silica gel with the same solvent (20 mL). The residue was then purified by flash chromatography on silica gel to provide the corresponding product. The pure product Se-phenyl dimethylcarbamoselenoate **4a** was obtained 1.96 g, 86% yield. More experimental details can be found in the Supplementary Materials.

4. Conclusions

In summary, a dual role of *N,N*-dimethylformamide participation in domino reactions has been developed. Starting from substituted halogenobenzenes and selenium powder, versatile biologically active Se-phenyl dimethylcarbamoselenoate derivatives were efficiently synthesized under mild reaction conditions. The reaction mechanism was studied by means of deuterium isotope experiments. These protocols involve a wider substrate scope and provide an economical approach toward C–selenium bond formation.

Supplementary Materials: The following supporting information can be downloaded at: https://www.mdpi.com/article/10.3390/molecules30030747/s1.

Author Contributions: Conceptualization, R.X. and J.X.; methodology, S.H. and L.W.; investigation, Y.N.; writing—review and editing, R.X. All authors have read and agreed to the published version of the manuscript.

Funding: This research was funded by Scientific Research Fund of Zhejiang Provincial Education Department grant number No. Y202454916 and the Huzhou Science and Technology Plan Project grant number No. 2024YZ11.

Institutional Review Board Statement: Not applicable.

Informed Consent Statement: Not applicable.

Data Availability Statement: All relevant data are within the paper.

Conflicts of Interest: The authors declare no conflict of interest.

References

1. Zingaro, R.A.; Cooper, W.C. *Selenium*; van Nostrand Reinhold Company: New York, NY, USA, 1974.
2. Begines, P.; Martos, S.; Lagunes, I.; Maya, I.; Padrón, J.M.; López, Ó.; Fernández-Bolaños, J.G. Chemoselective Preparation of New Families of Phenolic-Organoselenium Hybrids—A Biological Assessment. *Molecules* **2022**, *27*, 1315. [CrossRef]
3. Watanabe, A.; Nagatomo, M.; Hirose, A.; Hikone, Y.; Kishimoto, N.; Miura, S.; Yasutake, T.; Abe, T.; Misumi, S.; Inoue, M. Total Syntheses of Phorbol and 11 Tigliane Diterpenoids and Their Evaluation as HIV Latency-Reversing Agents. *J. Am. Chem. Soc.* **2024**, *146*, 8746–8756. [CrossRef] [PubMed]
4. Arora, A.; Singh, S.; Oswal, P.; Nautiyal, D.; Rao, G.K.; Kumar, S.; Kumar, A. Preformed Molecular Complexes of Metals with Organoselenium Ligands: Syntheses and Applications in Catalysis. *Coord. Chem. Rev.* **2021**, *438*, 213885. [CrossRef]
5. Kolay, S.; Wadawale, A.; Das, D.; Kisan, H.K.; Sunoj, R.B.; Jain, V.K. Cyclopalladation of Dimesityl Selenide: Synthesis, Reactivity, Structural Characterization, Isolation of an Intermediate Complex with C-H··· Pd Intra-molecular Interaction and Computational Studies. *Dalton Trans.* **2013**, *2*, 10828–10837. [CrossRef]
6. Zhou, M.; Frenking, G. Transition-metal Chemistry of the Heavier Alkaline Earth Atoms Ca, Sr, and Ba. *Acc. Chem. Res.* **2021**, *54*, 3071–3082. [CrossRef]
7. Chaudhary, V.; Ashraf, N.; Khalid, M.; Walvekar, R.; Yang, Y.; Kaushik, A.; Mishra, Y.K. Emergence of MXene-Polymer Hybrid Nanocomposites as High-performance Next-Generation Chemiresistors for Efficient Air Quality Monitoring. *Adv. Fun. Mat.* **2022**, *32*, 2112913. [CrossRef]
8. Benckendorff, C.M.M.; Sunde-Brown, P.; Cheallaigh, A.N.; Miller, G.J. Synthesis of Nucleoside Analogs Containing Sulfur or Selenium Replacements of the Ribose Ring Oxygen or Carbon. *J. Org. Chem.* **2024**, *89*, 16977–16989. [CrossRef] [PubMed]
9. Li, W.; Kaminski Schierle, G.S.; Lei, B.; Liu, Y.; Kaminski, C.F. Fluorescent nanoparticles for super-resolution imaging. *Chem. Rev.* **2022**, *122*, 12495–12543. [CrossRef]
10. Engl, S.; Reiser, O. Copper-photocatalyzed ATRA Reactions: Concepts, Applications, and Opportunities. *Chem. Soc. Rev.* **2022**, *51*, 5287–5299. [CrossRef]
11. Larock, R. *Comprehensive Organic Yransformations: A Guide to Functional Group Preparations*; John Wiley & Sons: New York, NY, USA, 1989.

12. Capperucci, A.; Petrucci, A.; Faggi, C.; Tanini, D. Click Reaction of Selenols with Isocyanates: Rapid Access to Selenocarbamates as Peroxide-Switchable Reservoir of Thiolperoxidase-Like Catalysts. *Adv. Synth. Catal.* **2021**, *363*, 4256–4263. [CrossRef]
13. Patel, R.I.; Sharma, S.; Sharma, A. Cyanation: A Photochemical Approach and Applications in Organic Synthesis. *Org. Chem. Front.* **2021**, *8*, 3166–3200. [CrossRef]
14. Gandeepan, P.; Müller, T.; Zell, D.; Cera, G.; Warratz, S.; Ackermann, L. 3d Transition Metals for C-H Activation. *Chem. Rev.* **2018**, *119*, 2192–2452. [CrossRef] [PubMed]
15. Nair, S.R.; Chinta, B.S.; Baire, B. A Domino One-Pot Approach to Functionalized Benzonitriles from 2-[(3-Hydroxy/acetoxy) propyn-1-yl] benzamides. *Synthesis* **2024**, *56*, 3001–3008. [CrossRef]
16. Xie, S.; Cai, F.; Liu, L.; Su, L.; Dong, J.; Zhou, Y. Copper-Mediated Selective Multiple Inert Chemical Bonds Cleavage for Cyanation of Indoles via Tandem Carbon and Nitrogen Atom Transfer. *Chin. J. Chem.* **2024**, *42*, 2299–2304.
17. Gao, H.; Zhou, L.; Wan, J.P.; Liu, Y. Rongalite as C1 Synthon in the Synthesis of Divergent Pyridines and Quinolines. *J. Org. Chem.* **2023**, *88*, 7188–7198.
18. Mondal, S.; Samanta, S.; Santra, S.; Bagdi, A.K.; Hajra, A. N,N-Dimethylformamide as a Methylenating Reagent: Synthesis of Heterodiarylmethanes via Copper-catalyzed Coupling Between Imidazo [1,2-a]pyridines and Indoles/N,N-dimethylaniline. *Adv. Synth. Catal.* **2016**, *358*, 3633–3641. [CrossRef]
19. Yang, K.; Zhang, F.; Fang, T.; Li, C.; Li, W.; Song, Q. Passerini-type Reaction of Boronic Acids Enables α-Hydroxyketones Synthesis. *Nat. Commun.* **2021**, *12*, 441. [CrossRef]
20. Zhang, Q.; Song, C.; Huang, H.; Zhang, K.; Chang, J. Cesium Carbonate Promoted Cascade Reaction Involving DMF as a Reactant for the Synthesis of Dihydropyrrolizino [3, 2-b] indol-10-ones. *Org. Chem. Front.* **2018**, *5*, 80–87. [CrossRef]
21. Duan, F.F.; Song, S.Q.; Xu, R.S. Iron (II)-catalyzed Sulfur Directed C (sp^3)-H Bond Amination/C-S Cross Coupling Reaction. *Chem. Commun.* **2017**, *53*, 2737–2739.
22. Cai, R.R.; Zhou, Z.D.; Chai, Q.Q.; Zhu, Y.E.; Xu, R.S. Copper-Catalyzed C-S Direct Cross-coupling of Thiols with 5-Arylpenta-2, 4-Dienoic Acid Ethyl Ester. *RSC Adv.* **2018**, *8*, 26828–26836. [CrossRef] [PubMed]
23. Cai, R.R.; Wei, Q.C.; Xu, R.S. A Nickel-catalyzed Tandem Reaction Involving Cyclic Esterification/C-S Bond Formation for Synthesizing 5-Oxa-11-thia-benzofluoren-6-ones. *RSC Adv.* **2020**, *10*, 26414–26417. [CrossRef]
24. Zhou, X.Y.; Xue, Y.Q.; Cheng, Y.Y.; Xu, R.S. Copper-catalyzed Tandem Reaction of Cyclic Esterification/selenoxidation for 11-Oxo-11H-5-oxa-11-selena-benzo [a] fluoren-6-ones Synthesis. *Arkivoc* **2021**, *4*, 119–129. [CrossRef]
25. Khan, D.; Kumari, B.; Alzahrani, A.Y.A.; Dua, N.; Shaily; Maurya, N. Microwave-assisted Synthesis of Pyrroles, Pyridines, Chromenes, Coumarins, and Betti Bases via Alcohol Dehydrogenation with Chroman-4-one Amino Ligands. *Curr. Org. Chem.* **2024**, *28*, 1593–1604. [CrossRef]
26. Wang, M.; Ren, H.Y.; Pu, X.Y.; Zhang, X.L.; Zhu, H.Y.; Wu, A.X.; Zhao, B.T. Rongalite/iodine-mediated C(sp^3)–H Bond Oximation and Thiomethylation Reaction of Methyl Ketones using Copper Nitrate as the [NO] Reagent: Synthesis of Thiohydroximic Acids. *Org. Biomol. Chem.* **2024**, *22*, 7623–7627. [CrossRef] [PubMed]
27. Yang, J.C.; Liao, M.L.; Li, P.G.; Zou, L.H. A Concise Protocol for the Synthesis of 2-Alkenylindoles through [4+1] Annulation of Aminobenzyl Phosphonium Salts with Acrylaldehydes. *Green. Chem.* **2024**, *26*, 9295–9299. [CrossRef]
28. Liu, J.M.; Zheng, X.H.; Luo, W.J.; Chen, Z.W.; Ling, F. TBAB-catalyzed Assisted C-C/C-N Bond Formations: An Efficient Approach to Dihydrobenzo[b][1,8]naphthyridin Derivatives via Metal Free Cascade Annulation. *Synth. Commun.* **2024**, *54*, 1252–1262. [CrossRef]

molecules

Article

Novel One-Step Total Synthesis of *trans*-Dehydroosthol and Citrubuntin

Zhiwen Liu [1,†], Baoyue Ge [1,†], Xushun Gong [1], Fusheng Wang [1], Ting Lei [1,2,*] and Shizhi Jiang [1,2,*]

1 College of Pharmacy, Dali University, Dali 671000, China; ldliuzhiwen@163.com (Z.L.); gby17662435129@163.com (B.G.); gongxushun@163.com (X.G.); wfsyn@163.com (F.W.)

2 Yunnan Provincial Key Laboratory of Entomological Biopharmaceutical R&D, Dali University, Dali 671000, China

* Correspondence: leiting@dali.edu.cn (T.L.); jiangshizhi@dali.edu.cn (S.J.)

† These authors contributed equally to this work.

Abstract: Efficient and simple syntheses of *trans*-dehydroosthol and citrubuntin were achieved in a single step by implementing a protecting-group-free, redox-neutral strategy that utilized readily available starting materials. In this approach, a practical one-pot (domino) Heck/dehydration reaction was carried out utilizing less reactive bromocoumarin, resulting in excellent stereoselectivity and atomic economy. Through the implementation of this new, efficient, and scalable synthesis method, the formal synthesis of a series of novel meroterpenoid natural products was successfully achieved.

Keywords: protecting-group-free; redox-neutral; one-pot (domino) Heck/dehydration reaction; isoprene; meroterpenoid

1. Introduction

Meroterpenoids are hybrid natural products and a fascinating class of compounds that possess diverse chemical structures and intriguing biological activities [1], including antimicrobial [2], antiviral [3], anticancer [4], anti-inflammatory [5], and antioxidant properties [6]. They are derived from the fusion of terpenoid and non-terpenoid moieties, which provide them with distinct properties and potential applications in various fields, including pharmaceutical, medicinal, and agricultural industries [7]. Meroterpenoids have a wide range of sources [8], including plants, marine organisms, and microorganisms. Their unique structures enable them to interact with specific targets in living systems, making them valuable candidates for drug discovery and development. The significant biological activities and unique chemical structures of meroterpenoids have attracted great interest from synthetic and biosynthetic chemists. However, current synthesis strategies are not straightforward owing to the complexes processes involved and strongly depend on the not easily available key intermediate and expensive starting materials to produce the target molecule.

Trans-dehydroosthol (**1**) and its structurally related compound citrubuntin (**2**) are a class of coumarin derivatives with the same unique isoprene side chain. These active natural products can be found in many commonly used medicinal plants and act as crucial intermediates in the synthesis of diverse meroterpenoids (Figure 1). *Trans*-dehydroosthol was originally isolated from the leaves of *Murraya exotica L.* in 1987 [9] and later isolated from *Citrus* plants in 1993 [10] and *Murraya paniculata* in 2019 [11]. The impact of *trans*-dehydroosthol on NO production in BV-2 microglial cells was investigated. The findings indicated that *trans*-dehydroosthol possesses noteworthy inhibitory properties, suggesting its potential anti-inflammatory and analgesic effects [11]. First reported in 1980, "citrubuntin" was formed by the dehydration of suberenol and named as "(*E*)-suberodiene" [12]. Even though "citrubuntin" had not yet been isolated from natural resources at that time, the existence of glenadiene and gleinene in nature indicated that this compound may occur naturally. Citrubuntin was isolated from *Citrus grandis* for the first time by Wu [13] in 1988 and then from *Micromelum falcatum* by Wang [14] in 2019. *Micromelum falcatum* is a traditional herbal remedy in China, Thailand, and Vietnam. Its leaves and roots are utilized in these regions for various medicinal purposes, such as treating infected wounds, relieving pain, addressing rheumatism and muscular atrophy, reducing fever, and alleviating discomfort caused by insect bites [15]. Notably, coumarin components, which have been extensively studied, are the main bioactive compounds responsible for these therapeutic properties [16]. This finding suggests that citrubuntin may also exhibit good efficacy.

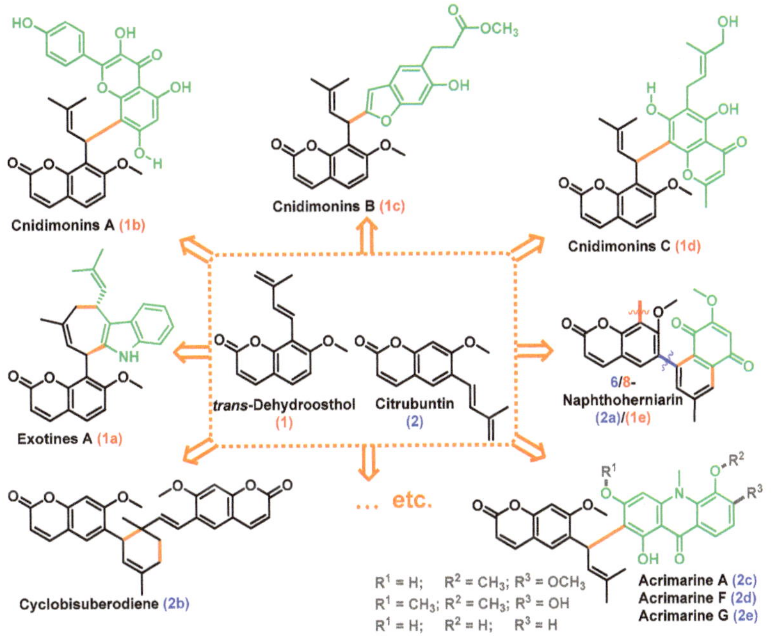

Figure 1. Structures of *trans*-dehydroosthol, citrubuntin, and several related meroterpenoids.

The chemical versatility of *trans*-dehydroosthol and citrubuntin enables the synthesis of various complex molecules with diverse biological activities and therapeutic potential. For example, synthetic chemists can modify and incorporate various dienophile (or conjugated diolefine), functional groups, and stereochemistry by strategically utilizing these two compounds as building blocks, streamlining synthesis paths toward numerous complex natural products. The total synthesis of these two isoprene-containing molecules has attracted the attention of numerous research groups [17–21], highlighting their significance in the field of meroterpenoid synthesis. Moreover, their synthesis aids in the quest for novel natural products with wide-ranging applications and contributes to the development of new drugs, flavors, and agricultural agents.

Given their significant pharmacological potential and unique structural features, trans-dehydroosthol and citrubuntin have emerged as compelling targets for synthetic exploration. These compounds belong to a broader class of biologically active meroterpenoids, which have attracted considerable attention in natural product synthesis. Recent studies have highlighted the structural diversity within this family, exemplified by notable examples such as exotines A (**1a**, indole-coumarin hybrid) [22], the cnidimonin series (**1b–d**, featuring flavonol-, benzofuran-, and chromone-coumarin frameworks) [23], 6/8-naphthoherniarin (**2a**/**1e**, quinone-coumarin conjugate) [24], cyclobisuberodiene (**2b**, coumarin dimer) [25], and the acrimarine group (**2c–e**, acridinone-coumarin hybrids) [26]. The development of efficient synthetic routes to these architecturally complex molecules remains crucial for advancing their biological evaluation and medicinal applications.

In 1988, Reisch and Murray [17,18] separately reported the initial total synthesis of *trans*-dehydroosthol, though the overall yields were not satisfactory. Their approach employed 8-iodo-7-methoxycoumarin as a crucial starting material. The highly reactive iodide was used as a coupling partner to introduce the 3-hydroxy-3-methyl-1-butenyl side chain, which served as a precursor for the isoprene unit. However, this method necessitated relatively high temperatures and extended reaction times (120 °C for 3 days; 90 °C for 24 hours under Jeffery conditions), even when using highly reactive iodides. Tedious dehydration reactions were performed using hazardous $POCl_3$ or *p*-TsCl as the acylation agent and hot pyridine (reflux) or DIPEA as the reaction medium to obtain *trans*-dehydroosthol, with overall yields of 23.8% and 29%, respectively (calculated from the corresponding iodo-coumarin). In 2018, Martin [19,20] achieved the synthesis of *trans*-dehydroosthol in a relatively high overall yield by integrating the advantages of Reisch and Murray's synthesis routes. Although this is a venerable transformation to the isoprene group in terms of yield (78%, two steps from iodo-coumarin; or 20%, four steps from 7-hydroxy coumarin), the use of highly active iodide cannot be avoided. According to the literature, the synthesis of 8-iodo-7-methoxycoumarin presents significant challenges. In the reported studies, inefficient processes such as iodination and subsequent methylation of the crude product were employed [27]. These methods resulted in very low conversions, necessitating the use of 7-hydroxycoumarin, which has a high structural similarity to the target compound. However, even with this approach, the desired iodide was obtained in yields of only 20%–30%, accompanied by a substantial amount of residual 7-methoxycoumarin. Furthermore, the instability of the iodide complicates its application, making the overall synthesis process highly complex.

Before being isolated and identified from the natural source, citrubuntin has been produced as an artificial molecule via $POCl_3$ and the pyridine-promoted dehydration of suberenol and named as (*E*)-suberodiene. In 1990, Reisch [21] published a report on the first total synthesis of citrubuntin, using challenging brominated substrate as the coupling substrate. The key Heck coupling reaction was conducted under Jeffery conditions [28], resulting in the formation of the coupling product in 62% yield. Following the above protocol, citrubuntin was successfully synthesized under strong heating conditions using hazardous *p*-TsCl as the acylating reagent and troublesome pyridine as the solvent. Although moderate yields of coupling product can be obtained under Jeffery conditions ($Pd(OAc)_2$, $NaHCO_3$, nBu_4NBr), which is considered "a major achievement" for the Heck reaction [29], the need for a phase-transfer catalyst for stoichiometry is essential and troublesome because nBu_4NBr is associated with inconvenience work-up and purification processes. Wastewater containing a non-negligible amount of a phase-transfer catalyst produced in the reactions also restricts the application of these reactions on an industrial scale. Efforts to develop efficient, scalable, and environmentally friendly synthesis strategies for these two compounds are imperative to advance research in meroterpenoid synthesis and broaden the applications of related molecules.

2. Results

Driven by the need for an efficient synthetic approach to produce trans-dehydroosthol and citrubuntin, which are crucial for the synthesis of numerous meroterpenoids, we sought an alternative strategy. Given the simplicity and efficiency of the one-pot (domino) Heck/dehydration reaction, we designed a novel retrosynthetic route as depicted in Scheme 1. We hypothesized that developing an effective catalyst system for the transition metal-catalyzed coupling of less reactive but cost-effective bromocoumarin would represent a significant improvement. This manuscript details our progress in achieving this goal.

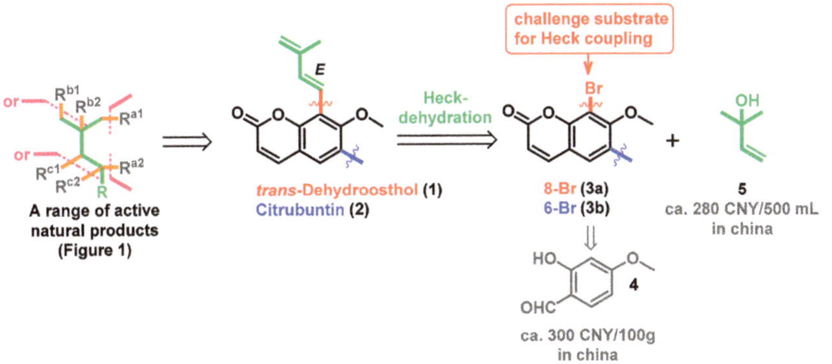

Scheme 1. Retrosynthetic analyses of trans-dehydroosthol, citrubuntin, and a series of natural products.

Although the isoprene side chain is a relatively uncommon biogenetic modification of prenyl residues, it frequently appears in the *trans*-configuration in many valuable natural and chemical compounds. Our interest in natural products with an isoprene group dates to our synthesis of several useful natural products [30–33]. A crucial step in this synthesis involves a streamlined one-pot (domino) Heck/dehydration reaction, where the corresponding bromine reacts with 1,1-dimethyl allyl alcohol in the presence of a slightly low loading of base (1.0 equiv. trialkylamine).

In our retrosynthesis analyses of *trans*-dehydroosthol (**1**) and citrubuntin (**2**), we identified the need for a coupling reaction with 8/6-bromo coumarin (**3a/3b**) and 1,1-dimethyl allyl alcohol (**5**), as shown in Scheme 2. This strategy appeared highly feasible owing to the easy availability of starting materials to synthesize these two natural products in a single step. Our synthesis commenced with brominated coumarin as the key material, which is commercially available and can also be prepared readily on a dekagram scale using inexpensive 4-methoxysalicylaldehyde **4** via the regioselective bromination and CsOAc-promoted Perkin reaction optimized by our group [33].

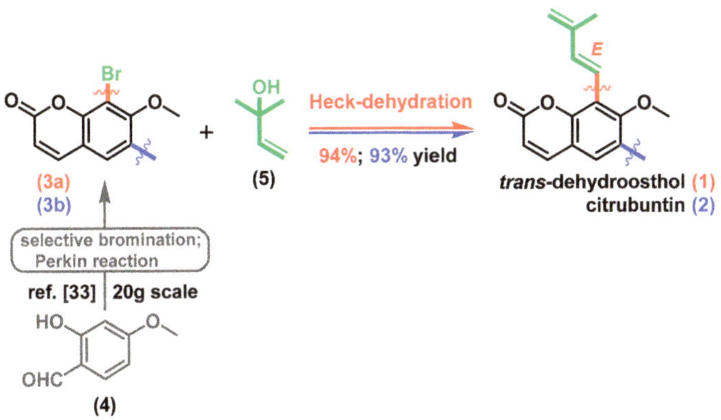

Scheme 2. One-step syntheses of *trans*-dehydroosthol and citrubuntin.

2.1. *Effect of the Bases*

After obtaining multigram quantities of the known compound **3a**, we focused on the crucial reaction for the introduction of isoprene moiety. Initially, we used the conditions roughly based on the previously reported synthesis of murraol—8-bromocoumarin, 1,1-dimethylallyl alcohol, $Pd(OAc)_2$, P(*o*-tol)$_3$, Et_3N (1.0 equiv.), toluene, and BHT (0.1 equiv.)—expecting that this low base and polymerization-inhibitor-containing version would facilitate the key C−C formation and the following cascade dehydration reaction. However, to our disappointment, this "standard" condition is completely ineffective, with only a trace of the desired product **1** observed after 3 h (Table 1, entry 1).

Table 1. Study on the effect of the bases.

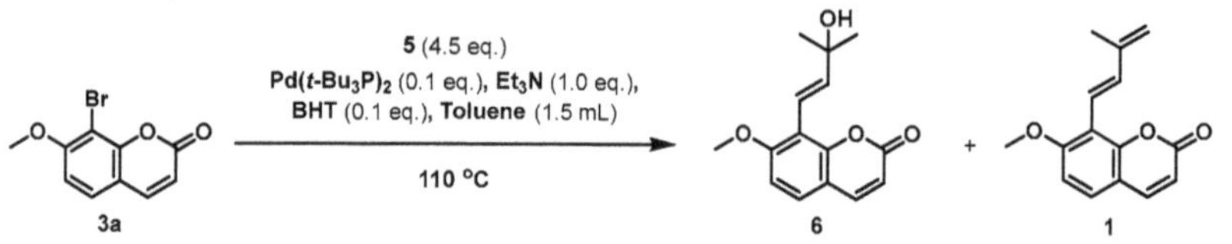

Entry	Variable	t[h]	3a (%) [a]	6 (%) [a]	1 (%) [a]
1 [b]	None	3 [b]/31	-	97/32	2/67
2 [b]	120 °C	10	-	63	35
3	Et_3N (0.9) [c]	18	-	31	68
4	(*n*-C_3H_7)$_3$N (1.0/0.9) [c]	21/29	-/-	31/22	69/77
5	(*n*-C_8H_{17})$_3$N (1.0/0.9) [c]	29/22	-/-	22/4	75/84
6	DIPEA	9	-	25	67
7	(Cy)$_2$NMe [d]	27	-	89	10
8	DABCO	13	-	67	32
9	DMAN [e] (0.85) [c]	31	4	39	56
10	N,N-Diethylaniline	5	64	-	28
11	2,6-Lutidine	10	71	-	27

"-" = Not detected. [a] Isolated yield. [b] Sealed tube. [c] The equiv. of the base. [d] *N,N*-Dicyclohexylmethylamine. [e] 1,8-Bis(dimethylamino)naphthalene.

Even when the reaction temperature was raised to 120°C, the coupling reaction still only achieved a 35% yield of the desired product **1** after 10 hours (entry 2). This indicates that the one-pot (domino) Heck/dehydration process involving this brominated substrate is highly challenging. The high temperature required for the dehydration of the 1,1-dimethylallyl alcohol intermediate is likely due to the relatively unreactive nature of the hydroxyl group at the allylic position. This issue is further complicated by the strong electron-donating effects of the oxygen atoms in the two phenoxy groups (located in the *ortho*-position) on the conjugated system. Consequently, the rate-limiting step for one-pot (domino) Heck/dehydration, which is the dehydration of the 1,1-dimethylallyl alcohol moiety to the diene group, is slowed down, leading to the deceleration of the entire cascade reaction. When the reaction time was inadvertently prolonged to 31 h and the amount of base was deliberately reduced to 0.9 equiv., the coupling reaction produced the desired diene **1** in 67% and 68% yields (entry 1–2 and entry 3), respectively. Considering that the synthesis process starts from a less reactive substrate and involves a sequence of successive reactions, these yields from one-pot (domino) Heck/dehydration may be considerably good.

Basing on the preceding analysis and considering that the nature and amount of the base tremendously influence the Heck coupling reaction and subsequent tandem dehydration reaction, we assumed that the Heck alkenylation of our brominated substrate required the addition of a suitable base that not only mediates the electronic properties and the steric hindrance of the Pd center, but also alters the dehydration conditions (catalyzed by corresponding $R_3N{\cdot}HBr$). Therefore, we tested several readily available bases and discovered that upon replacing the trialkylamine from Et_3N with $(n\text{-}C_3H_7)_3N$ and $(n\text{-}C_8H_{17})_3N$, the cascade reaction produced the desired product in 77% and 84% yields (entry 4–1 and entry 5–1), respectively. This phenomenon could be attributed to the more suitable electrical properties and steric hindrance nature of long alkyl-chain tertiary amines compared with triethylamine, possibly enhancing the reactivity of the oxidative insertion of the metal center into the deactivated Ar–Br bond. In addition, the increased steric demand of the catalyst complex also facilitates HBr dissociation in the reductive elimination step. The cascade dehydration reaction might also be enhanced. Conversely, other bases including DIPEA, $(Cy)_2NMe$, DABCO, and DMAN exhibited lower efficiencies (entries 6–9). Bases such as *N,N*-diethylaniline and 2,6-lutidine did not facilitate the one-pot (domino) Heck/dehydration reaction (entries 10–11).

2.2. *Effect of the Solvents*

Inspired by our recent comprehensive investigation on the one-pot (domino) Heck/dehydration reaction and its streamlined procedure, we screened different solvents in combination with $Pd(t\text{-}Bu_3P)_2$ and Et_3N to enhance the yield of this transformation. Among the solvents tested, a useful chloroalkane, DCE, yielded the best result (Table 2, entry 4). When the homolog of DCE, 1,3-DCP, was used as the reaction medium, a good yield was obtained after a short reaction time (90%, 10 h, entry 6–1). This optimization of solvent selection proved beneficial in improving the overall efficiency of the transformation. The use of other solvents, including xylene or chlorinated aromatics, chlorobenzene, and 2,4-DCT (entries 1–3), as well as CH_3CN, DMF, DMAC, NMP, DMSO, THF, 2-MeTHF, 1,4-dioxane, DME, DEE, and *n*-BuOAc (entries 7–17), resulted in a moderate to significant decrease in yield. When DMSO was used as the reaction medium, yields of diene and allyl alcohol were unsatisfactory, presumably attributed to the significant polymerization or decomposition of the isopentenyl moiety during the coupling reaction. These observations highlight the importance of solvent selection in achieving optimal reaction efficiency and the good performance of DCE and its homolog 1,3-DCP as a solvent in this process.

Following the preliminary optimization of the one-pot (domino) Heck/dehydration reaction conditions (Tables 1 and 2), we decided to combine the optimal bases with the best solvents to realize effective synthesis. According to the above experimental results (Table 2), the yield of diene **1** is relatively high when DCE and 1,3-DCP are used as the reaction media. Therefore, DCE and 1,3-DCP were selected as solvents and combined with $(n\text{-}C_3H_7)_3N$ or $(n\text{-}C_8H_{17})_3N$ to improve the yield. Under the combination of DCE and $(n\text{-}C_3H_7)_3N$, the yield of diene **1** reached up to 91% (or 93% yield on a Gram scale, Table 3, entry 2). However, the use of DCE (b.p. = 83.5 °C) as a solvent requires pressure-resistant equipment at a selected reaction temperature. In addition, the high boiling point of 1,3-DCP (b.p. = 120 °C–122 °C) facilitates various conventional heating reactions under normal atmospheric pressure. To further test the scalability of this methodology, we performed the reaction on a 1.2 g scale (4.7 mmol, Table 2, entries 6–2) with the suitable solvent–1,3-DCP. *Trans*-dehydroosthol was isolated in an excellent yield (94%) under atmospheric pressure, and the efficiency was greater than that obtained in the small-scale reaction (90%, Table 2, entries 6–1).

Table 2. Study on the effect of the solvents.

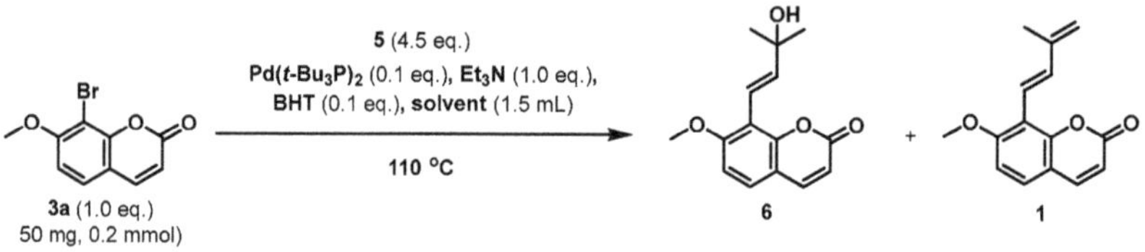

Entry	Variable	t[h]	3a (%) [a]	6 (%) [a]	1 (%) [a]
1	Xylene	27	-	78	20
2	Chlorobenzene	6	9	5	70
3	2,4-DCT [b]	22	36	21	27
4 [c]	DCE (1.0/0.9) [d]	21/8	-/-	4/-	82/86
5 [c]	1,2-DCP [e]	30	-	31	61
6	1,3-DCP [f] (1.0/0.9) [d]	10(10 [g])/14	-(-)/11	3(2)/16	90(94)/69
7 [c]	CH_3CN	21	-	61	36
8	DMF	17	-	47	48
9	DMAC	18	-	47	47
10	NMP	18	-	47	39
11	DMSO	19	-	12	26
12 [c]	THF	21	-	33	66
13 [c]	2-MeTHF [h]	22	-	38.1	51.8
14 [c]	1,4-Dioxane	15	-	15	77
15 [c]	DME	22	-	60.7	35.3
16	DEE [i]	20	-	58	30
17	*n*-BuOAc [j]	21	-	74	25

[a] Isolated yield. [b] 2,4-Dichlorotoluene. [c] Sealed tube. [d] The equiv. of the base. [e] 1,2-Dichloropropane. [f] 1,3-Dichloropropane. [g] Gram scale (1.2 g, 4.7 mmol). [h] 2-Methyltetrahydrofuran. [i] Ethylene glycol diethyl ether. [j] *n*-Butyl acetate.

Table 3. Study on the effect of the combination of solvents and bases.

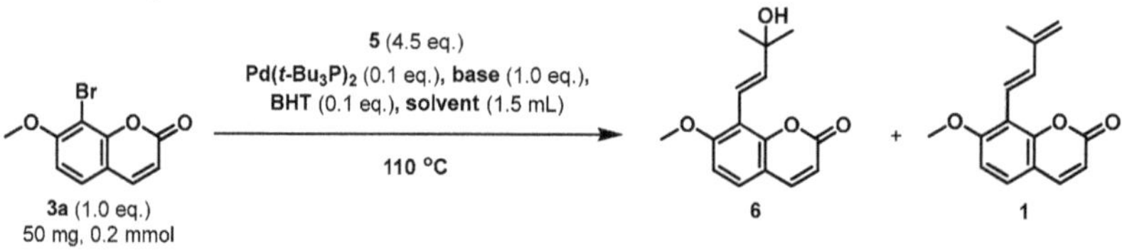

Entry	Variable	t[h]	3a (%) [a]	6 (%) [a]	1 (%) [a]
1 [b]	DCE, $(n\text{-}C_8H_{17})_3N$ (1.0/0.9) [c]	18/7	-/-	10/2	84/89
2 [b]	DCE, $(n\text{-}C_3H_7)_3N$ (1.0/0.9) [c]	14(14 [d])/11	-(-)/-	4(-)/7	91(93)/83
3	1,3-DCP, $(n\text{-}C_8H_{17})_3N$ (1.0/0.9) [c]	21.5/21	-/-	35/28	64/70
4	1,3-DCP, $(n\text{-}C_3H_7)_3N$ (1.0/0.9) [c]	26/16	-/-	15/23	78/67

[a] Isolated yield. [b] Sealed tube. [c] The equiv. of the base. [d] Gram scale (1.2 g, 4.7 mmol).

2.3. Further Application

Based on the aforementioned optimization of the one-pot (domino) Heck/dehydration reaction conditions, we synthesized analogs of trans-dehydroosthol and citrubuntin to evaluate their pharmacological activities and demonstrate the practicality of this synthetic approach. As illustrated in Table 4, the reaction proceeded very smoothly at 90 °C, yielding the desired diene **2** in excellent yield. The relatively low reaction temperature and time may be attributed to the reduced steric hindrance from the ortho-methoxy group (OMe) at the C-6 position of **3b**. While citrubuntin can be synthesized from (*E*)-suberenol via $POCl_3$ and pyridine-promoted dehydration, a method previously reported through Jeffery-modified Heck coupling from **3b** [12], this route is less efficient than the strategy employed by our group. Additionally, the reaction was highly efficient on a gram scale under atmospheric pressure, achieving a yield of 97% (Table 4, entries 1–2). The application of this methodology to a broad scope of useful natural products is currently underway in our laboratory and will be reported in the future.

Table 4. Study on the synthesis of citrubuntin (based on Table 2, entry 6-1 and Table 3, entry 2–1).

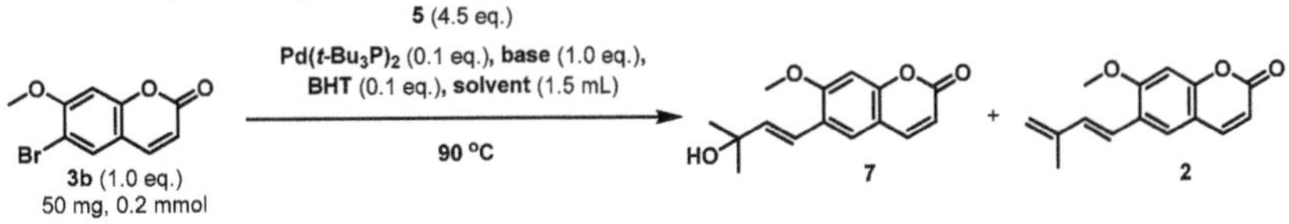

Entry	Variable	t[h]	3b (%) [a]	7 (%) [a]	2 (%) [a]
1	1,3-DCP, Et_3N	8/8 [c]	-/-	4/-	94/97
2 [b]	DCE, $(n\text{-}C_3H_7)_3N$	8/8 [c]	-/-	-/-	97/98

[a] Isolated yield. [b] Sealed tube, 110 °C. [c] Gram scale (1.2 g, 4.7 mmol).

With the efficient synthesis of *trans*-dehydroosthol and citrubuntin in hand and to further demonstrate the usefulness of the proposed synthesis method, we attempted to synthesize several valuable meroterpenoid natural products **1a**, **1b**, **1c**, **1d**, **1e**, **2a**, **2b**, **2c**, **2d**, and **2e** (Figure 1). These desired products could be prepared in a single step from commercially available or readily available substrates and *trans*-dehydroosthol (or citrubuntin), according to the literature [22–26]. Our laboratory is currently undertaking endeavors to enhance the synthesis efficiency of the abovementioned hybrid natural products, and we anticipate that the results of these endeavors will be reported in the future.

3. Materials and Methods

3.1. General Information

NMR spectra were acquired using a Bruker AVANCE III instrument (400 MHz for ^{1}H and 100 MHz for ^{13}C) in the specified solvent. Chemical shifts (δ) are reported in parts per million (ppm) relative to tetramethylsilane, with the solvent resonance serving as an internal reference. Deuterochloroform was used as the solvent in all cases. Coupling constants (J) are provided in Hertz (Hz). Multiplicity is described using the following abbreviations: s (singlet), d (doublet), t (triplet), q (quartet), dd (doublet of doublets), dt (doublet of triplets), AB q (AB-quartet), and m (multiplet). For ^{13}C-NMR, the number of contributing carbon nuclei is indicated in parentheses following the chemical shift value. Reaction progress was monitored by thin-layer chromatography on 0.2-0.25 mm silica gel plates (GF-254) using UV light (254 nm) for visualization. Phosphomolybdic acid (10 wt.% in EtOH) was used as the visualizing agent. Flash chromatography was conducted using silica gel (200-300 mesh).

Unless otherwise specified, all chemicals and solvents were used as received without further purification. All of the following solvents and chemicals were obtained from Innochem (Beijing, China): 2-Methyl-3-buten-2-ol (98%), Bis(tri-tert-butylphosphine)palladium(0) (98%), Phosphomolybdic acid hydrate (98%), Ethanol (99.7%), Triethylamine (99%), *N*,*N*-Dipropyl-1-propanamine (99%), Tri-n-octylamine (97%), *N*,*N*-Diisopropylethylamine (99%), *N*,*N*-Dicyclohexylmethylamine (98%), 1,8-Bis(dimethylamino)naphthalene (98%), 1,4-Diazabicyclo [2.2.2]octane (98%), 2,6-Lutidine(98%), *N*,*N*-Diethylaniline (99%), Butylated hydroxytoluene (99%). Acetonitrile (99.9%), *N*,*N*-Dimethylformamide (99.9%), and Dimethyl sulfoxide (99.8%) are extra dry solvents (with molecular sieves) and were used as received. In addition, Chlorobenzene (99%), Xylene (99%), Dichloroethane (98.9%), 1,2-Dichloropropane (99%), 1,3-Dichloropropane (99%), *N*,*N*-Dimethylacetamid ($\geq$99%), N-Methylpyrrolidone (99.5%), Ethylene glycol diethyl ether (98%), Dichloromethane

(≥99.5%), 1,2-Dimethoxyethane (99.5%), Tetrahydrofuran (99%), 1,4-Dioxane (99%), and 2-Methyltetrahydrofuran (99%) are all analytical reagents. An appropriate amount of calcium hydride was added and refluxed for 3 hours prior to use. Then, the fraction was taken out and degassed twice with a nitrogen-filled balloon. The resulting anhydrous and oxygen-free reagent was stored over molecular sieves under nitrogen. Petroleum ether and ethyl acetate were both industrial grade products that had been reevaporated using a rotary evaporator before use. The silica gel for the chromatography (0.2–0.25 mm, 50 × 100 mm, GF254) was obtained from Qingdao Haiyang Chemical Co., Ltd. (Qingdao, China).

3.2. *Synthesis of 3-Bromo-2-hydroxy-4-methoxybenzaldehyde and 5-Bromo-2-hydroxy-4-methoxybenzaldehyde*

3.2.1. Synthesis of 3-Bromo-2-hydroxy-4-methoxybenzaldehyde

Under a nitrogen atmosphere, a round-bottom flask equipped with a magnetic stir bar was charged with a solution of aldehyde **4** (20 g, 131 mmol) in dichloromethane (410 mL). The solution was cooled to −78 °C, followed by the dropwise addition of $TiCl_4$ (18 mL, 157 mmol, pure; or 157 mL of a 1 M solution in dichloromethane) over 20 min. Next, a solution of bromine (6.7 mL, 131 mmol) in dichloromethane (100 mL) was added dropwise over 30 min. The reaction mixture was stirred at −78 °C for 1 hour and then allowed to warm to room temperature over 2 hours. When TLC monitoring indicated a complete reaction (as monitored by TLC, about 5 h), a saturated aqueous solution of Na_2SO_3 (100 mL) was added to the resulting mixture and stirred for another 10 min. The mixture was separated, and the aqueous phase was extracted with CH_2Cl_2 (2 × 750 mL). The combined organic phases were washed with brine (100 mL), dried over Na_2SO_4, filtered, and concentrated in vacuo at 30 °C. After purification by flash column chromatography using petroleum ether/ethyl acetate (100:1 to 15:1) as the eluent, the title compound was obtained as a colorless solid (26.9 g, 89%), m.p. 115–117 °C. ^{1}H NMR (400 MHz, $CDCl_3$) δ_H: 11.93 (s, 1H), 9.71 (s, 1H), 7.51 (d, J = 8.7 Hz, 1H), 6.62 (d, J = 8.7 Hz, 1H), 3.99 (s, 3H); ^{13}C NMR (101 MHz, $CDCl_3$) δ_C: 194.43, 162.83, 160.20, 134.69, 116.19, 103.87, 99.69, 56.96; IR (KBr): 3731.00, 2991.06, 2873.84, 2348.90, 1637.36, 1479.51, 1361.26, 1200.23, 829.10, 763.08, 551.18 cm^{-1}; HRMS (EI) calcd for $C_8H_7BrO_3$ $[M-H]^-$ 228.9506, found 228.9506.

3.2.2. Synthesis of 5-Bromo-2-hydroxy-4-methoxybenzaldehyde

Under a nitrogen atmosphere, a round-bottom flask equipped with a magnetic stir bar was charged with a solution of aldehyde **4** (20 g, 131 mmol) in dichloromethane (410 mL). To this solution, bromine (6.7 mL, 131 mmol) dissolved in dichloromethane (100 mL) was added dropwise at room temperature over 30 minutes. The reaction mixture was stirred continuously, and progress was monitored by TLC until completion (approximately 3 hours). Upon completion, a saturated aqueous solution of Na_2SO_3 (100 mL) was added, and the mixture was stirred for an additional 10 minutes. The mixture was separated, and the aqueous phase was extracted with CH_2Cl_2 (2 × 750 mL). The organic phases were washed with brine (100 mL), dried over Na_2SO_4, filtered and concentrated in vacuo at 30 °C. After purification by flash column chromatography (petroleum ether (PE): ethyl acetate (EA) = 100:1 to 25:1), the title compound was obtained as a colorless solid (26.4 g, 87%), m.p. 126–128 °C. ^{1}H NMR (400 MHz, $CDCl_3$) δ_H: 11.43 (s, 1H), 9.68 (s, 1H), 7.67 (s, 1H), 6.47 (s, 1H), 3.94 (s, 3H); ^{13}C NMR (101 MHz, $CDCl_3$) δ_C: 193.80, 163.79, 162.66, 137.36, 115.85, 102.25, 100.50, 56.90; IR (KBr): 3423.16, 2949.95, 2849.27, 2347.53, 1635.93, 1499.15, 1361.11, 1289.78, 1240.24, 1062.87, 759.71, 645.90, 539.88 cm^{-1}; HRMS (EI) calcd for $C_8H_7BrO_3$ $[M-H]^-$ 228.9504, found 228.9506.

3.2.3. Synthesis of 8-Bromo-7-methoxy-2*H*-chromen-2-one-**3a**

Under a nitrogen atmosphere, a Heavy-Wall Pressure Vessel equipped with a magnetic stir bar was charged with 3-bromo-4-methoxysalicylaldehyde (20 g, 87 mmol), CsOAc (16.7 g, 87 mmol), and acetic anhydride (70 mL). The vessel was sealed and heated in an oil bath at 160 °C. The reaction progress was monitored by TLC and completed after approximately 12 h. The mixture was then cooled to room temperature, diluted with ethyl acetate (1000 mL), and washed sequentially with hot water (5 × 100 mL) and brine (120 mL). The organic layer was dried over sodium sulfate, filtered, and concentrated under reduced pressure at 40 °C to yield the crude product. After purification by flash column chromatography (PE:EA = 10:1 to 5:1), the title compound **3a** was obtained as a yellow powder solid (15.5 g, 70%), m.p. 165–167 °C. ^{1}H NMR (400 MHz, $CDCl_3$) δ_H: 7.62 (d, J = 9.5 Hz, 1H), 7.41 (d, J = 8.7 Hz, 1H), 6.87 (d, J = 8.7 Hz, 1H), 6.28 (d, J = 9.5 Hz, 1H), 3.99 (s, 3H); ^{13}C NMR (101 MHz, $CDCl_3$) δ_C: 160.31, 159.30, 152.43, 143.30, 127.68, 113.96, 113.91, 108.09, 99.87, 56.99; IR (KBr): 3426.02, 3061. 00, 2346.67, 1728.29, 1600.08, 1278.14, 1076.71, 925.20, 839.62, 632.05, 577.89 cm^{-1}; HRMS (EI) calcd for $C_{10}H_7O_3Br$ $[M + Na]^+$ 276.9497, found 276.9477.

3.2.4. Synthesis of 6-Bromo-7-methoxy-2*H*-chromen-2-one-**3b**

Under a nitrogen atmosphere, a Heavy-Wall Pressure Vessel equipped with a magnetic stir bar was charged with 5-bromo-4-methoxysalicylaldehyde (20 g, 87 mmol), CsOAc (16.7 g, 87 mmol), and acetic anhydride (70 mL). The vessel was sealed and heated in an oil bath at 160 °C. The reaction progress was monitored by TLC and completed after approximately 12 hours. The mixture was then cooled to room temperature, diluted with ethyl acetate (1000 mL), and washed sequentially with hot water (5 × 100 mL) and brine (120 mL). The organic layer was dried over sodium sulfate, filtered, and concentrated under reduced pressure at 40 °C to yield the crude product. After purification by flash column chromatography (PE:EA = 35:1 to 10:1), the title compound **3b** was obtained as a yellow powder solid (16.2 g, 73%), m.p. 196–198 °C. ^{1}H NMR (400 MHz, $CDCl_3$) δ_H: 7.66 (s, 1H), 7.59 (d, J = 9.5 Hz, 1H), 6.84 (s, 1H), 6.30 (d, J = 9.5 Hz, 1H), 3.97 (s, 3H); ^{13}C NMR (101 MHz, $CDCl_3$) δ_C: 160.60, 158.68, 155.03, 142.41, 131.51, 114.30, 113.40, 107.70, 100.31, 56.90; IR (KBr): 3420.10, 3285.39, 3066.57, 2344.55, 1731.58, 1601.17, 1371.41, 1261.69, 1211.35, 1036.02, 890.98, 693.81, 513.00 cm^{-1}; HRMS (EI) calcd for $C_{10}H_7O_3Br$ $[M + H]^+$ 254.9687, found 254.9651.

3.3. *General Procedure for Tables 1–4*

Under a nitrogen atmosphere, a double-neck round-bottom flask or a Heavy-Wall Pressure Vessel was equipped with a magnetic stir bar, a condenser, and charged with **3a** or **3b** (50 mg, 0.2 mmol, 1.0 eq.), Pd(t-$Bu_3P)_2$ (10 mg, 0.02 mmol, 0.1 eq.), BHT (4.3 mg, 0.02 mmol, 0.1 eq.), solvent (1.5 mL, degassed with nitrogen for 10 min prior to use), base (37 μL, 0.2 mmol, 1.0 eq.), and 1,1-dimethylallyl alcohol **5** (92 μL, 0.9 mmol, 4.5 eq.). The flask or vessel was then placed in an oil bath. Once the reaction was complete (monitored by TLC or at a predetermined time), the mixture was cooled to room temperature, and a saturated aqueous $NaHCO_3$ solution (1 mL) was added and stirred for an additional 5 min. The mixture was filtered through a pad of celite and washed with ethyl acetate (EA, 30 mL). The filtrate was diluted with EA (50 mL), washed with water and brine, dried over Na_2SO_4, filtered, and concentrated in vacuo at 30 °C to yield the crude product. Purification by flash column chromatography (PE: EA gradient from 8:1 to 2:1) afforded the desired compound.

3.3.1. Synthesis of *trans*-Dehydroosthol (**1**): Table 2, Entry 6–1 (Gram Scale)

Under a nitrogen atmosphere, a double-neck round-bottom flask or a Heavy-Wall Pressure Vessel was equipped with a magnetic stir bar, a condenser, and charged with **3a** (1.2 g, 4.7 mmol), Pd(t-$Bu_3P)_2$ (240 mg, 0.47 mmol), BHT (103.2 mg, 0.47 mmol), 1,3-Dichloropropane (36 mL, bubbled with nitrogen for 10 min prior to addition), Et_3N (653 µL, 4.7 mmol), and 1,1-dimethylallyl alcohol **5** (2.2 mL, 21 mmol). The flask was then immersed in an oil bath preheated to 110 °C. The reaction progress was monitored by TLC, and after approximately 10 hours, the mixture was cooled to room temperature. A saturated aqueous $NaHCO_3$ solution (10 mL) was added, and the mixture was stirred for 5 minutes. The resulting mixture was filtered through a celite pad and washed with ethyl acetate (100 mL). The filtrate was diluted with additional ethyl acetate (300 mL) and washed sequentially with water (240 mL) and brine (40 mL). The organic layer was dried over sodium sulfate, filtered, and concentrated under reduced pressure at 30 °C to yield the crude product. Purification by flash column chromatography (petroleum ether/ethyl acetate gradient, 8:1 to 2:1), the title compound *trans*-dehydroosthol was obtained as a yellow powder solid (1.07 g, 94% yield), m.p. 77–79 °C, and the compound **6** was obtained as a yellow powder solid (24.5 mg, 2%), m.p. 120–122 °C. Data for compound *trans*-dehydroosthol (**1**): ^{1}H NMR (400 MHz, $CDCl_3$) δ_H: 7.62 (d, J = 9.5 Hz, 1H), 7.49 (d, J = 16.5 Hz, 1H), 7.30 (d, J = 8.6 Hz, 1H), 6.90 (d, J = 16.5 Hz, 1H), 6.86 (d, J = 8.6 Hz, 1H), 6.27 (d, J = 9.5 Hz, 1H), 5.19 (d, J = 2.2 Hz, 1H), 5.14 (t, J = 1.8 Hz, 1H), 3.97 (s, 3H), 2.03 (d, J = 1.3 Hz, 3H); ^{13}C NMR (101 MHz, $CDCl_3$) δ_C: 161.12, 160.36, 152.67, 144.06, 143.20, 138.25, 127.08, 118.56, 117.28, 114.35, 113.22, 113.10, 107.68, 56.28, 18.47; IR (KBr): 3423.32, 3065.99, 2941.21, 2346.60, 1720.73, 1596.93, 1478.99, 1256.29, 1109.88, 1031.74, 840.74, 587.96, 474.00 cm^{-1}; HRMS (EI) calcd for $C_{15}H_{14}O_3$ $[M + Na]^+$ 265.0837, found 265.0835.

Data for compound **6**: ^{1}H NMR (400 MHz, $CDCl_3$) δ_H: 7.62 (d, 1H, J = 9.4 Hz), 7.30 (d, 1H, J = 8.6 Hz), 7.02 (d, 1H, J = 16.5 Hz), 6.93 (d, 1H, J = 16.5 Hz), 6.86(d, 1H, J = 8.6 Hz), 6.25(d, 1H, J = 9.4 Hz), 3.94 (s, 3H), 1.46(s, 6H); ^{13}C NMR (101 MHz, $CDCl_3$) δ_C: 161.14, 160.32, 152.69, 144.59, 144.07, 127.16, 114.40, 113.72, 113.12, 113.05, 107.66, 71.77, 56.24, 30.00; IR (KBr): 3735.67, 3466.37, 2960.23, 2347.90, 1707.97, 1598.36, 1471.26, 1252.81, 1182.87, 1087.44, 823.12, 703.70, 562.82 cm^{-1}; HRMS (EI) calcd for $C_{15}H_{16}O_4$ $[M + Na]^+$ 283.1038, found 283.1053.

3.3.2. Synthesis of Citrubuntin (**2**): Table 4, Entry 1–2 (Gram Scale)

Under a nitrogen atmosphere, a double-neck round-bottom flask or a Heavy-Wall Pressure Vessel was equipped with a magnetic stir bar, a condenser, and charged with **3b** (1.2 g, 4.7 mmol), Pd(t-$Bu_3P)_2$ (240 mg, 0.47 mmol), BHT (103.2 mg, 0.47 mmol), 1,3-Dichloropropane (36 mL, bubbled with nitrogen for 10 min prior to addition), Et_3N (653 µL, 4.7 mmol), and 1,1-dimethylallyl alcohol **5** (2.2 mL, 21 mmol). The flask was then immersed in an oil bath preheated to 90 °C. The reaction progress was monitored by TLC, and after approximately 8 hours, the mixture was cooled to room temperature. A saturated aqueous $NaHCO_3$ solution (10 mL) was added, and the mixture was stirred for 5 minutes. The resulting mixture was filtered through a celite pad and washed with ethyl acetate (100 mL). The filtrate was diluted with additional ethyl acetate (300 mL) and washed sequentially with water (240 mL) and brine (40 mL). The organic layer was dried over sodium sulfate, filtered, and concentrated under reduced pressure at 30 °C to yield the crude product. Purification by flash column chromatography (petroleum ether/ethyl acetate gradient, 15:1 to 5:1), the title compound citrubuntin was obtained as a yellow powder solid (1.07 g, 97% yield), m.p. 176–178 °C. ^{1}H NMR (400 MHz, $CDCl_3$) δ_H: 7.65 (d, J = 9.5 Hz, 1H), 7.55 (s, 1H), 6.87 (d, J = 16.3 Hz, 1H), 6.79 (d, J = 16.3 Hz, 1H), 6.78 (s, 1H), 6.27 (d, J = 9.5 Hz, 1H), 5.13 (d, J = 2.1 Hz, 1H), 5.10 (t, J = 1.7 Hz, 1H), 3.92 (s, 3H), 1.99 (d, J = 1.2 Hz, 3H); ^{13}C

NMR (101 MHz, $CDCl_3$) δ_C: 161.26, 160.05, 155.21, 143.63, 142.40, 133.21, 124.93, 124.37, 121.74, 117.94, 113.54, 112.43, 99.10, 56.17, 18.73; IR (KBr): 3427.83, 3063.80, 2930.04, 2345.77, 1725.98, 1610.08, 1368.16, 1270.11, 1123.71, 1001.52, 865.87, 819.85, 458.49 cm^{-1}; HRMS (EI) calcd for $C_{15}H_{14}O_3$ $[M + Na]^+$ 265.0837, found 265.0835.

Data for compound **7**, m.p. 172–174 °C: ^1H NMR (400 MHz, $CDCl_3$) δ_H: 7.63 (d, J = 9.5 Hz, 1H), 7.48 (s, 1H), 6.85 (d, J = 16.2 Hz, 1H), 6.77 (s, 1H), 6.36 (d, J = 16.2 Hz, 1H), 6.26 (d, J = 9.5 Hz, 1H), 3.90 (s, 3H), 1.44 (s, 6H); ^{13}C NMR (101 MHz, $CDCl_3$) δ_C: 161.30, 160.03, 155.22, 143.60, 139.30, 125.44, 123.88, 119.84, 113.49, 112.31, 99.05, 71.36, 56.11, 30.02; IR (KBr): 3838.15, 3732.92, 3433.47, 2932.10, 2345.14, 1728.08, 1611.93, 1356.06, 1210.07, 1020.71, 830.13, 675.92 cm^{-1}; HRMS (EI) calcd for $C_{15}H_{16}O_4$ $[M + Na]^+$ 283.0940, found 283.0941.

4. Conclusions

In summary, we developed a simple, practical method for preparing *trans*-dehydroosthol and citrubuntin in just one single step using the readily available starting materials. The naturally occurring compounds obtained in almost quantitative yield exhibited excellent stereoselectivity and atomic economy. This strategy offers several notable advantages: (1) the concise and efficient syntheses are characterized by a successful PGF (protecting group-free) approach and a redox-neutral strategy and (2) a highly active catalyst system has been developed for the one-pot (domino) Heck/dehydration reaction of deactivated coumarin substrates. This system is based on the electron-rich and bulky catalyst Pd[P(*t*-Bu)$_3$]$_2$, in combination with either Et_3N or the less commonly used trialkylamine (n-C_3H_7)$_3$N, and mediated by chlorinated solvents such as 1,3-DCP or DCE. Importantly, this synthetic approach not only enables the formal synthesis of novel dimeric natural products, including exotines A, cnidimonins A–C, 6/8-naphthoherniarin, cyclobi-suberodiene, and acrimarines A, F, and G, but also facilitates their overall synthesis. Ongoing efforts are focused on refining the practical, cost-effective conditions and methodologies for these dimeric compounds. The synthetic strategies reported in this study are being explored for potential application in related natural products. Further information on this development will be provided in the future.

Supplementary Materials: The following supporting information can be downloaded at https://www.mdpi.com/article/10.3390/molecules30051067/s1, Figures S1–S16: ^1H and ^{13}C NMR spectra of the products; Figures S17–S24: ^1H NMR Spectra for crude **6** and *trans*-dehydroosthol **(1)**; Tables S1–S4: ^1H and ^{13}C NMR spectral comparisons for compounds. References [9,17,21,27] are cited in the Supplementary Materials.

Author Contributions: Conceptualization, Z.L. and B.G.; methodology, X.G.; validation, Z.L. and B.G.; formal analysis, F.W.; investigation, Z.L.; resources, S.J. and T.L.; data curation, F.W.; writing—original draft preparation, B.G.; writing—review and editing, S.J.; visualization, Z.L.; supervision, S.J. and T.L.; project administration, T.L.; funding acquisition, S.J. and T.L. All authors have read and agreed to the published version of the manuscript.

Funding: This research was funded by National Natural Science Foundation of China (Grant No. 22361002), the Basic Research Special Project of Yunnan Provincial Department of Science and Technology-General Project (202201AT070175, 202401AT070071), and the Joint Special Fund Project for Basic Research of Local Undergraduate Universities (part of) in Yunnan Province (No. 202101AO070315).

Institutional Review Board Statement: Not applicable.

Informed Consent Statement: Not applicable.

Data Availability Statement: The data underlying this study are available in the published article and its online Supplementary Materials.

Conflicts of Interest: The authors declare no competing financial interests.

References

1. Geris, R.; Simpson, T.J. Meroterpenoids produced by fungi. *Nat. Prod. Rep.* **2009**, *26*, 1063–1094. [CrossRef] [PubMed]
2. Han, J.Y.; Zhang, J.Y.; Song, Z.J.; Zhu, G.L.; Liu, M.M.; Dai, H.Q.; Hsiang, T.; Liu, X.T.; Zhang, L.X.; Quinn, R.J.; et al. Genome-based mining of new antimicrobial meroterpenoids from the phytopathogenic fungus *Bipolaris sorokiniana* strain 11134. *Appl. Microbiol. Biotechnol.* **2020**, *104*, 3835–3846. [CrossRef] [PubMed]
3. Chang, J.L.; Gan, Y.T.; Peng, X.G.; Ouyang, Q.X.; Pei, J.; Ruan, H.L. Peniandranoids A–E: Meroterpenoids with antiviral and immunosuppressive activity from a *Penicillium* sp. *J. Nat. Prod.* **2023**, *86*, 66–75. [CrossRef]
4. Zbakh, H.; Zubía, E.; Reyes, C.; Calderón-Montaño, J.M.; López-Lázaro, M.; Motilva, V. Meroterpenoids from the brown alga *Cystoseira usneoides* as potential anti-inflammatory and lung anticancer agents. *Mar. Drugs* **2020**, *18*, 207. [CrossRef] [PubMed]
5. Jiang, M.H.; Guo, H.; Wu, Q.L.; Lu, X.; Zou, Y.T.; Fu, Q.Y.; Chen, S.H.; Liu, L.; Peng, B.; Chen, S.H. Anti-inflammatory acetylenic meroterpenoids from the ascidian-derived fungus *Amphichorda felina* SYSU-MS7 908. *Bioorg. Chem.* **2023**, *139*, 106715. [CrossRef] [PubMed]
6. Wang, C.F.; Liu, X.M.; Lian, C.L.; Ke, J.Y.; Liu, J.Q. Triterpenes and aromatic meroterpenoids with antioxidant activity and neuroprotective effects from *Ganoderma lucidum*. *Molecules* **2019**, *24*, 4353. [CrossRef] [PubMed]
7. Tomoda, H.; Nishida, H.; Kim, Y.K.; Obata, R.; Sunazuka, T.; Omura, S.; Bordner, J.; Guadliana, M.; Dormer, P.G.; Smith, A.B., III. Relative and Absolute Stereochemistry of Pyripyropene A, A Potent, Bioavailable Inhibitor of Acyl-CoA:Cholesterol Acyltransferase (ACAT). *J. Am. Chem. Soc.* **1994**, *116*, 12097–12098. [CrossRef]
8. Kuno, F.; Otoguro, K.; Shiomi, K.; Iwai, Y.; Omura, S. Arisugacins A and B, novel and selective acetylcholinesterase inhibitors from *Penicillium* sp. FO-4259. *J. Antibiot.* **1996**, *49*, 742–751. [CrossRef]
9. Ito, C.; Furukawa, H. Constituents of *Murraya exotica* L. structure elucidation of new coumarins. *Chem. Pharm. Bull.* **1987**, *35*, 4277–4285. [CrossRef]
10. Ito, C.; Ono, T.; Tanaka, E.; Takemura, Y.; Nakata, T.; Uchida, H.; Ju-Ichi, M.; Omura, M.; Furukawa, H. Structure of Pummeloquinoe, a new coumarin-Naphthoquinone dimer isolated from *Citrus* Plants. *Chem. Pharm. Bull.* **1993**, *41*, 205–207. [CrossRef]
11. Wang, X.T.; Liang, H.Z.; Zeng, K.W.; Zhao, M.B.; Tu, P.F.; Li, J.; Jiang, Y. Panitins A-G: Coumarin derivatives from *Murraya paniculata* from Guangxi Province, China show variable NO inhibitory activity. *Phytochemistry* **2019**, *162*, 224–231. [CrossRef] [PubMed]
12. Mock, J.R.; Senior, R.G.; Taylor, W.C. The chemical constituents of Australian *Zanthoxylum* species. VII. Some transformation products of suberosin. *Aust. J. Chem.* **1980**, *33*, 395–411. [CrossRef]
13. Wu, T.S. Alkaloids and coumarins of *Citrus grandis*. *Phytochemistry* **1988**, *27*, 3717–3718. [CrossRef]
14. Huang, S.; Luo, X.M.; Wang, J.H. Study on the chemical constituents from ethyl acetate extract of *Micromelum falcatum*. *J. Chin. Med. Mater.* **2013**, *36*, 744–746.
15. Suthiwong, J.; Sriphana, U.; Thongsri, Y.; Promsuwan, P.; Prariyachatigul, C.; Yenjai, C. Coumarinoids from the fruits of *Micromelum falcatum*. *Fitoterapia* **2014**, *94*, 134–141. [CrossRef] [PubMed]
16. Asghar, H.; Asghar, H.; Asghar, T. A Review on anti-urease potential of *Coumarins*. *Curr. Drug Targets* **2021**, *22*, 1926–1943. [CrossRef] [PubMed]
17. Reisch, J.; Bathe, A. Naturstoffchemie, 118[1)] synthese der cumarine 6- und 8-naphthoherniarin, dehydrogeijerin und Murraol. *Liebigs Ann. Chem.* **1988**, *1988*, 543–547. [CrossRef]
18. Murray, R.D.H.; Zeghdi, S. Synthesis of the natural coumarins, murraol (CM-c_2), *trans*-dehydroosthol and swietenocoumarin G. *Phytochemistry* **1989**, *28*, 227–230.
19. Lepovitz, L.T.; Martin, S.F. Biomimetically inspired synthesis of exotine A. *Org. Lett.* **2018**, *20*, 7875–7878. [CrossRef] [PubMed]
20. Lepovitz, L.T.; Martin, S.F. Biomimetically inspired, one-step synthesis of exotine A and exotine B. *J. Org. Chem.* **2021**, *86*, 10946–10953. [CrossRef] [PubMed]
21. Reisch, J.; Herath, H.M.T.B.; Kumar, N.S. ChemInform abstract: Natural product chemistry. Part 139. Synthesis of the natural coumarins (*E*)-suberenol, cyclobisuberodiene and two other related new coumarins. *Liebigs. Ann. Chem.* **1990**, *1990*, 931–933. [CrossRef]
22. Liu, B.Y.; Zhang, C.; Zeng, K.W.; Li, J.; Guo, X.Y.; Zhao, M.B.; Tu, P.F.; Jiang, Y. Exotines A and B, two heterodimers of isopentenyl-substituted indole and coumarin derivatives from *Murraya exotica*. *Org. Lett.* **2015**, *17*, 4380–4383. [CrossRef] [PubMed]

23. Su, F.Y.; Zhao, Z.; Ma, S.G.; Wang, R.B.; Li, Y.; Liu, Y.B.; Li, Y.H.; Li, L.; Qu, J.; Yu, S.S. Cnidimonins A–C, three types of hybrid dimer from *Cnidium monnieri*: Structural elucidation and semisynthesis. *Org. Lett.* **2017**, *19*, 4920–4923. [CrossRef] [PubMed]
24. Rozsa, Z.; Mester, I.; Reisch, J.; Szendrei, K. Naphthoherniarin: An unusual coumarin derivative from *Ruta graveolens*. *Planta Med.* **1989**, *55*, 68–69. [CrossRef] [PubMed]
25. Guise, G.B.; Ritchie, E.; Senior, R.G.; Taylor, W.C. The chemical constituents of Australian *Zanthoxylum* species. IV. Two new coumarins from *Z. suberosum* C. T. White (syn. *Z. dominianum* Merr. & Perry; *Z. ovalifolium* Wight). *Aust. J. Chem.* **1967**, *20*, 2429–2439.
26. Furukawa, H.; Ito, C.; Mizuno, T.; Ju-ichi, M.; Inoue, M.; Kajiura, I.; Omura, M. Spectrometric elucidation of acrimarines, the first naturally occurring acridone–coumarin dimers. *J. Chem. Soc. Perkin Trans.* **1990**, *1*, 1593–1599. [CrossRef]
27. Guthertz, A.; Leutzsch, M.; Wolf, L.M.; Gupta, P.; Rummelt, S.M.; Goddard, R.; Farès, C.; Thiel, W.; Fürstner, A. Half-sandwich ruthenium carbene complexes link *trans*-hydrogenation and *gem*-hydrogenation of internal alkynes. *J. Am. Chem. Soc.* **2018**, *140*, 3156–3169. [CrossRef]
28. Jeffery, T. *Advances in Metal-Organic Chemistry*; Liebeskind, L.S., Ed.; JAI: London, UK, 1996.
29. Diederich, F.; Stang, P.J. *Metal-Catalyzed Cross-Coupling Reactions*; Wiley-VCH: New York, NY, USA, 1998.
30. Wang, L.H.; Lei, T.; Wang, F.S.; Jiang, S.Z.; Yan, G.Y. Total synthesis of indiacen A using a practical one-pot reaction: Promoted by a key waste product, and its utility in natural products synthesis. *Tetrahedron Lett.* **2021**, *66*, 152822. [CrossRef]
31. Li, T.; Song, J.-J.; Wang, L.H.; Lei, T.; Jiang, S.Z.; Wang, F. A simple and efficient total synthesis of anticancer indole alkaloids TMC-205 and its analogues. *Tetrahedron Lett.* **2021**, *74*, 153137. [CrossRef]
32. Song, J.J.; Lu, G.D.; Yang, B.Q.; Bai, M.J.; Li, J.J.; Wang, F.S.; Lei, T.; Jiang, S.Z. A concise first total synthesis of luteoride A and luteoride B. *Tetrahedron* **2022**, *122*, 132933. [CrossRef]
33. Gong, X.S.; Bai, M.J.; Lu, G.D.; Yang, B.Q.; Lei, T.; Jiang, S.Z. Total synthesis of murraol, (*E*)-suberenol and toward the collective total synthesis of exotines A, cnidimonins A-Cetc. *Tetrahedron* **2022**, *126*, 133061. [CrossRef]

molecules

MDPI

Article

Design, Synthesis, and Biological Evaluation of 5,8-Dimethyl Shikonin Oximes as SARS-CoV-2 M^{pro} Inhibitors

Jiahua Cui [1,2,*,†], Shouyan Xiang [1,3,†], Qijing Zhang [4], Shangqing Xiao [1], Gaoyang Yuan [1], Chenwu Liu [1] and Shaoshun Li [4]

[1] School of Pharmacy, Gannan Medical University, Ganzhou 341000, China; tc1423177159@sjtu.edu.cn (S.X.); gmuxsq@163.com (S.X.); ygy17630814755@163.com (G.Y.); 18579009691@163.com (C.L.)

[2] Jiangxi Province Key Laboratory of Pharmacology of Traditional Chinese Medicine, Gannan Medical University, Ganzhou 341000, China

[3] School of Chemistry and Chemical Engineering, Shanghai Jiaotong University, Shanghai 200240, China

[4] School of Pharmacy, Shanghai Jiaotong University, Shanghai 200240, China; lianyi0810@163.com (Q.Z.); ssli@sjtu.edu.cn (S.L.)

* Correspondence: cpucjh@sjtu.edu.cn; Tel./Fax: +86-21-34204775

† These authors contributed equally to this work.

Abstract: We have designed, synthesized, and characterized a small library of shikonin derivatives and demonstrated their inhibitory activity against the main protease, M^{pro}, of SARS-CoV-2. One analog, 5,8-dimethyl shikonin oxime (**15**), exhibited the highest activity against SARS-CoV-2 M^{pro} with an IC_{50} value of 12.53 ± 3.59 μM. It exhibited much less toxicity as compared with the parent compound, shikonin, in both in vitro and in vivo models. Structure–activity relationship analysis indicated that the oxime moieties on the naphthalene ring and the functional groups attached to the oxygen atom on the side chain play a pivotal role in enzymatic inhibitory activity. Molecular docking results implied that the inhibitor **15** is perfectly settled in the core of the substrate-binding pocket of M^{pro} by possibly interacting with three catalytic residues, His41, Cys145, and Met165. Overall, the shikonin oxime derivative **15** deserves further investigation as an antiviral agent against SARS-CoV-2.

Keywords: SARS-CoV-2 M^{pro}; shikonin; dimethyl shikonin oximes; inhibitors; COVID-19

1. Introduction

The severe acute respiratory infectious disease caused by a new coronavirus (SARS-CoV-2) led to the outbreak of pneumonia (COVID-19), which has seriously endangered the world's public health [1,2]. According to the data from WHO, by 1 December 2024, there were more than 776.97 million diagnosed COVID-19 cases and 7.07 million confirmed deaths, making it one of the deadliest pandemics in human history [3]. From December 2021, the number of cases appears to be rapidly increasing due to the rapid epidemic expansion of the SARS-CoV-2 Omicron variant. Therefore, it is an urgent need to develop highly effective drugs against the ongoing pandemic coronavirus disease [4].

The new coronavirus is a single-strand positive-sense RNA virus with high homology to SARS-CoV and MERS-CoV [5]. After entry of the coronavirus into host cells, nuclear acids were released within the host cytoplasm and the ORF1a/b region of the viral genome translated into two polyprotein precursors (pp1a and pp1ab), which were cleaved to virus structural and non-structural proteins under the action of main protease (M^{pro}) [6,7]. M^{pro} was also called the 3C-like protease because its cleavage site specificity was similar to that of picornavirus 3C protease. The non-structural proteins produced by M^{pro} were involved in the synthesis of viral subgene RNA and also four structural proteins vital for the viral reproduction. Since the main protease plays a pivotal role in the life cycle of coronavirus, and there are no homologous proteins within the host cells, M^{pro} is an ideal target for antiviral drug research and development [8,9]. Although dozens of distinct vaccines have been authorized for use against COVID-19, certain variants with mutations on their spike proteins might escape from the immune responses of vaccination [10,11].

Natural active compounds are a wellspring of lead compounds for antiviral drug screening [12]. Shikonin (Figure 1), a natural naphthoquinone isolated from *Lithospermum erythrorhizon* Sieb. et Zucc., exhibited striking antiviral, antibacterial, anti-inflammatory, and anticancer activity. Within concentrations from 0.0156 μM to 1 μM, the naphthoquinone showed inhibitory effects against adenovirus through down-regulation of viral hexon protein and prohibition of cellular apoptosis induced by the virus [13]. Its acetyl derivative potently inhibited both infection and replication of Coxsackievirus A16 in vitro and in vivo [14]. In recent studies, it was identified as a potent inhibitor of SARS-CoV-2 M^{pro} with its IC_{50} value of 15.75 ± 8.22 μM [8].

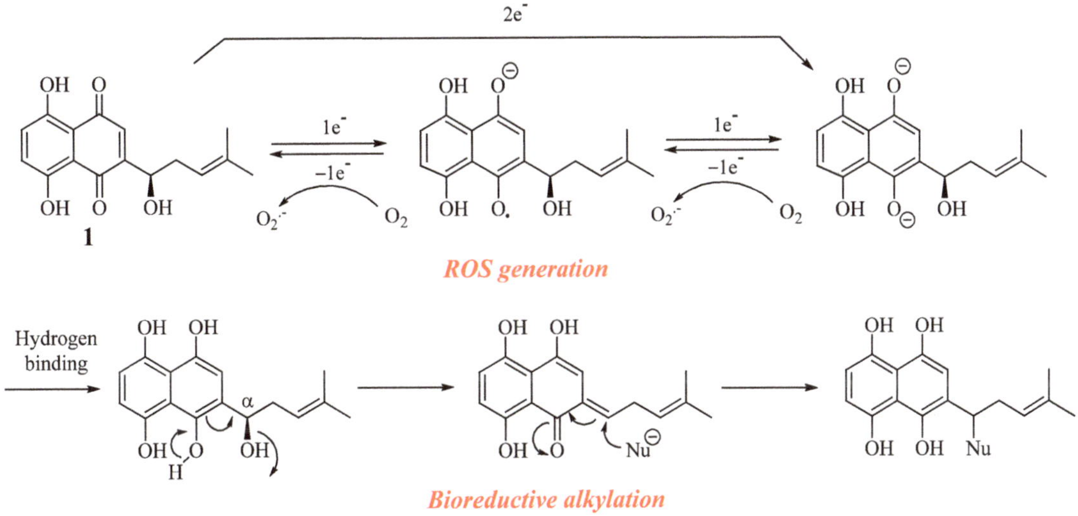

Figure 1. Generation of ROS from naphthazarin nucleus and bioreductive alkylation of shikonin with nucleophiles.

In spite of the potent antiviral activity, it has not been used in clinical trials mainly ascribed to the non-specific cytotoxicity both in vivo and in vitro. From the chemical point of view, the naphthazarin nucleus contributed to ROS generation and bioreductive alkylation of the hallmark molecule, leading to high toxicity (Figure 1) [15]. Therefore, rational structural modifications of the naphthoquinone scaffold of **1** could prevent the cytotoxicity and also provide antiviral candidates with few side effects.

The study that focused on the crystal structure of SARS-CoV-2 M^{pro} in complex with shikonin implied that the inhibitor formed multiple interactions with the target enzyme [16] (Figure 2). The phenolic hydroxyl group on the naphthazarin nucleus hydrogen bonded with protease polar triad Cys145 and His164 amino acid residues. A π–π interaction between the shikonin naphthazarin moieties with His41 on the S1 subsite also contributed to the tight binding affinity of the inhibitor with M^{pro}. These findings suggested that exchange of phenolic hydroxyl groups on the A-ring of shikonin with certain hydroxyl group-contained functional groups possibly maintained the enzymatic inhibition activity.

In addition, carbonyl/hydroxyl groups on the naphthazarin nucleus should be masked to avoid the generation of ROS, since ROS accumulation was correlated to the cytotoxicity of resulting compounds. The electron-withdrawing groups were not preferred since the decrease in electron density of the naphthalene ring might lead to weakened π–π interaction of prepared compounds with the side chain of His41. All of these studies motivated us to prepare 5,8-dimethyl shikonin oximes (Figure 3) and also test their enzymatic inhibition activity against SARS-CoV-2 M^{pro}.

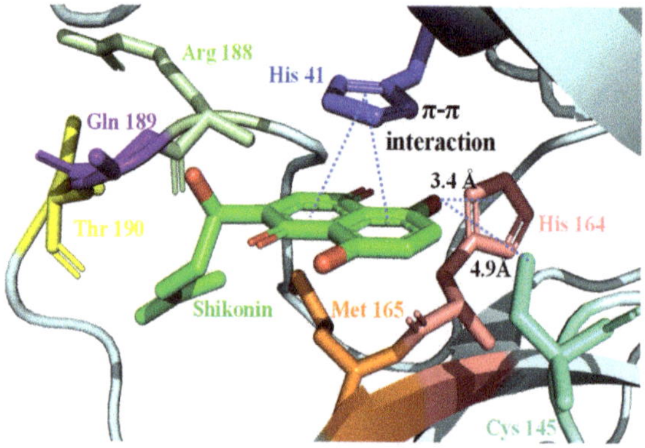

Figure 2. X-ray cocrystal structure of shikonin–M^{pro} complex (PDB ID: 7CA8). Shikonin in magenta color was shown in sticks. His41 (blue), His164 (yellow), and Cys145 (orange) were shown in lines.

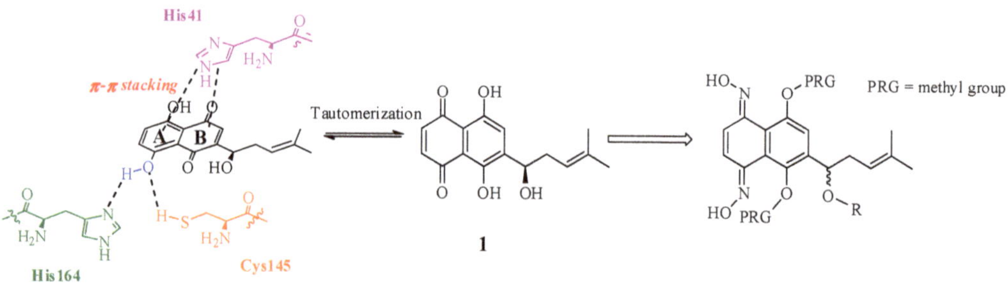

Figure 3. Overlooked strategy for M^{pro} inhibitor design.

2. Results and Discussion

2.1. Synthetic Studies

Racemic 4-methyl-1-(1,4,5,8-tetramethoxynaphthalen-2-yl)pent-3-en-1-ol (**2**), which was prepared according to the reported procedures [17], was employed as the starting material in the study. The secondary alcoholic hydroxyl group of starting material was first etherified using sodium hydride and brominated isoamyl to afford compound **3** in high yield with potassium iodine as the catalyst (Scheme 1). Then, the methyl groups of **3** were cleaved by cerium ammonium nitrate (CAN)-mediated oxidation under mild conditions to afford a pair of isomers, among which naphthoquinone **4** was separated through column chromotography. Oximation of the quinone moiety of the substrate (**4**) using hydroxyl amine hydrochloride and pyridine in alcoholic solutions gave the target compound (**5**) with a high yield. Further esterification of the oxime hydroxyl group of **5** produced the ester (**6**).

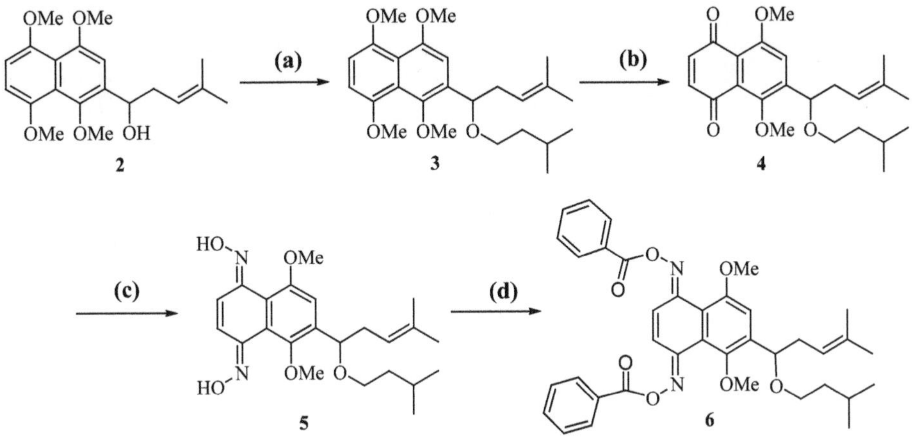

Scheme 1. Reagents and conditions: (**a**) isoamyl bromide, NaH, KI, DMF, 0 °C, 20 min, then 60 °C, overnight; yield: 88.3%. (**b**) CAN, DCM/ACN, 0 °C, 10 min; yield: 38.7%. (**c**) $NH_2OH{\cdot}HCl$, Py, EtOH, 50 °C, 24 h; yield: 90.4%. (**d**) PhCOOH, EDCI, DMAP, DCM, overnight; yield: 83.2%.

Methylated shikonin analogues (**7** and **8**) were prepared by the same synthetic strategy using tetrahydropyranyl (THP) group-protected bromohydrin as a reactant instead of the brominated isopentane (Scheme 2). Acidic hydrolysis of the THP-protecting group and further oxidation–oximation reactions afforded 5,8-dimethyl shikonin oxime derivatives (**9** and **10**). Compound **12** was prepared by esterification of the secondary alcoholic hydroxyl group of **2** with cinnamoyl acid and subsequent oxidation–oximation reactions (Scheme 2).

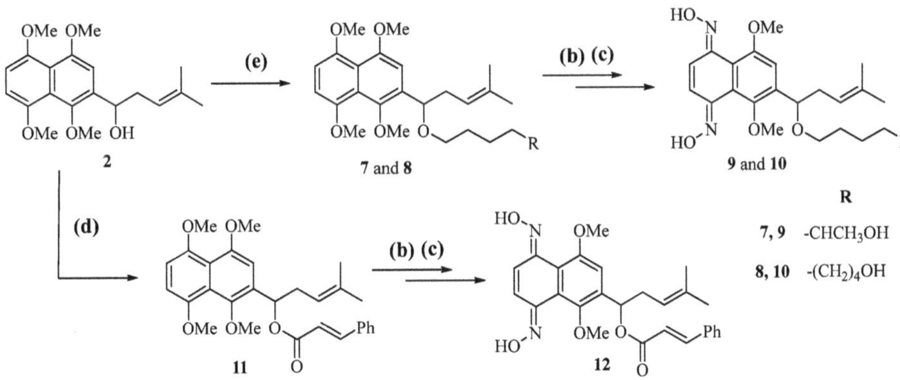

Scheme 2. Reagents and conditions: (**e**) THP-protected bromohydrin, NaH, KI, DMF, 60 °C, overnight; then HCl, CH_3OH, r.t., 2 h; yield for compound **7**: 81.4%; yield for compound **8**: 85.8%. (**b**)–(**d**) were the same with counterparts illustrated in Scheme 1.

In the preparation of enantiomeric secondary alcohols (**2-*R*** and **2-*S***), the racemate **2** was first subject to moderate Dess–Martin oxidation to afford ketone **13** in high yield (Scheme 3). Further asymmetric hydrogenation of ketone **13** produced the enantiomeric alcohols **2-*R*** and **2-*S*** in excellent enantiomeric excess values using diisopinocampheyl chloroborane (+)-DIP-Cl and (−)-DIP-Cl as the reducing agent, respectively. Due to the steric hindrance of the α-pinenyl substituent, the substituted borane only hydroborates unhindered substrates, and the hydroboration reactions proceeded through the formation of six-member cyclic rings [18,19]. As shown in Scheme 4, the smaller six-carbon side chain faced the axial 2′-methyl group, while the bulky substituted naphthalene ring occupied the equatorial-like orientation in the preferred transition-state intermediate (**16**). The *cis*-elimination of boron moiety and hydrogen probably resulted in the formation of the secondary alcohol (**2-*S***) with *S*-configuration. In the disfavored intermediate (**17**), the steric repulsion between the axial 2′-methyl group and 1,4,5,8-tetramethoxy naphthalene ring prohibited the formation of *R*-enantiomer (**2-*R***).

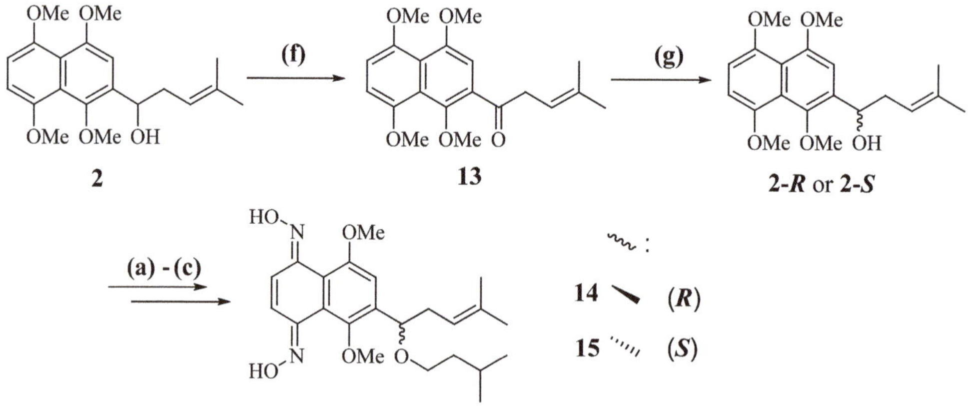

Scheme 3. Reagents and conditions: (**f**) Dess–Martin periodinane, DCM, −15 °C, 2 h; yield: 84.5%. (**g**) (+)-DIP-Cl or (−)-DIP-Cl, −30 °C, overnight; (+)-DIP-Cl for **2-*R*** and (−)-DIP-Cl for **2-*S***. (a)–(c) were the same with counterparts illustrated in Scheme 1.

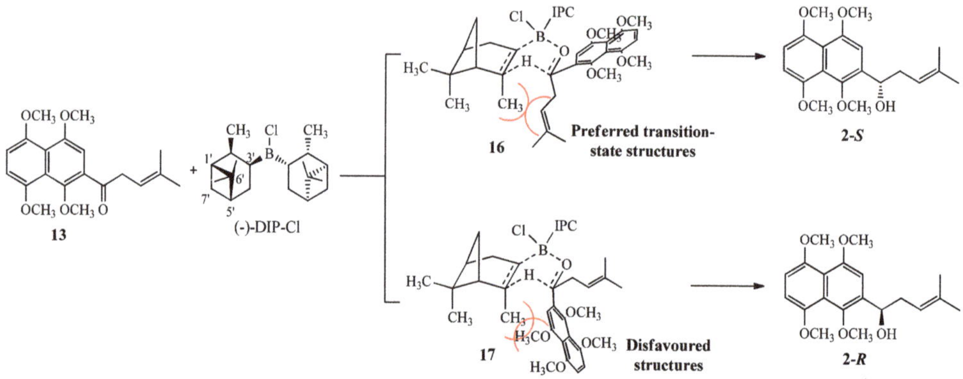

Scheme 4. Transition-state model for (−)-DIP-Cl-mediated hydroboration of compound **13**.

Similarly, the reduction of ketone **13** using (+)-DIP-Cl preferentially afforded the alcohol **2-*R*** with the chiral center in *R*-configuration, and the reaction proceeded via the formation of a boat-like bicyclic transition-state intermediate (**18**, Figure 4).

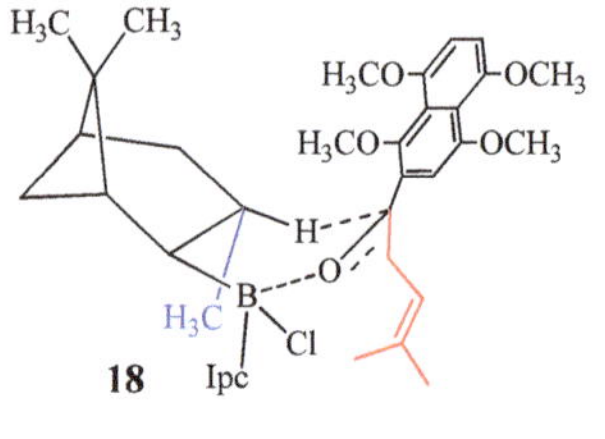

Figure 4. Structure of favored transition-state intermediate for (+)-DIP-Cl-mediated hydroboration.

The configuration of products in campheylborane DIP-Cl-mediated hydroboration of **13** as a substrate was different from the reported hydrogenation of the methylene acetal-protected analogue (**19**) using DIP-Cl [20,21] (Scheme 5). The results from previous studies indicated that the reduction of ketone intermediate **19** using (+)-DIP-Cl afforded corresponding alcohol (**20**) with the chiral center in *S*-configuration, and the (−)-DIP-Cl provided *R*-alcohol (**21**). The methoxyl group-substituted naphthalene ring of ketone **13** should be bigger in size as compared with the methylene acetal-protected naphthalene moiety of **19**. The steric repulsion between the pinocampheyl methyl group and naphthalene ring should be much weaker in intermediate **22** than that in the transition state of intermediate **17**. According to the classical theories [19,20] on DIP-Cl-mediated hydroboration reactions, there might be additional interactions between the oxygen atoms in methylene acetal-protecting groups with the boron atom, which contributed to the stabilization of transition-state intermediate **22**.

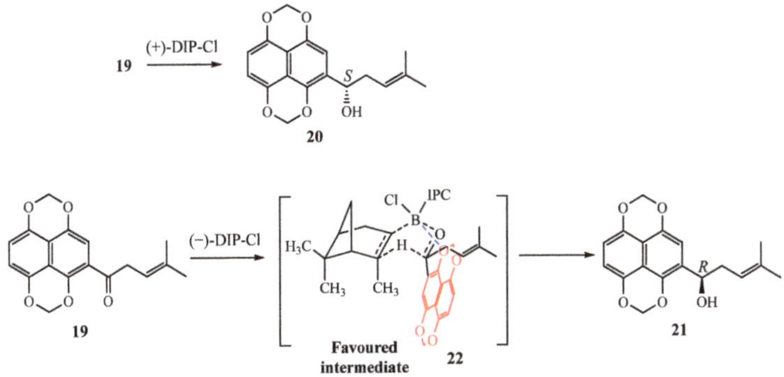

Scheme 5. Asymmetric reduction of ketone intermediate **19** with organoborane DIP-Cl and plausible mechanisms.

The optical purities for chiral alcohols (**2-*R*** and **2-*S***) were determined by established chiral chromatography using the Chiralpak OD-H column with *n*-hexane-isopropanol (6:4, V/V) as the eluent [22]. The optical purity was 96% and 95% for compound **2-*R*** and **2-*S***, respectively (see Supplementary Materials). The absolute configuration of chiral centers for two optical isomers was confirmed by comparing the chromatographic retention times of two compounds with the optical intermediate obtained by Ru(II)-catalyzed asymmetric hydrogenation [23]. In the synthesis of chiral compounds **14** and **15**, no racemization reactions were involved with **2-*R*** and **2-*S*** as the starting material. The purity of target compounds (**14** and **15**) was confirmed by the chiral liquid chromatography with amylose tris[(S)-α-methylbenzylcarbamate] (CHIRALPAK® IH, 250 × 4.6 mm, 5 μm) as the stationary phase and *n*-hexane/*i*-PrOH (9:1, V/V) as the mobile phase (compound **14**, 96% *e.e.*; compound **15**, 95% *e.e.*).

2.2. Enzymatic Inhibition Assay

The M^{pro} inhibition activity of prepared compounds was measured employing the reported Fluorescence Resonance Energy Transfer (FRET) method [24], in which the fluorescent MCA and Dnp were used as the donor and the acceptor, respectively. In the primary screening, compounds (**4–6**, **9**, **10**, and **12**) and shikonin as the positive control were tested at the concentration of 10 μM and the fluorescence intensity of each well in the enzymatic assay was monitored upon incubation for 5 min. Since racemic compound **5** was a relatively more potent inhibitor within tested 5,8-dimethyl shikonin analogues in the primary screening, compounds **14** and **15** as enantiomers and the lead shikonin were then determined for their IC_{50} values, which were in the range from 11.26 to 22.75 μM.

2.3. Structure–Activity Relationship Studies

The results from the preliminary enzymatic inhibition assay indicated that the substitutions on the naphthazarin moiety of shikonin and the functional groups attached to the oxygen atom on the side chain played pivotal roles in the activity (Table 1). Oximation of the quinone ring led to an increase in inhibitory activity since compound **5** was nearly a three-fold more potent inhibitor to the parent compound **4** with a quinoidal scaffold. However, benzoylation of the oxime hydroxyl group (**6**) resulted in complete loss of activity in screening. During modification of the ether linkage on the side chain, elongation of the isopentane branched chain (**5**) to an *n*-octane backbone (**10**) caused a drop in enzyme inhibition efficacy. Exchange of the isopentane group of **5** to a hexan-2-ol moiety (**9**) was also not preferred. Additionally, 5,8-dimethyl shikonin oxime (**12**) with the enzymatic inhibition rate of 28% at the concentration of 10 μM was less potent as compared with the ether derivative **5**. In the preliminary screening, the racemic compound **5** was identified as the most potent one among the tested shikonin derivatives with an enzymatic inhibition rate of about 36%.

Table 1. Enzymatic inhibition rates of tested compounds in the primary screening.

No. of Compd.	Enzymatic Inhibition Rate (%)
4	10.6
5	35.8
6	−6.9
9	10.7
10	11.3
12	28.0
1	51.4

Since most enantiomers of racemic drugs displayed marked differences in pharmacological activities [25,26], the enantiomers of compound **5** prepared through enantioselective hydrogenation were tested for their enzymatic inhibition efficacy. As shown in Table 2, *S*-enantiomer **15** was characterized as the eutomer with respect to inhibition of SARS-CoV-2 M^{pro} with the IC_{50} value of 12.53 ± 3.59 μM. It was equally potent, as compared with shikonin, as the lead (IC_{50} = 11.26 ± 2.35 μM). The eutomer **15** was a 1.8-fold more potent inhibitor as compared with the distomer (**14**). The results implied that there might be some positive or negative interactions between the isoamylene moiety on the chiral center and the isopentane substituent attached to the oxygen atom, and the combined effects influenced the M^{pro} inhibitory activity.

2.4. Molecular Docking Studies

To further understand the putative binding modes of compound **15** against SARS-CoV-2 M^{pro}, we performed a molecular docking study using the MOE 2008 software (Chemical Computing Group Inc., Montreal, QC, Canada). The X-ray crystal structure of SARS-CoV-2 M^{pro} (PDB: 7CA8) complexed with shikonin in the substrate-binding site was obtained from the RSC Protein Data Bank (Figure 5). The active site cavity was defined as amino acid residues within an 8 Å spherical radius to shikonin. In the system adaptability test of docking studies, shikonin as the native ligand was docked back to the original model (7CA8) from PDB. The result from validation studies indicated that shikonin in the predicted binding model with the lowest binding energy (−16.0859 Kcal/mol) posed a similar conformation and orientation in the active site cavity as compared with the original model. Employing the established molecular docking algorithm, compound **15** was successfully docked in the shikonin-binding pocket in SARS-CoV-2 M^{pro} with a binding energy of −16.8006 Kcal/mol. Molecular formulas, Lipinski's rule of five, binding affinities (Kcal/mol), and binding active amino acid residues are shown in Table 3.

Table 2. IC_{50} values of selected enantiomers against SARS-CoV-2 M^{pro}.

No. of Compd.	Chemical Structure	IC_{50} (μM)
14	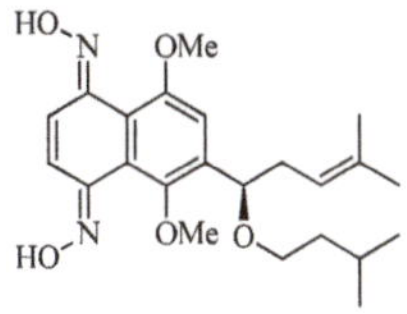	22.75 ± 4.61
15	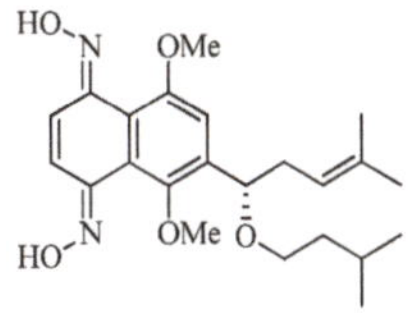	12.53 ± 3.59
1	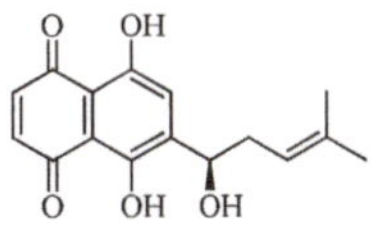	11.26 ± 2.35

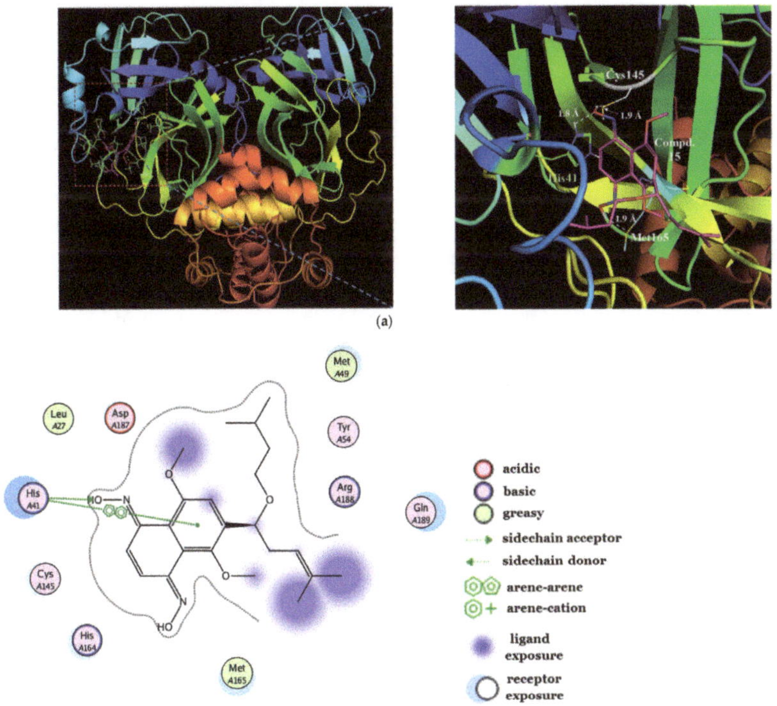

(a)

(b)

Figure 5. (**a**) The predicted binding model of the top-hit compound (shown as magenta sticks) in the substrate-binding pocket of SARS-CoV-2 M^{pro}. White dotted lines represent hydrogen bonds with amino acid residues. (**b**) Representation of the interactions between compound **15** and surrounding amino acid residues in the SARS-CoV-2 M^{pro}-binding pocket.

Table 3. Properties, Lipinski's rule of five, binding affinities, and active amino acid residues in docking studies.

Compd.	Molecular Formula	Lipinski's Rule of Five		Calculated Binding Energy (Kcal/mol)	Binding Amino Acid Residues
15	$C_{23}H_{32}N_2O_5$	Molecular weight (<500 DA)	416.51	−16.8006	**His41, Cys145, His164, Met165, Thr190, Arg188, Gln189**
		LogP (<5)	4.29 *		
		H-bond donor (5)	2		
		H-Bond acceptor (10)	7		
Shikonin	$C_{16}H_{16}O_5$	Molecular weight (<500 DA)	288.30	−16.0859	**His41, Cys145, His164, Met165, Tyr54, Arg188,** Asp187, **Gln189,** Met49
		LogP (<5)	0.92 *; 1.08 $^{\Delta}$		
		H-bond donor (5)	3		
		H-Bond acceptor (10)	5		

Note: * the data were predicted by ChemDraw Ultra 12.0 software; $^{\Delta}$ stands for the experimental value [27].

In the proposed binding modes (Figure 5), the inhibitor **15** was well placed in the SARS-CoV-2 M^{pro} catalytic triad region, forming hydrogen bonding with the polar Cys145 located on the S1 subsite with a distance of only 1.9 Å. In addition, the aromatic naphthalene ring in the structure of shikonin formed a π–π interaction with His41 amino acid residue on the S2 subsite. The oxygen atom on the oxime moiety also formed one hydrogen bond with the His41 imidazole functional group (bond length of 1.8 Å), contributing to the tight binding affinity. The hydrophobic interactions between the isopentene side chain and Met165 together with the hydrogen bonding between one oxime hydroxyl group and Met165 sulfur atom also confirmed the tight binding affinity of compound **15** with the substrate-binding site.

2.5. Surface Plasmon Resonance Assay

The real-time binding profile between SARS-CoV-2 M^{pro} protein and the inhibitor **15** was identified by the standard surface plasmon resonance (SPR) assay. SARS-CoV-2 M^{pro} proteins were immobilized to a CM5 sensorchip. For affinity analysis, compound **15** was dissolved in a PBS solution supplemented with 0.05% Tween-20 and 5% DMSO at concentrations of 1.0 μM, 2.0 μM, 4.0 μM, 8.0 μM, and 16.0 μM, respectively. We used the Biacore^{TM} insight evaluation software to calculate multi-cycle kinetics for samples. As shown in Figure 6, the binding rate constant (ka) of 0.220 $M^{-1}\cdot s^{-1}$ confirmed binding affinity of inhibitor **15** with the target enzyme.

2.6. Cytotoxicity Evaluations

Shikonin as the lead compound and 5,8-dimethyl shikonin oxime **15** were tested for their cytotoxicity using the standard MTT assay described in the Experimental Section. The results implied that shikonin was highly toxic towards the tested human normal HFF-1 and African green monkey Vero E6 cells with CC_{50} values of 1.31 ± 0.09 μM and 1.48 ± 0.06 μM (Table 4), respectively.

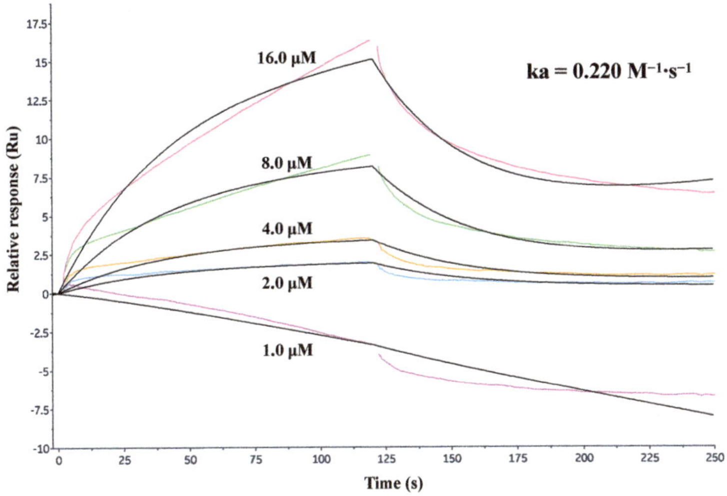

Figure 6. The real-time binding profile between SARS-CoV-2 M^{pro} and shikonin oxime **15**.

Table 4. Cytotoxic activity of shikonin and compound **15** against selected mammalian cell lines.

No. of Compd.	Chemical Structures	CC_{50} Values	
		HFF-1	Vero E6
15	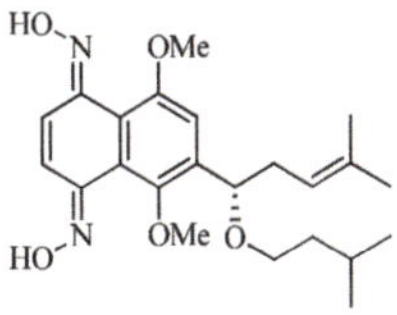	85.6 ± 5.9 μM	96.7 ± 8.3 μM
1	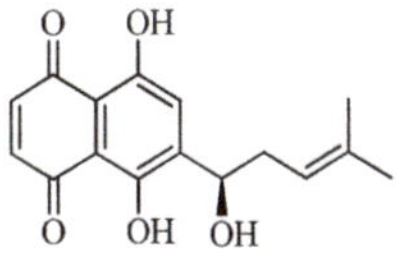	1.31 ± 0.09 μM	1.48 ± 0.06 μM

On the contrary, 5,8-dimethyl shikonin oxime **15** exhibited rather low cytotoxicity towards these two cell lines with CC_{50} values much higher than 50 μM. The observations were in accordance with previously published research results that the cytotoxicity of natural shikonin greatly decreased upon modifications of the naphthazarin core scaffold [28,29].

2.7. In Vitro Antiviral Activity

In order to determine the antiviral potential of synthesized 5,8-dimethyl shikonin oximes, we further examined the effects of compound **15** against wildtype SARS-CoV-2 replicating in Vero E6 cells. Culture supernatant was collected after treatment of the infected cells by shikonin oxime **15** at concentrations of 12.5, 25, 50, and 75 μM, respectively. Then supernatant from cell cultures was collected and SARS-CoV-2 copies were measured by qRT-PCR assay [8]. The results indicated that compound **15** at the concentration of 75 μM suppressed viral replications by about 50% in host Vero E6 cells through the quantitative RT-PCR assay (Figure 7).

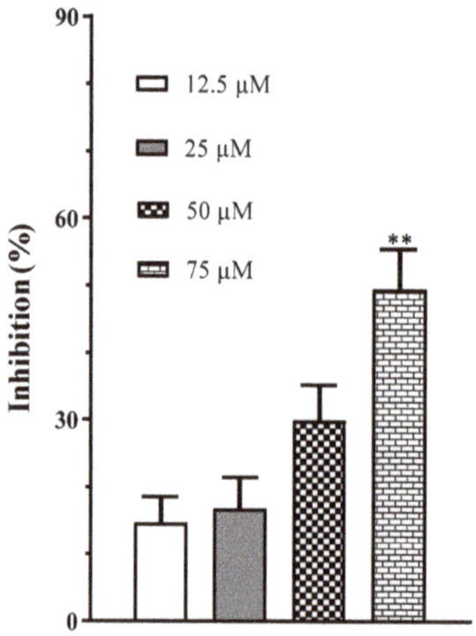

Figure 7. Compound **15** inhibited live SARS-CoV-2 replication in Vero E6 cells (** $p < 0.01$).

Further immunofluorescence assays for viral N proteins were conducted to confirm the anti-viral efficacy of targeted compounds. As shown in Figure 8, cells treated with shikonin and compound **15** exhibited significantly decreased expression of viral N proteins than the untreated cells. However, due to the high toxicity of shikonin, the blue fluorescence from the live cell nucleus in the shikonin-treated group was almost invisible. All of the results implied that the shikonin oxime derivative **15** deserved further development as a potential antiviral drug candidate for the treatment of SARS-CoV-2 infections.

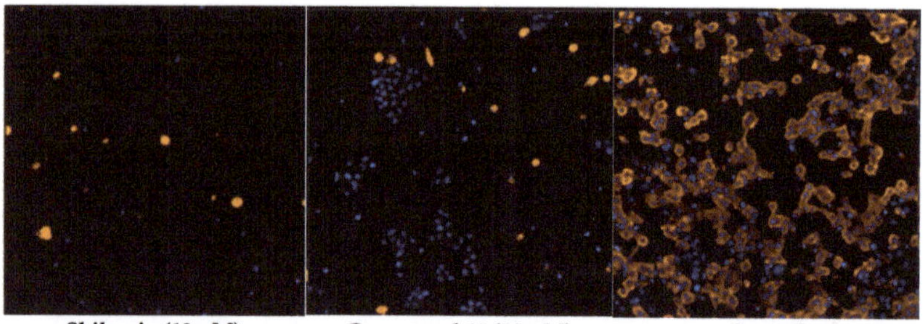

Figure 8. Immunofluorescent assay was used to detect the expression of SARS-CoV-2 N proteins. The yellow lights indicated viral N proteins, while the blue fluorescence from DAPI stands for nucleus of live cells.

The therapeutic index was defined as the ratio between the antiviral EC_{50} values and the cytotoxicity. Although the shikonin analog **15** had slightly decreased enzymatic inhibitory activity than shikonin, its therapeutic index (about 0.78) was much less than that of shikonin (>1.0/0.8 ± 0.0) [30]. It deserves further investigation as an antiviral drug candidate against SARS-CoV-2.

2.8. In Vivo Toxicity Evaluation of 5,8-Dimethyl Shikonin Oxime 15 and Shikonin in Balb/c Mice

We performed the in vivo toxicity study of 5,8-dimethyl shikonin oxime (**15**) and lead compound shikonin in Balb/c mice by repeatedly intravenous administration of compound **15** (30 mg/kg, i.v.) (Figure 9) or shikonin (10 mg/kg, i.v.) for sive times on every other day. We monitored toxicity symptoms like loss of weight by 15% for three consecutive days, loss of appetite, slowness in activity, and treatment-related mortality, if any, from day 1 to day 13, plus two more days after the last administration. Repeated administration of compound **15** (30 mg/kg) alone did not induce any mortality or toxicity symptoms. However, the intravenous administration of shikonin (10 mg/kg) was not tolerable since all the animals died within six days after the first treatment (Figure 10). All of these observations suggested that 5,8-dimethyl shikonin oxime **15** was much less toxic in murine as compared with the parent compound shikonin, and oxime derivative **15** had certain advantages in efficacy evaluations in animals.

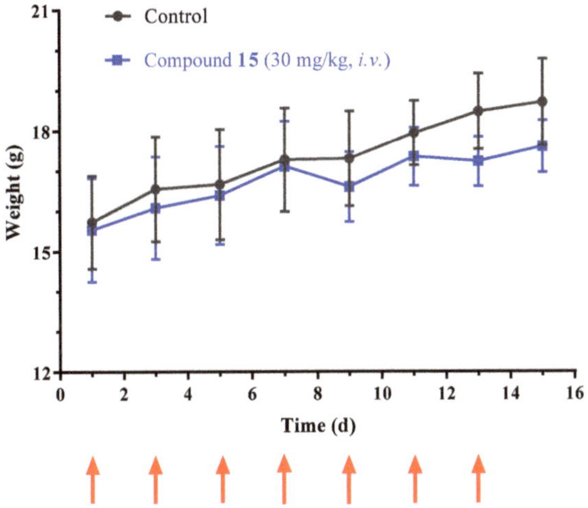

Figure 9. Body weight changes of animals upon treatment by compound **15**. (Arrows stands for the date of compound administration).

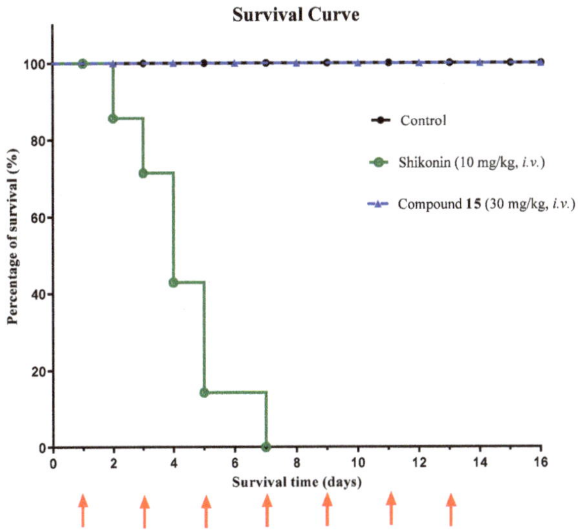

Figure 10. Survival curve of animals for compound **15** and shikonin group.

3. Experimental

3.1. Chemistry

Reagents and solvents in reagent grade were obtained from Shanghai Titan Scientific Co. Ltd. (Shanghai, China) and used without further purification unless otherwise stated. Melting points were determined on a WRR digital melting point apparatus (40–280 °C, Shanghai INESA Physical-Optical Instrument Co., Ltd., Shanghai, China). All NMR spectra were recorded on a Bruker Advance 400 MHz spectrometer (ideaoptics, Shanghai, China) at 400 MHz for ^{1}H and 101 MHz for ^{13}C or an Agilent 300 MHz spectrometer at 300 MHz for ^{1}H and 75 MHz for ^{13}C. All NMR measurements were carried out at room temperature and the chemical shifts are reported as parts per million (ppm) in units relative to the resonance of $CDCl_3$ (7.26 ppm in the ^{1}H and 77.16 ppm for the central line of the triplet in the ^{13}C modes, respectively) and DMSO-d_6 (2.50 ppm in the ^{1}H and 39.52 ppm for the central line of the septet in the ^{13}C modes, respectively). The plates used for thin-layer chromatography (TLC) were E. Merck Silica Gel 60F254 (0.25 mm thickness), and they were visualized under short (254 nm) and long (365 nm) UV light. Chromatographic purifications were carried out using MN silica gel 60 (230–400 mesh). The purity of tested compounds was determined by HPLC, which was performed by using the Agilent 1100 series (Agilent Technologies Deutschland GmbH Hewlett-Packard-Strasse 8, Waldbronn, Germany) installed with an analytic column, the Agilent Zorbax C18 column (4.6 mm × 250 mm, 5 μm), at UV detection of 318 nm (reference at 450 nm) with acetonitrile (60%)/Milli-Q water (40%) at a flow rate of 1.0 mL/min. All tested compounds were shown to >98% purity according to HPLC analysis.

3.1.1. Synthesis of 2-(1-(Isopentyloxy)-4-methylpent-3-en-1-yl)-1,4,5,8-tetramethoxy Naphthalene (**3**)

The 4-methyl-1-(1,4,5,8-tetramethoxynaphthalen-2-yl)pent-3-en-1-ol (**2**, 3.0 g, 8.7 mmol) was dissolved in dry DMF (30 mL) under water–ice cooling, and NaH in mineral oil (60%, 1.0 g, 25 mmol) was added in portions. After the addition, the mixture was stirred for 20 min. Then, bromoisopentane (2.6 g, 17.2 mmol) and a catalytic amount of potassium iodine were added. The reaction mixture was further headed at 60 °C overnight. After completion of the reaction, the reaction mixture was poured on ice and the mixture was extracted with dichloromethane (20 mL × 4). The combined organic layer was washed with brine, dried over anhydrous sodium sulphate, and evaporated under reduced pressure to give a brown oil, which was subjected to flash column chromatography on silica gel with 10% ethyl acetate in petroleum ether as the eluent to furnish the desired product as a light-yellow oil (3.2 g), obtaining a yield of 88.3% as well as the following: ^{1}H NMR (400 MHz, $CDCl_3$) δ 6.98 (s, 1H), 6.83 (s, 2H), 5.26 (t, J = 7.2 Hz, 1H), 4.87 (t, J = 6.6 Hz, 1H), 3.97–3.88 (m, 9H), 3.74 (s, 3H), 3.40–3.25 (m, 2H), 2.54–2.40 (m, 2H), 1.77–1.68 (m, 1H), 1.66 (s, 3H), 1.54 (s, 3H), 1.52–1.37 (m, 2H), 0.86 (d, J = 6.6 Hz, 3H), 0.81 (d, J = 6.6 Hz, 3H).

3.1.2. Synthesis of 6-(1-(Isopentyloxy)-4-methylpent-3-en-1-yl)-5,8-dimethoxy Naphthalene-1,4-dione (**4**)

To a solution of 2-(1-(isopentyloxy)-4-methylpent-3-en-1-yl)-1,4,5,8-tetramethoxynaphthalene **3** (2.0 g, 4.8 mmol) in a mixture of dichloromethane–acetonitrile (3:1, 10 mL) under water–ice cooling, a solution of ammonium cerium nitrate (CAN, 5.8 g, 10.6 mmol) in water (8 mL) was added. After the addition, the mixture was stirred for 10 min until consumption of compound **3** as the starting material. Then, the reaction mixture was extracted with ethyl acetate (10 mL × 4), and the combined organic phase was washed with brine, dried over anhydrous sodium sulfate, and concentrated under vacuum. Finally, the residue was purified by flash chromatography on silica gel with gradient elution (20% ethyl acetate in petroleum ether to 35% ethyl acetate in petroleum ether) to furnish the desired product as a yellow-orange oil (0.72 g), with a yield of 38.7% as well as the following: ^{1}H NMR (400 MHz, $CDCl_3$) δ 7.72 (s, 2H), 7.22 (s, 1H), 5.26 (s, 1H), 4.77 (s, 1H), 4.04 (s, 3H), 3.71 (s, 3H), 3.39 (t, *J* = 6.6 Hz, 2H), 2.45 (s, 2H), 1.81–1.72 (m, 1H), 1.70 (s, 3H), 1.56 (s, 3H), 1.50 (q, *J* = 6.9 Hz, 2H), 0.91 (d, *J* = 6.7 Hz, 3H), 0.88 (d, *J* = 6.7 Hz, 3H).

3.1.3. (1E,4E)-6-(1-(Isopentyloxy)-4-methylpent-3-en-1-yl)-5,8-dimethoxynaphthal-ene-1,4-dione Dioxime (**5**)

Hydroxylamine hydrochloride (716 mg, 10.3 mmol) and pyridine (815 mg, 10.3 mmol) were added to a solution of naphthoquinone **4** (500 mg, 1.29 mmol) in anhydrous ethanol (20 mL). The mixture was stirred at 50 °C for 24 h under nitrogen atmosphere. After completion of the reaction, solvent was evaporated under reduced pressure. Then, the residue was poured into cold water and the yellow precipitate was collected by simple filtration. The obtained filter cake was recrystallized in ethanol to afford the title compound as a light-yellow solid (487 mg), obtaining the following: yield: 90.4%; M.P. > 205 °C (decomposed); Rf value of 0.73 (50% ethyl acetate in petroleum ether); ^{1}H NMR (400 MHz, DMSO-d_6) δ 12.02 (s, 2H), 7.42–7.28 (m, 2H), 7.05 (s, 1H), 5.23–5.13 (m, 1H), 4.68–4.55 (m, 1H), 3.74 (s, 3H), 3.55 (s, 3H), 3.30–3.19 (m, 2H), 2.32–2.26 (m, 2H), 1.74–1.65 (m, 1H), 1.60 (s, 3H), 1.47 (s, 3H), 1.40–1.28 (m, 2H), 0.88–0.65 (m, 6H); ^{13}C NMR (101 MHz, DMSO-d_6) δ 153.8, 149.0, 148.0, 147.7, 138.1, 133.0, 124.4, 121.1, 120.1, 119.5, 119.4, 110.9, 75.9, 67.1, 61.2, 56.5, 38.7, 36.1, 26.0, 24.9, 23.0, 22.7, 18.1; ESI-HRMS: calcd. for $C_{23}H_{32}N_2NaO_5^+$: 439.22034, found: 439.2199 [M+Na]$^+$.

3.1.4. (1E,4E)-6-((R)-1-(Isopentyloxy)-4-methylpent-3-en-1-yl)-5,8-dimethoxy Naphthalene-1,4-dione Dioxime (**14**)

Compound **14** as a light-yellow solid was prepared by using the above-mentioned synthetic procedures for compound **5** (Scheme 1, from ***a*** to ***c***), in which (*R*)-4-methyl-1-(1,4,5,8-tetramethoxynaphthalen-2-yl)pent-3-en-1-ol (**2-*R***) was used instead of the racemic 4-methyl-1-(1,4,5,8-tetramethoxynaphthalen-2-yl)pent-3-en-1-ol (**2**) in the etherification reaction (***a***), obtaining the following: total yield: 31.9%; M.P. > 205 °C (decomposed); Rf value of 0.73 (50% ethyl acetate in petroleum ether); ^{1}H NMR (400 MHz, DMSO-d_6) δ 12.03 (s, 2H), 7.38 (s, 2H), 7.08 (s, 1H), 5.20 (t, *J* = 7.2 Hz, 1H), 4.65 (t, *J* = 6.3 Hz, 1H), 3.78 (s, 3H), 3.59 (s, 3H), 3.31–3.29 (m, 2H), 2.39–2.29 (m, 2H), 1.79–1.66 (m, 1H), 1.64 (s, 3H), 1.51 (s, 3H), 1.46–1.32 (m, 2H), 0.86 (d, *J* = 6.6 Hz, 3H), 0.81 (d, *J* = 6.6 Hz, 3H); ^{13}C NMR (101 MHz, DMSO-d_6) δ 153.4, 148.6, 147.3, 137.7, 132.5, 124.0, 120.7, 119.7, 119.1, 110.7, 75.4, 66.7, 60.7, 56.2, 38.3, 35.6, 25.5, 24.5, 22.5, 22.3, 17.6; ESI-HRMS: calcd. for $C_{23}H_{32}N_2NaO_5^+$: 439.22034, found: 439.2206 [M+Na]$^+$.

3.1.5. (1E,4E)-6-((S)-1-(Isopentyloxy)-4-methylpent-3-en-1-yl)-5,8-dimethoxy Naphthalene-1,4-dione Dioxime (**15**)

Compound **15** as a light-yellow solid was synthesized by using (*S*)-4-methyl-1-(1,4,5,8-tetramethoxynaphthalen-2-yl)pent-3-en-1-ol (**2-*S***) as the starting material, instead of the racemic 4-methyl-1-(1,4,5,8-tetramethoxynaphthalen-2-yl)pent-3-en-1-ol (**2**) in the synthesis, obtaining the following: total yield: 32.6%; M.P. > 205 °C (decomposed); Rf value of 0.73 (50% ethyl acetate in petroleum ether); ^{1}H NMR (400 MHz, $CDCl_3$) δ 11.86 (s, 2H), 7.77–7.63 (m, 2H), 7.20 (s, 1H), 5.30–5.22 (m, 1H), 4.77 (dd, *J* = 7.1, 5.7 Hz, 1H), 4.01 (s, 3H), 3.71 (s, 3H), 3.39 (t, *J* = 6.7 Hz, 2H), 2.45 (s, 2H), 1.81–1.71 (m, 1H), 1.70 (s, 3H), 1.56 (s, 3H), 1.50 (q, *J* = 6.7 Hz, 2H), 0.91 (d, *J* = 6.6 Hz, 3H), 0.88 (d, *J* = 6.6 Hz, 3H); ^{13}C NMR (101 MHz, DMSO-d_6) δ 153.4, 148.6, 147.6, 147.3, 137.7, 132.6, 124.0, 120.7, 119.7, 119.1, 110.6, 75.4, 66.7, 60.8, 56.2, 38.3, 35.6, 25.6, 24.5, 22.6, 22.3, 17.7; ESI-HRMS: calcd. for $C_{23}H_{32}N_2NaO_5^+$: 439.22034, found: 439.2210 [M+Na]$^+$.

3.1.6. (1E,4E)-6-(1-((5-Hydroxyhexyl)oxy)-4-methylpent-3-en-1-yl)-5,8-dimethoxy Naphthalene-1,4-dione Dioxime (**9**)

The title compound as a yellow solid was prepared by CAN-mediated oxidation (Scheme 2, ***b***) and further oximation (***c***) with compound **7** as the starting material, obtaining the following: yield: 32.5%; M.P. > 205 °C (decomposed); Rf value of 0.38 (50% ethyl acetate in petroleum ether); ^{1}H NMR (400 MHz, DMSO-d_6) δ 11.98 (s, 2H), 7.43–7.38 (m, 2H), 7.05 (s, 1H), 5.18 (t, J = 6.4 Hz, 1H), 4.61 (t, J = 6.4 Hz, 1H), 4.23 (d, J = 4.6 Hz, 1H), 3.74 (s, 3H), 3.58 (s, 3H), 3.53–3.48 (m, 1H), 3.26–3.20 (m, 2H), 2.34–2.28 (m, 2H), 1.60 (s, 3H), 1.46 (s, 3H), 1.46–1.40 (m, 2H), 1.40–1.32 (m, 4H), 1.08–1.02 (m, 3H); ^{13}C NMR (101 MHz, DMSO-d_6) δ 153.9, 149.0, 148.0, 147.8, 138.2, 132.9, 124.4, 121.1, 120.1, 119.5, 111.2, 75.8, 68.9, 66.2, 61.2, 56.7, 39.2, 36.1, 30.0, 26.0, 24.0, 22.6, 18.1; ESI-HRMS: calcd. for $C_{24}H_{34}N_2NaO_6^+$: 469.23091, found: 469.2315 [M+Na]$^+$.

3.1.7. (1E,4E)-6-(1-((8-Hydroxyoctyl)oxy)-4-methylpent-3-en-1-yl)-5,8-dimethoxy Naphthalene-1,4-dione Dioxime (**10**)

The title compound as a yellow solid was prepared by CAN-mediated oxidation (***b***) and further oximation (***c***) with compound **8** as the starting material, obtaining the following: yield: 31.6%; M.P. > 205 °C (decomposed); Rf value of 0.38 (50% ethyl acetate in petroleum ether); ^{1}H NMR (400 MHz, DMSO-d_6) δ 11.98 (s, 2H), 7.38–7.32 (m, 2H), 7.04 (s, 1H), 5.18 (t, J = 6.3 Hz, 1H), 4.60 (t, J = 6.3 Hz, 1H), 4.24–4.16 (m, 1H), 3.74 (s, 3H), 3.55 (s, 3H), 3.34–3.28 (m, 2H), 3.25–3.18 (m, 2H), 2.32–2.24 (m, 2H), 1.59 (s, 3H), 1.46 (s, 3H), 1.48–1.38 (m, 12H); ^{13}C NMR (101 MHz, DMSO-d_6) δ 153.8, 149.0, 148.0, 147.8, 138.2, 132.9, 124.4, 121.2, 120.1, 119.5, 111.1, 75.8, 68.8, 61.2, 61.2, 56.6, 36.1, 33.0, 29.8, 29.4, 29.3, 26.2, 26.0, 25.9, 18.0; ESI-HRMS: calcd. for $C_{26}H_{38}N_2NaO_6^+$: 497.26221, found: 497.2621 [M+Na]$^+$.

3.1.8. 1-((5E,8E)-5,8-bis(Hydroxyimino)-1,4-dimethoxy-5,8-dihydronaphthalen-2-yl)-4-methylpent-3-en-1-yl Cinnamate (**12**)

4-Methyl-1-(1,4,5,8-tetramethoxynaphthalen-2-yl)pent-3-en-1-ol (**2**, 3.46 g, 10 mmol) was first esterified by cinnamic acid (2.22 g, 15 mmol), EDCI (2.88 g, 15 mmol), and DMAP (20 mg) using the same synthetic procedure for the preparation of compound **6**. Further CAN-mediated oxidation and oximation reactions furnished the title compound as a yellow solid (1.8 g), obtaining the following: total yield: 38.2%; M.P. > 188 °C (decomposed); Rf value of 0.62 (50% ethyl acetate in petroleum ether); ^{1}H NMR (400 MHz, DMSO-d_6) δ 12.08 (m, 2H), 7.89–7.61 (m, 3H), 7.54–7.26 (m, 5H), 7.14 (s, 1H), 6.73 (d, J = 16.0 Hz, 1H), 6.29–6.06 (m, 1H), 5.17 (s, 1H), 3.79 (s, 3H), 3.68 (s, 3H), 2.66–2.55 (m, 2H), 1.65 (s, 3H), 1.58 (s, 3H); ^{13}C NMR (101 MHz, DMSO-d_6) δ 165.61, 153.36, 147.92, 147.43, 147.20, 144.96, 135.56, 134.32, 133.96, 130.54, 128.90, 128.41, 124.15, 119.70, 119.10, 119.01, 118.01, 110.97, 70.36, 60.54, 56.47, 33.86, 25.51, 17.70; ESI-HRMS: calcd. for $C_{27}H_{28}N_2NaO_6^+$: 499.18396, found: 499.1843 [M+Na]$^+$.

3.1.9. Synthesis of (1E,4E)-6-(1-(Isopentyloxy)-4-methylpent-3-en-1-yl)-5,8 -dimethoxynaphthalene-1,4-dione O,O-Dibenzoyl Dioxime (**6**)

A mixture of 5,8-dimethyl shikonin oxime **5** (208 mg, 0.5 mmol), benzoic acid (195 mg, 1.6 mmol), EDCI (307, 1.6 mmol), and catalytic amount of DMAP (20 mg) were dissolved in dry dichloromethane, and the mixture was stirred at room temperature overnight. After completion of the reaction, the mixture was diluted with cold water and extracted by DCM (10 mL × 4). The usual work-up including washing and solvent evaporation afforded a residue, which was subject to flash chromatography with 10% ethyl acetate in petroleum ether as the eluent to furnish the ester **6** as a yellow solid (260 mg), obtaining the following: yield: 83.2%; M.P. > 230 °C (decomposed); Rf value of 0.82 (50% ethyl acetate in petroleum ether); ^{1}H NMR (400 MHz, $CDCl_3$) δ 8.16–8.12 (m, 2H), 8.11 (dd, J = 2.9, 1.4 Hz, 2H),

7.71–7.63 (m, 2H), 7.65–7.59 (m, 2H), 7.54–7.48 (m, 4H), 7.25 (s, 1H), 6.11 (dd, J = 17.6, 10.8 Hz, 1H), 4.96 (dd, J = 10.8, 1.4 Hz, 1H), 4.79 (dd, J = 17.6, 1.5 Hz, 1H), 4.52 (s, 1H), 4.01 (s, 3H), 3.99 (s, 3H), 3.34–3.28 (m, 2H), 1.77–1.71 (m, 1H), 1.46–1.40 (m, 2H), 1.14 (s, 3H), 0.94 (s, 3H), 0.90 (s, 3H), 0.85 (s, 3H); ^{13}C NMR (101 MHz, $CDCl_3$) δ 163.3, 163.2, 154.2, 153.9, 153.4, 151.6, 144.5, 139.3, 133.6, 133.5, 129.7, 129.7, 128.8, 128.7, 128.7, 128.7, 123.3, 122.8, 122.8, 117.6, 115.9, 112.4, 82.1, 68.1, 62.1, 56.9, 42.6, 38.8, 25.2, 25.0, 22.7, 22.6; ESI-HRMS: calcd. for $C_{37}H_{40}N_2NaO_7^+$: 647.27277, found: 647.2732 [M+Na]$^+$.

3.1.10. Synthesis of 6-((4-Methyl-1-(1,4,5,8-tetramethoxynaphthalen-2-yl)pent-3-en-1-yl)oxy)hexan-2-ol (**7**) and 8-((4-Methyl-1-(1,4,5,8-tetramethoxynaphthalen-2-yl)pent-3-en-1-yl)oxy)octan-1-ol (**8**)

4-Methyl-1-(1,4,5,8-tetramethoxynaphthalen-2-yl)pent-3-en-1-ol (**2**, 0.5 g, 1.4 mmol) in dry DMF (15 mL) was treated with NaH (0.45 g, 60% in mineral oil, 18.8 mmol) at 5 °C. Then, the mixture was stirred for 20 min and 2-((6-bromohexan-2-yl)oxy)tetrahydro-2H-pyran (0.74 g, 2.8 mmol) and potassium iodine (46 mg) were added. The reaction mixture was heated at 60 °C for 12 h and poured on ice after consumption of compound **2** as the starting material. The usual extraction work-up using dichloromethane and further concentration afforded a yellow oil, which was purified by flash column chromatography on silica gel with 10% ethyl acetate in petroleum ether as the eluent to furnish the THP protected intermediate (0.68 g). The intermediate was digested in a mixture of concentrated hydrochloric acid–methanol (1:10, V/V, 11 mL) and the resulting solution was stirred for 2 h at room temperature. Then, the solution was diluted with dichloromethane (10 mL) and carefully neutralized by a saturated sodium bicarbonate solution. The separated organic layer was separated, washed with brine, dried over sodium sulphate anhydrous, and concentrated. The residue was purified by flash chromatography on silica gel with gradient elution (20% ethyl acetate in petroleum ether to 35% ethyl acetate in petroleum ether) to furnish the desired product as a light-yellow oil (0.51 g), obtaining the following: yield: 81.4%; ^{1}H NMR (400 MHz, $CDCl_3$) δ 6.92 (s, 1H), 6.78–6.74 (m, 2H), 5.22–5.18 (m, 1H), 4.85–4.81 (m, 1H), 4.03–4.00 (m, 1H), 3.94–3.61 (m, 12H), 3.32–3.18 (m, 2H), 2.46–2.40 (m, 2H), 2.03–1.96 (m, 1H), 1.62 (s, 3H), 1.48 (s, 3H), 1.45–1.11 (m, 6H), 1.10–1.02 (m, 3H); ^{13}C NMR (101 MHz, $CDCl_3$) δ 153.4, 151.4, 150.2, 147.4, 133.1, 132.7, 122.4, 120.7, 108.2, 107.6, 105.8, 75.2, 68.7, 67.7, 62.7, 57.7, 57.0, 56.9, 56.8, 39.0, 36.1, 29.7, 25.7, 23.3, 22.5, 17.9.

Compound **8** was prepared using 2-((8-bromooctyl)oxy)tetrahydro-2H-pyran instead of 2-((6-bromohexan-2-yl)oxy)tetrahydro-2H-pyran as the starting material in the synthetic procedure for compound **7** (Scheme 2), obtaining the following: yield: 85.8%; ^{1}H NMR (400 MHz, $CDCl_3$) δ 6.89 (s, 1H), 6.72–6.66 (m, 2H), 5.21–5.15 (m, 1H), 4.82–4.74 (m, 1H), 3.82 (s, 3H), 3.79 (s, 3H), 3.75 (s, 3H), 3.63 (s, 3H), 3.46–3.40 (m, 2H), 3.25–3.16 (m, 2H), 2.80–2.71 (m, 1H), 2.44–2.35 (m, 2H), 1.55 (s, 3H), 1.43 (s, 3H), 1.40–1.34 (m, 2H), 1.31–1.08 (m, 10H); ^{13}C NMR (101 MHz, $CDCl_3$) δ 153.3, 151.3, 150.1, 147.3, 132.9, 132.7, 122.4, 120.8, 120.1, 108.2, 107.6, 105.8, 75.2, 68.8, 62.5, 62.4, 57.6, 56.8, 56.8, 36.1, 32.6, 29.8, 29.3, 29.2, 26.1, 25.6, 20.8, 17.8.

3.1.11. Synthesis of 4-Methyl-1-(1,4,5,8-tetramethoxynaphthalen-2-yl)pent-3-en-1-one (**13**)

2-(1-Hydroxy-4-methyl-3-pentenyl)-1,4,5,8-tetramethoxynaphthalene (**2**, 5.0 g, 14.4 mmol) was dissolved in dry CH_2Cl_2 (50 mL) cooled in a salt-ice bath at −15 °C. Dess–Martin periodinane (DMP, 7.3 g, 17.3 mmol) was added in portions, and the mixture was stirred for 2 h. After the consumption of the substrate, the excessive oxidant was removed by filtration, and the filtrate was concentrated under reduced pressure. The residue was purified by column chromatography with 20% ethyl acetate in petroleum ether as the eluent to obtain 4.2 g of the ketone **13** as a pale-yellow oil, obtaining the following: yield: 84.5%; ^{1}H NMR (400 MHz, $CDCl_3$) δ 6.83 (d, J = 2.3 Hz, 1H), 6.72–6.64 (m, 2H), 5.38–5.30 (m, 1H), 3.77–3.72

(m, 6H), 3.70 (d, J = 6.9 Hz, 2H), 3.67 (s, 3H), 3.60 (s, 3H), 1.57 (s, 3H), 1.48 (s, 3H); ^{13}C NMR (101 MHz, $CDCl_3$) δ 202.7, 153.1, 151.0, 150.9, 150.0, 134.8, 130.3, 122.3, 122.1, 116.8, 110.5, 108.0, 105.6, 63.7, 57.5, 56.6, 56.5, 42.8, 25.6, 18.0.

3.1.12. Synthesis of (S)-4-Methyl-1-(1,4,5,8-tetramethoxynaphthalen-2-yl)pent-3-en-1-ol (**2-S**) and (R)-4-Methyl-1-(1,4,5,8-tetramethoxynaphthalen-2-yl)pent-3-en-1-ol (**2-R**)

The 4-methyl-1-(1,4,5,8-tetramethoxynaphthalen-2-yl)pent-3-en-1-one (**13**, 5.0 g, 14.4 mmol) was dissolved in anhydrous THF (60 mL) and the solution was stirred for 5 min at −30 °C temperature under nitrogen atmosphere. Then, (−)-DIP-Cl (1.7 M in *n*-hexane, 12.8 mL, 21.8 mmol) was dropwise added to the solution and the mixture was maintained at −30 °C overnight. After the completion of reaction, a few drops of cold acetone were added. The quenched reaction mixture was poured into a saturated NH_4Cl solution and extracted with ethyl acetate (30 mL × 5). The organic layer was washed with brine, dried over anhydrous sodium sulphate, and concentrated under reduced pressure. The residue was purified by column chromatography with 35% ethyl acetate in petroleum ether as the eluent to obtain compound (**2-*S***) as a yellow oil (4.5g), obtaining the following: yield: 89.5%; ^{1}H NMR (300 MHz, $CDCl_3$) δ 7.02 (s, 1H), 6.82 (s, 2H), 5.32–5.19 (m, 2H), 3.95 (s, 3H), 3.93 (s, 3H), 3.89 (s, 3H), 3.77 (s, 3H), 2.53 (t, J = 7.0 Hz, 2H), 2.32 (s, br, 1H), 1.73 (s, 3H), 1.65 (s, 3H).

Compound (**2-*R***) as a yellow oil was prepared by asymmetric hydrogenation of 4-methyl-1-(1,4,5,8-tetramethoxynaphthalen-2-yl)pent-3-en-1-one (**13**) using (+)-DIP-Cl, obtaining the following: yield: 87.3%; ^{1}H NMR (400 MHz, $CDCl_3$) δ 7.02 (s, 1H), 6.82 (s, 2H), 5.25 (q, J = 7.7, 7.0 Hz, 2H), 3.95 (s, 3H), 3.94 (s, 3H), 3.90 (s, 3H), 3.77 (s, 3H), 2.53 (t, J = 7.1 Hz, 2H), 2.33 (s, br, 1H), 1.73 (s, 3H), 1.65 (s, 3H).

3.2. *Biological Activity Evaluations*

Methyl thiazolyl tetrazolium (MTT) was purchased from Sigma-Aldrich. DMEM, fetal bovine serum (FBS), and penicillin/straptomycin were obtained from Hyclone. The recombinant SARS-CoV-2 M^{pro} was expressed and purified from an *Escherichia coli* expression system [8]. Shikonin (purity in HPLC > 98%, *e.e.* value of 96%) as the positive control in the enzymatic assay was synthesized by the reported procedures [23].

3.2.1. Enzymatic Inhibition Assay

The inhibitory potency of the tested naphthoquinones against SARS-CoV-2 M^{pro} was evaluated according to the reported FRET detection method [8,12], using fluorescently labeled peptide MCA-AVLQSGFR-Lys(Dnp)-Lys-NH_2 as the substrate. Upon incubation, the fluorescence intensity of each well was determined by a FlexStation3 microplate reader (Molecular Device, Silicon Valley, CA, USA) with the excitation and emission filter set at 320 and 405 nm, respectively.

3.2.2. Molecular Docking

Molecular docking studies were carried out using MOE 2008 software and taking SARS-CoV-2 M^{pro} as the target enzyme. The protein was downloaded from the RSC Protein Data Bank (PDB ID: 7CA8). Before docking studies, ligands and water molecules are removed from the downloaded protein, and then gasteiger charges are calculated after addition of polar hydrogens. The chemical structures of shikonin and compound **15** was generated by ChemDraw Ultra 12.0 software and structural energy minimization was conducted using Chem3D Pro 12.0. For docking, we used default values of parameters in MOE 2008, except for the first scoring function, where ASE scoring was used instead of the defaulting London dG. The type of post-placement refinement and the rescoring algorithm were set as forcefield and ASE, respectively. Then, the obtained optimal binding modes of shikonin and compound **15** in active site cavities of SARS-CoV-2 M^{pro} were employed to evaluate the reasonability of the predicted interactions.

3.2.3. Surface Plasmon Resonance Analysis

The surface plasmon resonance (SPR)-based measurements were performed by the Biacore 8K apparatus. Briefly, the SARS-CoV-2 M^{pro} proteins were immobilized to an activated CM5 sensorchip (Cytiva) using an amino group coupling kit. For affinity analysis, the inhibitor was dissolved in a PBS buffered solution (PBS-T) containing 0.05% Tween-20 (V/V) and 5% DMSO (V/V) at final concentrations of 1.0 μM, 2.0 μM, 4.0 μM, 8.0 μM, and 16.0 μM. Each sample that was bound to the target enzyme was dissociated by the PBS-T buffer solution for 120 s at a flow rate of 20 μL/min. Regeneration of sensor chips was performed for 30 s using a regeneration buffer solution (pH 2.0). The binding profile for each concentration and the binding rate constant (ka) were determined by the Biacore (Cytiva) apparatus.

3.2.4. Cell Lines

The human HFF-1 and monkey Vero E6 cells were provided by Cell Bank in Shanghai, Chinese Academy of Sciences. HFF-1 cells were cultured in DMEM complete medium containing 15% FBS, 100 U/mL penicillin, and 100 μg/mL of streptomycin, while Vero E6 cells were maintained in DMEM complete medium containing 10% FBS. They were maintained at 37 °C in a humidified atmosphere with 5% CO_2 (V/V).

3.2.5. Cytotoxicity Evaluation

The in vitro cytotoxicity of compounds was determined by the standard MTT assay according to our reported procedure. Briefly, well-cultured cells were seeded in 96-well plates at a density of 5×10^3 cells per well. After being cultured overnight in a 37 °C humidified incubator (5% CO_2, V/V), cells were incubated with tested compounds for 48 h. Then, cells in each well were treated with MTT in PBS (5 mg/mL) for 4 h at 37 °C, and formazan crystals in viable cells were dissolved by dimethyl sulfoxide (150 μL) at ambient temperature. The absorbance of solubilized formazan was measured by the Synergy multimode reader (BioTek, Winooski, VT, American) at the wavelength of 490 nm.

3.2.6. In Vitro Antiviral Activity Evaluation

The in vitro antiviral activity of compound **15** at concentrations of 12.5 μM, 25 μM, 50 μM, and 75 μM against SARS-CoV-2 was evaluated according to the reported qRT-PCR assay [8]. To further confirm the anti-SARS-CoV-2 activity of the target compound, we perform more anti-viral assays through viral N-protein detection. Human Vero E6 cells were infected by live SARS-CoV-2 at an MOI value of 0.01. Cells were then washed 3 times with PBS to remove the free virus after 2 h-infection and then maintained in DMEM culture medium containing compound **15** (50 μM) or shikonin (10 μM) and 2% FBS for 48 h. Then, cells in each group were collected and the immunofluorescence assay was used to detect the expression of viral N protein, and the result was analyzed by high-content screening.

3.2.7. In Vivo Toxicity Evaluation of Compound 15 in Balb/c Mice

Five- to six-week-old female Balb/c mice, weighing between 14 and 16 g, were obtained from Charles River Laboratories in China. After arrival, these Balb/c mice were quarantined for 3 days before housing in a germ-free environment with a 12 h-of-light and 12 h-of-dark cycle. All investigation procedures were performed according to the regulation of the Animals Ethics Subcommittee of Shanghai Jiao Tong University (A2019113).

The stock solution of compound **15** (9 mg/mL) for in vivo experiments was prepared by dissolving the powder of compound **15** (90 mg) in N-methyl-2-pyrrolidone (NMP,

5.0 mL), followed by addition of Cremophor EL in an equal volume (5.0 mL). The stock solution was diluted by sterilized saline to afford compound **15** formulation (1.8 mg/mL). In the formulation, the ratio of NMP, Cremophor EL, and saline was 1:1:8. The stock solution of shikonin (6 mg/mL) for in vivo experiments was prepared by dissolving shikonin (98%, 60 mg) in a mixture of ethanol–Cremophor EL (1:1, V/V, 10 mL). The formulation (1 mg/mL) was obtained by dilution of the stock solution with a 5-fold volume of saline.

In the in vivo toxicity evaluations, six-week-old female Balb/c mice were randomized into 3 groups, with 7 mice per group. Groups 1–3 were as follows: (**1**) compound **15** solvent; (**2**) compound **15** (30 mg/kg); (**3**) shikonin (10 mg/kg). In addition, 5,8-dimethyl shikonin oxime **15** was intravenously administrated (i.v.) on every other day for a consecutive 14 days. Administration of shikonin (i.v.) was also conducted on every other day for 7 times from day 1 to day 14. During the treatment, the body weight and activity of mice were monitored. Low activity, body weight loss of more than 15% for 3 consecutive days, or treatment-related mortality were regarded as toxicity symptoms. Mice were observed for 2 more days after the end of treatment for any delayed toxicity.

4. Conclusions and Future Perspectives

The research results from previous studies indicated that the natural bioactive compound shikonin was a strong inhibitor of SARS-CoV-2 M^{pro} [8,16]. Cross-validation studies have shown that shikonin only inhibited M^{pro} in the absence of a reducing reagent such as DTT, suggesting that shikonin is a non-specific cysteine protease inhibitor, leading to cytotoxicity towards host cells. In addition, the generation of reactive oxygen species (ROS) and bioreductive alkylation reactions with biomolecules were considered as the roots for its pervasive toxicity. Apparently, modification of the shikonin naphthazarin scaffold might provide a good template for the discovery of viral M^{pro} inhibitors.

We have designed, synthesized, and characterized a small library of shikonin derivatives and demonstrated that they are inhibitory in vitro against the main protease of SARS-CoV-2 (M^{pro}), which causes COVID-19, a serious disease epidemic in 280 countries worldwide. Compound **15** as the most active one showed an IC_{50} value of 12.53 ± 3.59 μM against SARS-CoV-2 M^{pro} as a key antiviral drug target. The results of molecular docking studies indicated that inhibitor **15** is perfectly settled in the core of the substrate-binding pocket of M^{pro} by possibly interacting with three catalytic residues, His41, Cys145, and Met165. The target compound **15** exhibited much less toxicity as compared with the lead shikonin both in vivo and in vitro. The antiviral activity of the compound was assessed against SARS-CoV-2 where it exhibited strong inhibition at the concentration of 75 μM. The unique chemical structure and its strong enzymatic inhibition potency, coupled with the favorable safety data both in vivo and in vitro, emphasized that the shikonin oxime derivative **15** deserves further development as an antiviral drug candidate against SARS-CoV-2 in the future. Additionally, taking compound **15** as a new lead compound, we would possibly obtain more safe and effective antiviral agents to combat infection caused by SARS-CoV-2.

Supplementary Materials: The following supporting information can be downloaded at https://www.mdpi.com/article/10.3390/molecules30061321/s1: Figures S1–S11. Representative ^{1}H & ^{13}C-NMR Spectra; HPLC trace for chiral separation of 2-R and 2-S as the key intermediates; HPLC trace for compound 15.

Author Contributions: Conceptualization, J.C. and S.L.; Software, J.C. and G.Y.; Formal analysis, J.C. and S.X. (Shouyan Xiang); Investigation, J.C., S.X. (Shouyan Xiang), Q.Z. and C.L.; Data curation, J.C.; writing—original draft preparation, J.C., S.X. (Shouyan Xiang) and Q.Z.; writing—review and editing, J.C., S.X. (Shangqing Xiao), Q.Z., G.Y. and C.L. All authors have read and agreed to the published version of the manuscript.

Funding: This research was funded by Medical and Engineering Interdisciplinary Research Fund of Shanghai Jiao Tong University (Grant No. 20X190020002) and the APC was funded by the same grant (No. 20X190020002).

Institutional Review Board Statement: The animal study protocol was approved by the Animals Ethics Subcommittee of Shanghai Jiao Tong University (A2019113).

Informed Consent Statement: Not applicable.

Data Availability Statement: The raw data supporting the conclusions of this article will be made available by the authors on request.

Acknowledgments: We would like to thank Hong Liu and Yechun Xu at the Shanghai Institute of Materia Medica, Chinese Academy of Sciences, for their generous help in the biological evaluation.

Conflicts of Interest: All authors declare that they have no competing interests.

References

1. Zhu, N.; Zhang, D.; Wang, W.; Li, X.; Yang, B.; Song, J.; Zhao, X.; Huang, B.; Shi, W.; Lu, R.; et al. A Novel Coronavirus from Patients with Pneumonia in China, 2019. *N. Engl. J. Med.* **2020**, *382*, 727–733. [CrossRef] [PubMed]
2. Zhou, P.; Yang, X.-L.; Wang, X.-G.; Hu, B.; Zhang, L.; Zhang, W.; Si, H.-R.; Zhu, Y.; Li, B.; Huang, C.-L.; et al. A pneumonia outbreak associated with a new coronavirus of probable bat origin. *Nature* **2020**, *579*, 270–273. [CrossRef]
3. World Health Organization. Coronavirus Disease (COVID-19) Weekly Epidemiological Update and Weekly Operational Update. 2024, 862, p. 478. Available online: https://www.who.int/emergencies/diseases/novel-coronavirus-2019/situation-reports (accessed on 24 December 2024).
4. Garcia-Beltran, W.F.; St Denis, K.J.; Hoelzemer, A.; Lam, E.C.; Nitido, A.D.; Sheehan, M.L.; Berrios, C.; Ofoman, O.; Chang, C.C.; Hauser, B.M.; et al. mRNA-based COVID-19 vaccine boosters induce neutralizing immunity against SARS-CoV-2 Omicron variant. *Cell* **2022**, *185*, 457–466. [CrossRef] [PubMed]
5. Schmidt, N.; Lareau, C.A.; Keshishian, H.; Ganskih, S.; Schneider, C.; Hennig, T.; Melanson, R.; Werner, S.; Wei, Y.; Zimmer, M.; et al. The SARS-CoV-2 RNA–protein interactome in infected human cells. *Nat. Microbiol.* **2021**, *6*, 339–353. [CrossRef]
6. Zhang, L.; Lin, D.; Sun, X.; Curth, U.; Drosten, C.; Sauerhering, L.; Becker, S.; Rox, K.; Hilgenfeld, R. Crystal structure of SARS-CoV-2 main protease provides a basis for design of improved α-ketoamide inhibitors. *Science* **2020**, *368*, 409–412. [CrossRef] [PubMed]
7. Dai, W.; Zhang, B.; Jiang, X.-M.; Su, H.; Li, J.; Zhao, Y.; Xie, X.; Jin, Z.; Peng, J.; Liu, F.; et al. Structure-based design of antiviral drug candidates targeting the SARS-CoV-2 main protease. *Science* **2020**, *368*, 1331–1335. [CrossRef]
8. Jin, Z.; Du, X.; Xu, Y.; Deng, Y.; Liu, M.; Zhao, Y.; Zhang, B.; Li, X.; Zhang, L.; Peng, C.; et al. Structure of Mpro from SARS-CoV-2 and discovery of its inhibitors. *Nature* **2020**, *582*, 289–293. [CrossRef]
9. Sezer, A.; Halilović-Alihodžić, M.; Vanwieren, A.R.; Smajkan, A.; Karić, A.; Djedović, H.; Šutković, J. A review on drug repurposing in COVID-19: From antiviral drugs to herbal alternatives. *J. Genet. Eng. Biotechnol.* **2022**, *20*, 78. [CrossRef]
10. Chakraborty, C.; Sharma, A.R.; Bhattacharya, M.; Lee, S.-S. A Detailed Overview of Immune Escape, Antibody Escape, Partial Vaccine Escape of SARS-CoV-2 and Their Emerging Variants with Escape Mutations. *Front. Immunol.* **2022**, *13*, 801522. [CrossRef]
11. Jung, C.; Kmiec, D.; Koepke, L.; Zech, F.; Jacob, T.; Sparrer, K.M.J.; Kirchhoff, F. Omicron: What Makes the Latest SARS-CoV-2 Variant of Concern So Concerning? *J. Virol.* **2022**, *96*, e0207721. [CrossRef]
12. Cui, J.; Jia, J. Discovery of juglone and its derivatives as potent SARS-CoV-2 main proteinase inhibitors. *Eur. J. Med. Chem.* **2021**, *225*, 113789. [CrossRef] [PubMed]
13. Gao, H.; Liu, L.; Qu, Z.-Y.; Wei, F.-X.; Wang, S.-Q.; Chen, G.; Qin, L.; Jiang, F.-Y.; Wang, Y.-C.; Shang, L.; et al. Anti-adenovirus Activities of Shikonin, a Component of Chinese Herbal Medicine in Vitro. *Biol. Pharm. Bull.* **2011**, *34*, 197–202. [CrossRef] [PubMed]
14. Liu, X.; Zhang, X.; Li, J.; Zhou, H.; Carr, M.J.; Xing, W.; Zhang, Z.; Shi, W. Effects of Acetylshikonin on the Infection and Replication of Coxsackievirus A16 in Vitro and in Vivo. *J. Nat. Prod.* **2019**, *82*, 1089–1097. [CrossRef] [PubMed]
15. Zhang, X.; Cui, J.-H.; Meng, Q.-Q.; Li, S.-S.; Zhou, W.; Xiao, S. Advance in Anti-tumor Mechanisms of Shikonin, Alkannin and their Derivatives. *Mini-Rev. Med. Chem.* **2018**, *18*, 164–172. [CrossRef]
16. Li, J.; Zhou, X.; Zhang, Y.; Zhong, F.; Lin, C.; McCormick, P.J.; Jiang, F.; Luo, J.; Zhou, H.; Wang, Q.; et al. Crystal structure of SARS-CoV-2 main protease in complex with the natural product inhibitor shikonin illuminates a unique binding mode. *Sci. Bull.* **2021**, *66*, 661–663. [CrossRef]
17. Zhao, L.-M.; Xu, D.-F.; Zhou, W.; Li, S.-S. Concise Formal Synthesis of (±)-Shikonin Via a Highly α-Regioselective Prenylation of 1, 4, 5, 8-Tetramethoxynaphthalene-2-Carbaldehyde. *Lett. Org. Chem.* **2008**, *5*, 234–236. [CrossRef]

18. Giagou, T.; Meyer, M.P. Kinetic Isotope Effects in Asymmetric Reactions. *Chem. Eur. J.* **2010**, *16*, 10616–10628. [CrossRef]
19. Stafford, S.E.; Meyer, M.P. Experimental transition state for the B-chlorodiisopinocampheylborane (DIP-Cl) reduction. *Tetrahedron Lett.* **2009**, *50*, 3027–3030. [CrossRef]
20. Nicolaou, K.C.; Hepworth, D. Concise and Efficient Total Syntheses of Alkannin and Shikonin. *Angew. Chem. Int. Ed.* **1998**, *37*, 839–841. [CrossRef]
21. Zheng, X.; Hu, H.; Xu, D. A new synthetic method toward a key intermediate in the total synthesis of alkannin and shikonin. *J. Chem. Res.* **2021**, *45*, 831–834. [CrossRef]
22. Xu, Y.; Cui, J.; Wang, R.; Li, S. Asymmetric synthesis of shikonin and alkannin. *J. Shenyang Pharm. Univ.* **2014**, *31*, 440–443.
23. Wang, R.; Guo, H.; Cui, J.; Li, S. A novel and efficient total synthesis of shikonin. *Tetrahedron Lett.* **2012**, *53*, 3977–3980. [CrossRef]
24. Su, H.-X.; Yao, S.; Zhao, W.-F.; Li, M.-J.; Liu, J.; Shang, W.-J.; Xie, H.; Ke, C.-Q.; Hu, H.-C.; Gao, M.-N.; et al. Anti-SARS-CoV-2 activities in vitro of Shuanghuanglian preparations and bioactive ingredients. *Acta Pharmacol. Sin.* **2020**, *41*, 1167–1177. [CrossRef]
25. Alkadi, H.; Jbeily, R. Role of Chirality in Drugs: An Overview. *Infect. Disord. Drug Targets* **2018**, *18*, 88–95. [CrossRef] [PubMed]
26. Nguyen, L.A.; He, H.; Pham-Huy, C. Chiral drugs: An overview. *Int. J. Biomed. Sci.* **2006**, *2*, 85–100. [PubMed]
27. Ordoudi, S.A.; Tsermentseli, S.K.; Nenadis, N.; Assimopoulou, A.N.; Tsimidou, M.Z.; Papageorgiou, V.P. Structure-radical scavenging activity relationship of alkannin/shikonin derivatives. *Food Chem.* **2011**, *124*, 171–176. [CrossRef]
28. Zhou, W.; Zhang, X.; Xiao, L.; Ding, J.; Liu, Q.-H.; Li, S.-S. Semi-synthesis and antitumor activity of 6-isomers of 5, 8-O-dimethyl acylshikonin derivatives. *Eur. J. Med. Chem.* **2011**, *46*, 3420–3427. [CrossRef]
29. Wang, R.; Zhang, X.; Song, H.; Zhou, S.; Li, S. Synthesis and evaluation of novel alkannin and shikonin oxime derivatives as potent antitumor agents. *Bioorg. Med. Chem. Lett.* **2014**, *24*, 4304–4307. [CrossRef]
30. Ma, C.; Hu, Y.; Townsend, J.A.; Lagarias, P.I.; Marty, M.T.; Kolocouris, A.; Wang, J. Ebselen, Disulfiram, Carmofur, PX-12, Tideglusib, and Shikonin Are Nonspecific Promiscuous SARS-CoV-2 Main Protease Inhibitors. *ACS Pharmacol. Transl. Sci.* **2020**, *3*, 1265–1277. [CrossRef]

molecules

MDPI

Article

Design, Synthesis and Herbicidal Activity of 5-(1-Amino-4-phenoxybutylidene)barbituric Acid Derivatives Containing an Enamino Diketone Motif

Ke Chen [1], Shumin Wang [2], Shuyue Fu [2], Yuxiao Zhang [2], Wei Gao [2], Jin Liu [3], Rui Liu [1,*] and Kang Lei [2,*]

[1] Department of Biotechnology, The University of Suwon, Hwaseong 18323, Gyeonggi-Do, Republic of Korea; chenke_sd@163.com
[2] School of Pharmaceutical Sciences and Food Engineering, Liaocheng University, Liaocheng 252059, China; 13686366329@163.com (S.W.); fsyue1213@163.com (S.F.); zhangyuxiao0515@163.com (Y.Z.); gaowei@lcu.edu.cn (W.G.)
[3] Shandong Academy of Innovation and Development, Jinan 250101, China; lliujin7294@163.com
* Correspondence: liurcau@suwon.ac.kr (R.L.); leikang@lcu.edu.cn (K.L.)

Abstract

In continuation of our efforts to identify novel herbicide lead compounds, twenty new 5-(1-amino-4-phenoxybutylidene)barbituric acid derivatives containing an enamino diketone motif were synthesized and evaluated for their herbicidal activities. The greenhouse bioassay results indicated that several of the target compounds, including **BA-1**, **BA-2**, **BA-5**, **BA-18**, and **BA-20**, exhibited notable post-emergence herbicidal activity, with sum inhibition rates exceeding 70% at a dosage of 150 g ha^{-1}, which was superior to that of the commercial herbicide flumiclorac-pentyl (FP). The structure–activity relationship analysis demonstrated that the steric and electronic effects of the R group, as well as the lipophilicity of the target compounds, significantly influenced herbicidal activity. Among these, **BA-1** was identified as a promising herbicide lead compound due to its high total herbicidal efficacy, broad-spectrum activity, and favorable crop safety profile. Molecular simulation studies indicated that **BA-1** binds effectively to *Nicotiana tabacum* protoporphyrinogen IX oxidase (*Nt*PPO), suggesting its potential as a novel PPO inhibitor. This study highlights **BA-1** as a promising lead compound for the development of novel PPO-inhibiting herbicides.

Keywords: barbituric acid; enamino diketone; herbicides; protoporphyrinogen IX oxidase

1. Introduction

As essential tools in the prevention and control of weeds in agricultural production, herbicides play a crucial role in maintaining stable agricultural yields and enhancing economic efficiency [1–3]. It is estimated that the absence of herbicides would result in a 34% reduction in global crop yields due to weed infestation [4]. However, the extensive and indiscriminate use of herbicides has led to various adverse effects, including significant environmental issues and the development of herbicide-resistant weed species [5–9]. The development of new herbicides encounters considerable challenges, such as an extended development cycle, substantial financial investment, and low success rates [10]. Identifying novel lead scaffolds for herbicides is still a key step in the development of new pesticide agents [11–14].

The enamino diketone represents a fundamental structural motif present in some natural products (Figure 1A) [15,16]. Meanwhile, compounds containing the enamino diketone motif (Figure 1B) have demonstrated significant utility in the pharmaceutical and agrochemical fields due to their antimicrobial [17,18], antibacterial [19–21], anticancer [22–26], herbicidal [27–29], antifungal [30–32], and anti-*toxoplasma gondii* activities [33]. The distinctive structural and biological properties of the enamino diketone motif underscore its potential utility in the development of novel pesticidal agents.

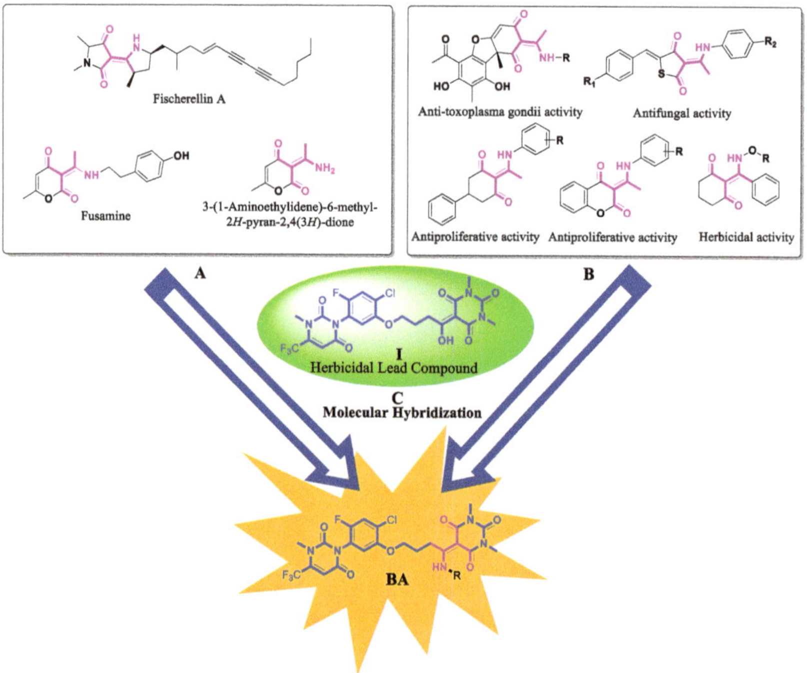

Figure 1. Design of target compound **BA** based on the molecular hybridization strategy. (**A**) Natural products with enamino diketone moiety; (**B**) Bioactive compounds with enamino diketone moiety; (**C**) Reported lead compound **I**.

Recently, during our investigation into novel compounds with potential herbicidal applications, we identified a promising lead structure, designated as compound **I** (Figure 1C) [34,35]. Notably, compound **I** contains a diketone moiety that is structurally similar to those found in enamino diketone derivatives. Based on this observation, we hypothesized that converting the carbonyl group of the acyl moiety in compound **I** into an imine, followed by isomerization to the enamine form, could facilitate the construction of compounds featuring the naturally occurring enamino diketone motif. Such structural modifications are expected to possess herbicidal activity. Accordingly, twenty new 5-(1-amino-4-phenoxybutylidene)barbituric acid derivatives (**BA**) containing an enamino diketone motif were designed, synthesized, and their herbicidal activities were evaluated. This report presents the synthesis, structure-activity relationship (SAR) analysis, and molecular simulation studies of **BA derivatives**.

2. Results and Discussion

2.1. Chemistry

The target compounds **BA-1~BA-20** were prepared through an eight-step synthetic pathway, as illustrated in Scheme 1, and their chemical structures are presented in Figure 2. The calculated oil/water partition coefficients (Clog *P*) are predicted using ChemBioDraw

14.0. The synthetic route commenced with a base-promoted nucleophilic substitution reaction between 2-chloro-4-fluoro-5-nitrophenol and ethyl 4-bromobutanoate. Briefly, the 2-chloro-4-fluoro-5-nitrophenol reacted with ethyl 4-bromobutanoate in DMF by using K_2CO_3 as a base to generate intermediate **1**. The nitro group in intermediate **1** was then chemically reduced by using iron powder in glacial acetic acid at room temperature to yield intermediate **2**, which subsequently underwent a cyclization reaction with ethyl (Z)-3-(3,3-dimethylureido)-4,4,4-trifluorobut-2-enoate to produce intermediate **3**. Methylation of compound **3** with iodomethane produced intermediate **4**, which was hydrolyzed by heating under acidic conditions to form carboxylic acid **5**. Carboxylic acid **5** was readily converted to the corresponding acid chloride **6** on treatment with thionyl chloride. The key intermediate **7** could then be smoothly synthesized by reaction of acid chloride **6** with barbituric acid. Finally, the target compounds **BA-1~BA-20** were obtained in yields ranging from 16% to 93% through condensation reactions between intermediate **7** and corresponding amines in ethanol. The structures of all the target compounds were identified using ^1H and ^{13}C NMR spectroscopy and HRMS.

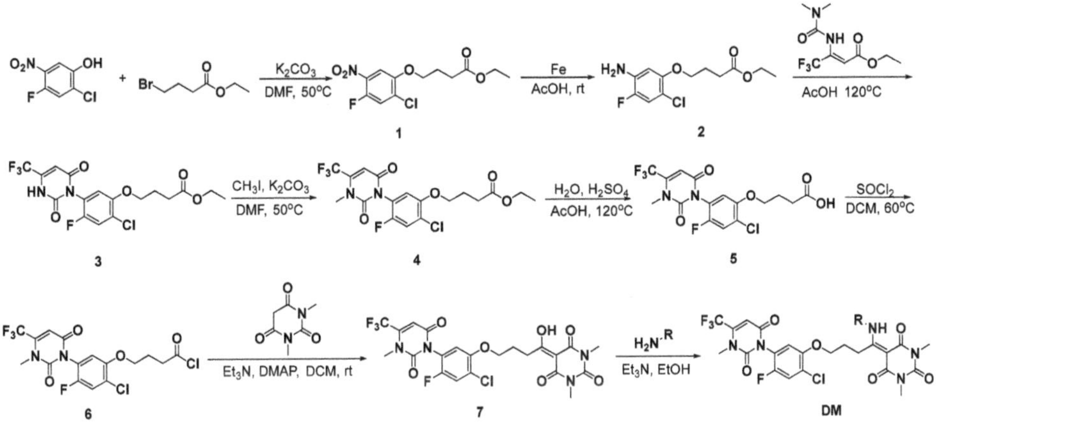

Scheme 1. General synthetic pathway for the target compounds **BA-1~BA-20**.

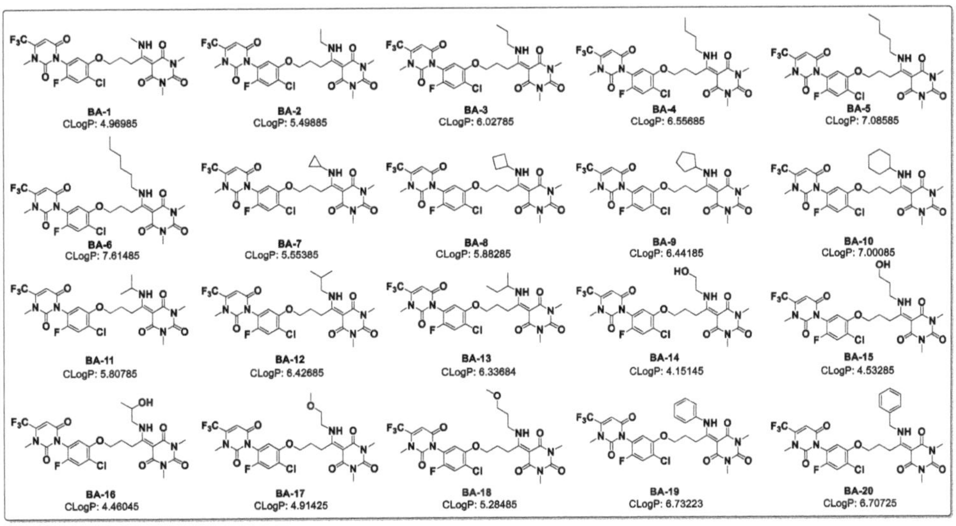

Figure 2. The structures of target compounds **BA-1~BA-20**.

2.2. Herbicidal Activity and SAR

To evaluate the herbicidal activity of the newly synthesized target compounds **BA-1~BA-20**, greenhouse trials were conducted at a post-emergence application rate of 150 g ha^{-1}. Commercial herbicide flumiclorac-pentyl (FP) was employed as the positive control. As observed in Figure 3, most of the target compounds exhibited moderate to good herbicidal activity against the four tested weeds. Among them, target compounds **BA-1**, **BA-2**, **BA-5**, and **BA-20** demonstrated complete inhibition against *Brassica campestris* (Figure 3A). Apart from **BA-3**, **BA-6**, **BA-8**, and **BA-12~BA-16**, all other target compounds demonstrated complete inhibitory activity against *Amaranthus tricolor*, showing efficacy comparable to that of the commercial herbicide FP (Figure 3B). Furthermore, it was found that some of the newly synthesized target compounds, such as **BA-1** and **BA-2**, exhibited stronger herbicidal activity against *Echinochloa crus-galli* (Figure 3C) and *Digitaria sanguinalis* (Figure 3D) than the commercial herbicide FP. To better understand the herbicidal activity, the total effects of the target compounds **BA-1~BA-20** on the loss of plant weight at the dosage of 150 g ha^{-1} were calculated, and the results shown in Figure 4. It was easy to observe that some of the target compounds, such as **BA-1**, **BA-2**, **BA-5**, **BA-18**, and **BA-20**, demonstrated higher sum inhibition rate (SIR) than that of the commercial herbicide FP. These promising results indicated that the series target compound **BA** was effectively designed.

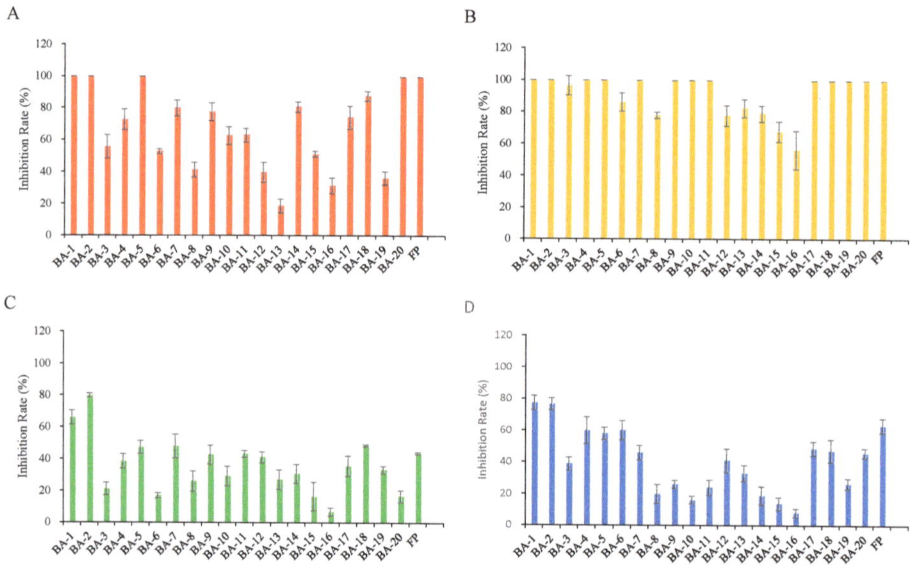

Figure 3. Effects (% inhibition) of the target compounds **BA-1~BA-20** on the loss of plant weight at a dosage of 150 g ha^{-1} under the post-emergence condition; (**A**) *B. campestris*; (**B**) *A. retroflexus*; (**C**) *E. crus-galli*; (**D**) *D. sanguinalis*.

Based on the total herbicidal inhibition rate at the dosage of 150 g ha^{-1}, the structure-activity relationship (SAR) of the target compounds was investigated. It was found that, among the target compounds containing straight-chain alkyl groups (i.e., compounds **BA-1~BA-6**), **BA-1** (R = Me) and **BA-2** (R = Et) exhibited higher SIR than those with longer alkyl chains (i.e., compounds **BA-3~BA-6**). When cycloalkyl groups (i.e., compounds **BA-7~BA-10**) or branched-chain alkyl groups (i.e., compounds **BA-11** and **BA-13**) were introduced on the nitrogen atom of target compounds, the target compounds (excluding **BA-7**) exhibited lower SIR than the corresponding straight-chain compounds. For instance, the target compound **BA-4** (R = *n*-butyl) exhibited a total inhibitory effect against the four tested weeds with an SIR of 66%, which is higher than that of **BA-8** (SIR = 36%), **BA-12** (SIR = 42%) and **BA-13** (SIR = 26%). Based on the above analysis, it was speculated that the introduction of smaller substituents on the nitrogen atoms of the target compounds may enhance herbicidal activity. However, through a comparative analysis of the herbicidal activities of compounds **BA-3~BA-6** and **BA-8~BA-10**, it was found that the SIR increased with the extension of carbon chain and expansion of carbon ring, and the trend terminated at compound **BA-5** (R = pentyl) and **BA-8** (R = cyclopentyl), respectively. This finding contradicts the aforementioned speculation, suggesting that the steric effect of the R group is not the sole factor influencing herbicidal activity.

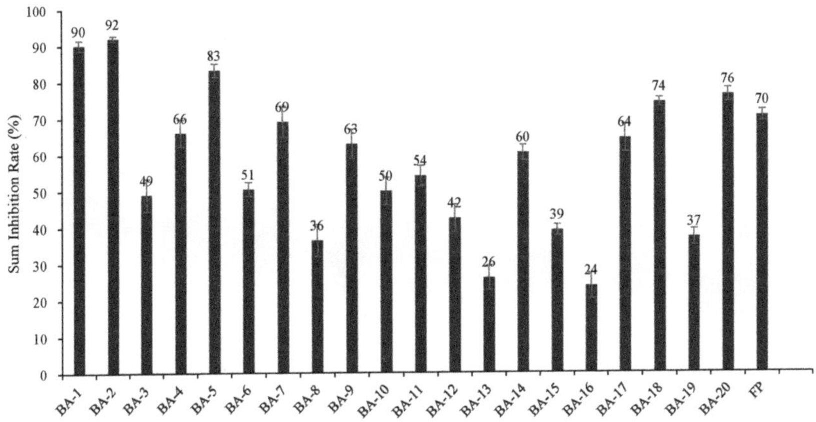

Figure 4. Total effects (% inhibition) of the target compounds **BA-1~BA-20** on the loss of plant weight at a dosage of 150 g ha^{-1} under the post-emergence condition.

Previous studies have revealed that lipophilicity is an important parameter affecting the absorption of pesticides by plants, and appropriate lipophilicity is essential for biological activity [36]. Thus, lipophilicity as Clog *P* was predicted by ChemBioDraw 14.0 as shown in Figure 2. It was found that there are some extent correlations between herbicidal activity and lipophilicity of the target compounds. For instance, for the target compounds **BA-3~BA-6**, as the Clog *P* value increases, the herbicidal activities of the target compounds **BA-3** (Clog *P* = 6.0, SIR = 49%), **BA-4** (Clog *P* = 6.5, SIR = 66%), and **BA-5** (Clog *P* = 7.0, SIR = 83%) progressively enhance; With the continuous increase in the Clog *P* value, target compound **BA-6** (Clog *P* = 7.6, SIR = 51%) exhibited lower total herbicidal inhibition efficiency than compound **BA-5**, which may be caused by the poor uptake and translocation of **BA-6** in plants due to relatively high lipophilicity. A similar trend is also evident in target compounds **BA-8~BA-10**. Furthermore, the introduction of hydroxyl groups onto the alkyl chains attached to the nitrogen atoms of the target compounds **BA-2** and **BA-3** resulted in reduced herbicidal activity among compounds **BA-14** (Clog *P* = 4.1, SIR = 60%), **BA-15** (Clog *P* = 4.5, SIR = 39%), and **BA-16** (Clog *P* = 4.4, SIR = 24%). Therefore, it can be concluded that the introduction of hydrophilic substituents on the nitrogen atom of the target compounds does not enhance herbicidal activity. The herbicidal activity of compounds **BA-17** and **BA-18** supported this hypothesis. When the hydroxyl group in **BA-14** and **BA-15** was replaced by a methoxy group, the herbicidal activity of **BA-17** (Clog *P* = 4.9, SIR = 64%) and **BA-18** (Clog *P* = 5.2, SIR = 74%) was enhanced. These findings indicate that increasing the lipophilicity of target compounds to a certain extent is beneficial to improving the herbicidal activity; However, if the Clog *P* value is excessively low or high, the herbicidal efficiency decreases.

When a benzene ring was introduced on the nitrogen atom of target compounds, **BA-19** (SIR = 37%) exhibited lower herbicidal activity compared to **BA-6** (SIR = 51%). However, inserting a straight-chain alkyl group between the benzene ring and the nitrogen atom significantly enhanced herbicidal activity, as demonstrated by compound **BA-20** (SIR = 76%) relative to **BA-19**. These results suggest that, in addition to steric effects and lipophilicity, electronic effects also have a crucial influence on the herbicidal activities of these compounds.

To further investigate the herbicidal activity of the target compounds, five compounds, i.e., **BA-1**, **BA-2**, **BA-5**, **BA-18**, and **BA-20**, that demonstrated a higher SIR compared to the commercial herbicide FP, were selected for dose–response analysis through serial two-fold dilutions. As shown in Table 1, reducing the dosage from 75 to 18.8 g ha^{-1} resulted in a progressive decline in the herbicidal activity of all tested compounds. Moreover, the tested compounds demonstrated greater efficacy against dicotyledonous weed species compared to monocotyledonous plant species. For instance, compound **BA-1** achieved herbicidal activities of 84% and 100% against *B. campestris* and *A. tricolor*, respectively, at a dosage of 18.8 g ha^{-1}, whereas the inhibition rates against *E. crus-galli* and *D. sanguinalis* were only 18% and 11%, respectively. Notably, among the evaluated compounds, **BA-1**, **BA-2**, and **BA-18** exhibited strong herbicidal activity even at a dosage of 18.8 g ha^{-1}, achieving SIRs of 64%, 51%, and 50%, respectively, which exceeded the commercial herbicide FP. These findings suggest that these newly synthesized compounds hold promise as potential lead candidates for the development of novel herbicides.

Table 1. Effects (% inhibition) of the target compounds **BA-1**, **BA-2**, **BA-5**, **BA-18**, and **BA-20** on the loss of plant weight at different dosages in greenhouse testing [a].

Comp.	Dosage (g ha^{-1})	Inhibition Rate (%)				SIR
		B. campestris	*A. tricolor*	*E. crus-galli*	*D. sanguinalis*	
BA-1	75	100	100	57 ± 5	62 ± 2	87 ± 1
	37.5	94 ± 3	100	23 ± 4	16 ± 2	72 ± 3
	18.8	84 ± 2	100	18 ± 4	11 ± 4	64 ± 2
BA-2	75	92 ± 2	100	62 ± 8	44 ± 4	78 ± 2
	37.5	80 ± 5	100	51 ± 7	0 ± 0	66 ± 5
	18.8	58 ± 3	100	42 ± 5	0 ± 2	51 ± 4
BA-5	75	100	100	15 ± 1	35 ± 2	77 ± 1
	37.5	79 ± 3	100	11 ± 5	8 ± 6	59 ± 1
	18.8	40 ± 7	100	2 ± 6	0 ± 0	32 ± 6
BA-18	75	71 ± 8	100	42 ± 6	29 ± 10	63 ± 4
	37.5	70 ± 1	100	28 ± 9	6 ± 1	57 ± 3
	18.8	63 ± 1	100	21 ± 5	0 ± 4	50 ± 1
BA-20	75	74 ± 2	100	18 ± 13	2 ± 2	56 ± 3
	37.5	61 ± 3	72 ± 3	7 ± 6	0 ± 5	45 ± 3
	18.8	54 ± 4	56 ± 4	0 ± 3	0 ± 0	39 ± 1
FP	75	88 ± 4	100	52 ± 2	48 ± 3	77 ± 3
	37.5	53 ± 4	100	50 ± 3	42 ± 3	54 ± 4
	18.8	37 ± 6	90 ± 3	51 ± 6	13 ± 4	40 ± 2

[a] Each value represents the mean ± SD of three experiments.

2.3. Herbicidal Spectrum and Crop Safety of Target Compound **BA-1**

Based on the results of the above two rounds of screening, compound **BA-1** was selected for further evaluation of its herbicidal spectrum due to its pronounced herbicidal activity. As shown in Figure 5, compound **BA-1** exhibited substantial herbicidal efficacy against the majority of tested dicotyledonous weed species, including *B. campestris*, *A. tricolor*, *Lactuca indica*, *Portulaca oleracea*, *Taraxacum mongolicum*, *Chenopodium album*, and *Ipomoea nil*, with inhibition rates exceeding 85%. In contrast, compound **BA-1** displayed relatively limited inhibitory effects against the monocotyledonous plant species tested, indicating a degree of selectivity toward dicotyledonous weeds. Furthermore, a crop safety assessment was conducted to evaluate the potential application of **BA-1** as an herbicide. The results presented in Table 2 indicated that among the four tested crops treated with **BA-1**, *Triticum aestivum* and *Zea mays* exhibited relatively high tolerance, whereas *Gossypium hirsutum* and *Glycine max* were more susceptible under the same experimental conditions, with injury rates of 44% and 47%, respectively. Collectively, these findings suggest that compound **BA-1** holds promise for development as a post-emergence herbicide for the control of dicotyledonous weeds in fields of *T. aestivum* and *Z. mays*.

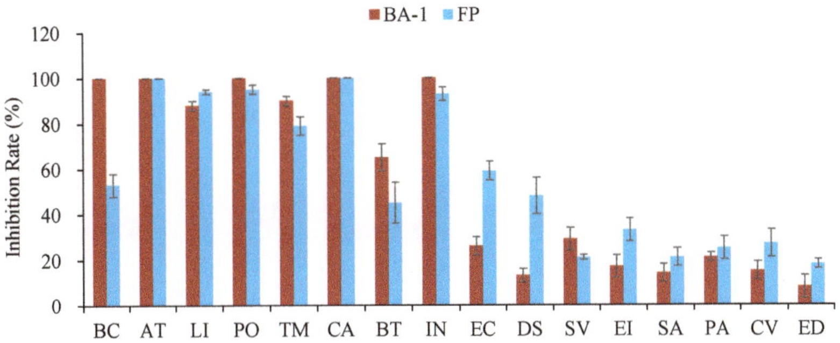

Figure 5. Herbicidal spectrum testing of compound **BA-1** under the post-emergence conditions at the dosage of 37.5 g ha^{-1}; Abbreviation: BC: *B. campestris*, AT: *A. tricolor*, LI: *L. indica*, PO: *P. oleracea*, TM: *T. mongolicum*, CA: *C. album*, BT: *Bidens tripartita*, IN: *I. nil*, EC: *E. crus-galli*, DS: *D. sanguinalis*, SV: *Setaria viridis*, EI: *Eleusine indica*, SA: *Spartina alterniflora*, PA: *Pennisetum alopecuroides*, CV: *Chloris virgata*, and ED: *Elymus dahuricus*.

Table 2. Post-emergence crop selectivity of **BA-1** and FP at the dosage of 37.5 g ha^{-1} (Injury %) [a].

Comp.	Injury (%)			
	T. aestivum	*Z. mays*	*G. hirsutum*	*G. max*
BA-1	4 ± 2	2 ± 2	44 ± 2	47 ± 3
FP	5 ± 2	3 ± 1	33 ± 4	14 ± 1

[a] Each value represents the mean ± SD of three experiments.

2.4. *Molecular Simulation Analysis of* **BA-1**

Given that **BA-1** possesses pyrimidinedione moiety like the commercial herbicide saflufenacil, it is reasonable to hypothesize that **BA-1** may function as a protoporphyrinogen IX oxidase (PPO) inhibitor. To verify the above speculation, a molecular docking study was performed to confirm the interactions between **BA-1** or FP and *Nicotiana tabacum* PPO (*Nt*PPO). As shown in Figure 6, **BA-1** and FP had some identical interacting amino acid residues, such as Arg98, Leu356, Leu372, and Phe392. The pyrimidinedione ring of **BA-1** (Figure 6A,C) and the maleimide ring of FP (Figure 6B,D) engage in π–π stacking interactions with Phe392, respectively. Additionally, the benzene rings of **BA-1** and FP participate in π–σ interactions with Leu356 and Leu372, respectively, which are conserved residues among *Nt*PPO enzymes. Furthermore, Arg98 forms a hydrogen bond with **BA-1**, like the interaction observed with FP. Notably, the barbiturate structure in **BA-1** shapes π-cation stacking interactions with Arg98 to enhance the binding with *Nt*PPO active cavity. To assess the binding stability of the complex formed between **BA-1** and *Nt*PPO,

50 ns molecular dynamics (MD) simulations were conducted using the GROMACS 2023.3 software package. FP was employed as the positive control. As illustrated in Figure 7, both the ligand (Figure 7A) and the protein structure (Figure 7B) exhibited stable conformational behavior throughout the 50 ns simulation period, with root-mean-square deviation (RMSD) fluctuations consistently below 0.5 Å. These findings indicate that compound **BA-1** forms a stable interaction with *Nt*PPO.

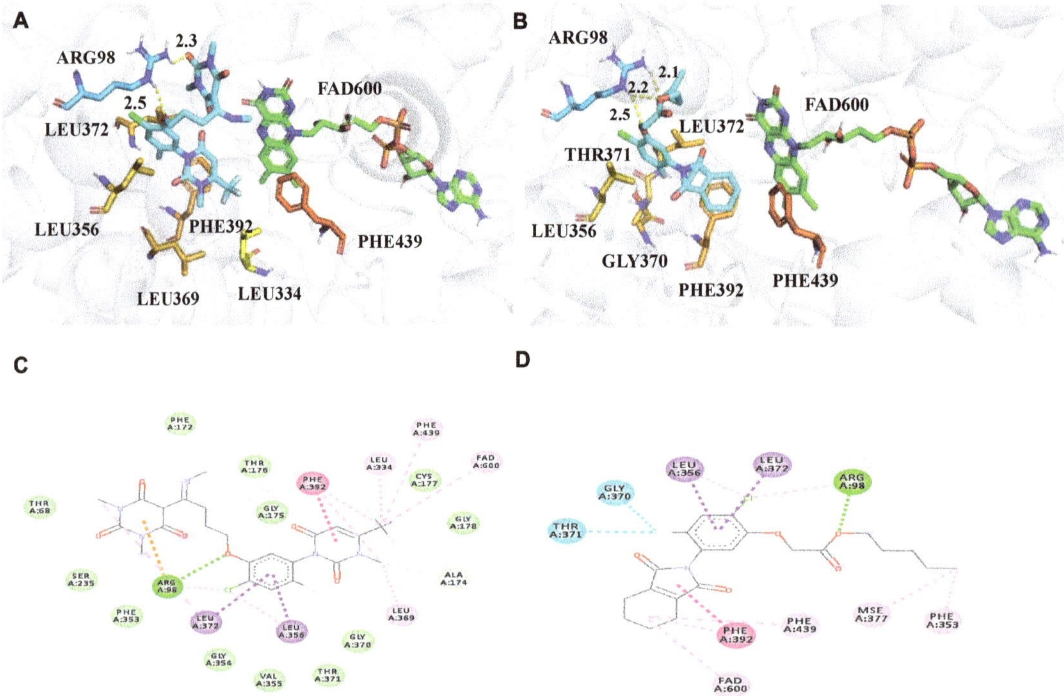

Figure 6. Docking analysis between **BA-1** or FP and *Nt*PPO. (**A**) 3D of molecular docking between **BA-1** and *Nt*PPO; (**B**) 3D of molecular docking between FP and *Nt*PPO; (**C**) 2D of molecular docking between **BA-1** and *Nt*PPO; (**D**) 2D of molecular docking between FP and *Nt*PPO.

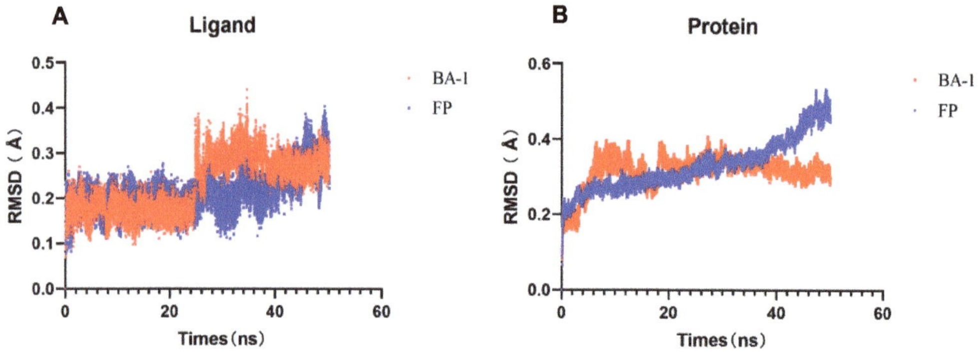

Figure 7. RMSD of protein (**A**) and ligand (**B**) plots of protein–ligand complexes during 50 ns MD simulations.

3. Materials and Methods

3.1. Chemical Synthesis Procedures

Detailed synthetic procedures for the intermediates and target compounds are described below; however, the reaction yields have not been optimized.

3.1.1. Synthesis of Intermediates **1–7**

The intermediates **1–7** was synthesized according to a previously reported method [11].

3.1.2. General Procedure for the Synthesis of Target Compounds **BA-1** to **BA-20**

The target compounds **BA-1~BA-20** were synthesized according to a previously reported method [34,35]. A representative example for the synthesis of **BA-1** is described as follows: The intermediate **7** (281 mg, 0.5 mmol) was dissolved in 10 mL of ethanol followed by the addition of methylamine hydrochloride (40.8 mg, 0.6 mmol), and the mixture was refluxed at 90 °C for 12 h. After cooling to room temperature, the resulting solid was collected by filtration, recrystallized with ethanol to give target compound **BA-1** as a white solid (84.5 mg, yield: 29.4%). The target compounds **BA-2~BA-20** were prepared by a procedure like that for **BA-1**. The spectrum of ^{1}H NMR, ^{13}C NMR, and HRMS of all target compounds **BA-1~BA-20** can be found in Supplementary Materials (Figures S1–S60), and the data as follows:

5-(4-(2-Chloro-4-fluoro-5-(3-methyl-2,6-dioxo-4-(trifluoromethyl)-3,6-dihydropyrimidin-1(2*H*)-yl)phenoxy)-1-(methylamino)butylidene)-1,3-dimethylpyrimidine-2,4,6(1*H*,3*H*,5*H*)-trione (**BA-1**): white solid, yield 29.4%, m.p. 191–194 °C; ^{1}H NMR (500 MHz, $CDCl_3$) δ 12.57 (s, 1H), 7.32 (d, *J* = 8.8 Hz, 1H), 6.80 (d, *J* = 6.3 Hz, 1H), 6.38 (s, 1H), 4.13 (t, *J* = 5.4 Hz, 2H), 3.57 (s, 3H), 3.41–3.35 (m, 2H), 3.32 (s, 3H), 3.30 (s, 3H), 3.26 (d, *J* = 5.2 Hz, 3H), 2.16 (m, 2H); ^{13}C NMR (125 MHz, $CDCl_3$) δ 177.25 (s), 166.69 (s), 162.54 (s), 159.94 (s), 152.43 (s), 151.45 (d, *J* = 248.0 Hz), 151.34 (s), 151.01 (d, *J* = 2.4 Hz), 150.69 (s), 141.79 (q, *J* = 34.6 Hz), 124.53 (d, *J* = 9.4 Hz), 120.67 (d, *J* = 14.9 Hz), 119.37 (q, *J* = 275.4 Hz), 118.49 (d, *J* = 24.1 Hz), 113.53 (s), 103.11 (q, *J* = 5.4 Hz), 89.93 (s), 68.88 (s), 32.74 (q, *J* = 3.4 Hz), 30.06 (s), 27.93 (s), 27.65 (s), 26.65 (s), 26.61 (s); HRMS, m/z calcd. for $C_{23}H_{23}ClF_4N_5O_6^+$ [M + H]$^+$ 576.12675, found 576.12628.

5-(4-(2-Chloro-4-fluoro-5-(3-methyl-2,6-dioxo-4-(trifluoromethyl)-3,6-dihydropyrimid in-1(2*H*)-yl)phenoxy)-1-(ethylamino)butylidene)-1,3-dimethylpyrimidine-2,4,6(1*H*,3*H*,5*H*)-trione (**BA-2**): white solid, yield 31%, m.p. 212–215 °C; ^{1}H NMR (500 MHz, $CDCl_3$) δ 12.56 (s, 1H), 7.33 (d, *J* = 8.8 Hz, 1H), 6.80 (d, *J* = 6.3 Hz, 1H), 6.38 (s, 1H), 4.12 (t, *J* = 5.4 Hz, 2H), 3.70–3.61 (m, 2H), 3.57 (s, 3H), 3.39–3.29 (m, 8H), 2.16 (m, 2H), 1.38 (t, *J* = 7.3 Hz, 3H); ^{13}C NMR (125 MHz, $CDCl_3$) δ 176.03 (s), 166.73 (s), 162.60 (s), 159.94 (s), 151.44 (d, *J* = 248.0 Hz), 151.37 (s), 151.03 (d, *J* = 2.2 Hz), 150.70 (s), 141.80 (q, J = 34.6 Hz), 124.49 (d, *J* = 9.5 Hz), 120.69 (d, *J* = 14.9 Hz), 119.37 (q, *J* = 275.2 Hz), 118.49 (d, *J* = 24.1 Hz), 113.51 (s), 103.11 (q, *J* = 5.6 Hz), 89.60 (s), 68.91 (s), 38.38 (s), 32.74 (q, *J* = 3.2 Hz), 27.93 (s), 27.65 (s), 27.11 (s), 26.79 (s), 14.90 (s); HRMS, m/z calcd. for $C_{24}H_{25}ClF_4N_5O_6^+$ [M + Na]$^+$ 590.14240, found 590.14178.

5-(4-(2-Chloro-4-fluoro-5-(3-methyl-2,6-dioxo-4-(trifluoromethyl)-3,6-dihydropyrimid in-1(2*H*)-yl)phenoxy)-1-(propylamino)butylidene)-1,3-dimethylpyrimidine-2,4,6(1*H*,3*H*,5*H*)-trione (**BA-3**): white solid, yield 93%, m.p. 225–227 °C; ^{1}H NMR (500 MHz, $CDCl_3$) δ 12.63 (s, 1H), 7.33 (d, *J* = 8.8 Hz, 1H), 6.80 (d, *J* = 6.3 Hz, 1H), 6.38 (s, 1H), 4.12 (t, *J* = 5.4 Hz, 2H), 3.62–3.53 (m, 5H), 3.40–3.28 (m, 8H), 2.16 (m, 2H), 1.81–1.71 (m, 2H), 1.06 (t, *J* = 7.4 Hz, 3H); ^{13}C NMR (125 MHz, $CDCl_3$) δ 176.15 (s), 166.74 (s), 162.58 (s), 159.92 (s), 151.42 (d, *J* = 248.0 Hz), 151.36 (s), 151.01 (d, *J* = 2.4 Hz), 150.68 (s), 141.77 (q, *J* = 34.4 Hz), 124.46 (d, *J* = 9.4 Hz), 120.69 (d, *J* = 14.9 Hz), 119.37 (q, *J* = 275.3 Hz), 118.46 (d, *J* = 24.1 Hz), 113.48 (s),

103.10 (q, *J* = 5.4 Hz), 89.63 (s), 68.86 (s), 45.15 (s), 32.73 (q, *J* = 3.5 Hz), 27.92 (s), 27.65 (s), 27.07 (s), 26.81 (s), 22.88 (s), 11.40 (s); HRMS, *m*/*z* calcd. for $C_{25}H_{27}ClF_4N_5O_6^+$ [M + H]$^+$ 604.15805, found 604.15729.

5-(1-(Butylamino)-4-(2-chloro-4-fluoro-5-(3-methyl-2,6-dioxo-4-(trifluoromethyl)-3,6-dihydropyrimidin-1(2*H*)-yl)phenoxy)butylidene)-1,3-dimethylpyrimidine-2,4,6(1*H*,3*H*,5*H*)-trione (**BA-4**): white solid, yield 75%, m.p. 217–219 °C; ^{1}H NMR (500 MHz, $CDCl_3$) δ 12.61 (s, 1H), 7.32 (d, *J* = 8.8 Hz, 1H), 6.80 (d, *J* = 6.3 Hz, 1H), 6.38 (s, 1H), 4.12 (t, *J* = 5.4 Hz, 2H), 3.60 (dd, *J* = 14.6, 8.9 Hz, 5H), 3.40–3.28 (m, 8H), 2.15 (m, 2H), 1.78–1.67 (m, 2H), 1.47 (m, 2H), 0.98 (t, *J* = 7.3 Hz, 3H); ^{13}C NMR (125 MHz, $CDCl_3$) δ 176.09 (s), 166.74 (s), 162.58 (s), 159.92 (s), 151.43 (d, *J* = 248.1 Hz), 151.36 (s), 151.02 (d, *J* = 2.5 Hz), 150.69 (s), 141.78 (q, *J* = 34.6 Hz), 124.47 (d, *J* = 9.4 Hz), 120.69 (d, *J* = 14.8 Hz), 119.37 (q, *J* = 275.3 Hz), 118.46 (d, *J* = 24.2 Hz), 113.49 (s), 103.10 (q, *J* = 5.3 Hz), 89.63 (s), 68.89 (s), 43.28 (s), 32.73 (q, *J* = 3.4 Hz), 31.54 (s), 27.92 (s), 27.66 (s), 27.08 (s), 26.84 (s), 20.05 (s), 13.69 (s); HRMS, *m*/*z* calcd. for $C_{26}H_{29}ClF_4N_5O_6^+$ [M + H]$^+$ 618.17370, found 618.17316.

5-(4-(2-Chloro-4-fluoro-5-(3-methyl-2,6-dioxo-4-(trifluoromethyl)-3,6-dihydropyrimidin-1(2*H*)-yl)phenoxy)-1-(pentylamino)butylidene)-1,3-dimethylpyrimidine-2,4,6(1*H*,3*H*,5*H*)-trione (**BA-5**): white solid, yield 36%, m.p. 205–207 °C; ^{1}H NMR (500 MHz, $CDCl_3$) δ 12.61 (s, 1H), 7.33 (d, *J* = 8.8 Hz, 1H), 6.80 (d, *J* = 6.3 Hz, 1H), 6.38 (s, 1H), 4.12 (t, *J* = 5.4 Hz, 2H), 3.59 (dd, *J* = 11.4, 5.7 Hz, 5H), 3.41–3.28 (m, 8H), 2.15 (m, 2H), 1.79–1.68 (m, 2H), 1.46–1.34 (m, 4H), 0.93 (t, *J* = 7.0 Hz, 3H); ^{13}C NMR (125 MHz, $CDCl_3$) δ 176.06 (s), 166.73 (s), 162.60 (s), 159.93 (s), 151.43 (d, *J* = 248.0 Hz), 151.37 (s), 151.02 (d, *J* = 2.6 Hz), 150.69 (s), 124.47 (d, *J* = 9.3 Hz), 120.69 (d, *J* = 14.8 Hz), 119.38 (q, *J* = 275.4 Hz), 118.46 (d, *J* = 24.4 Hz), 113.49 (s), 103.10 (q, *J* = 5.4 Hz), 89.62 (s), 68.88 (s), 43.56 (s), 32.73 (q, *J* = 3.2 Hz), 29.24 (s), 28.91 (s), 27.92 (s), 27.66 (s), 27.07 (s), 26.85 (s), 22.28 (s), 13.88 (s); HRMS, *m*/*z* calcd. for $C_{27}H_{31}ClF_4N_5O_6^+$ [M + H]$^+$ 632.18935, found 632.18842.

5-(4-(2-Chloro-4-fluoro-5-(3-methyl-2,6-dioxo-4-(trifluoromethyl)-3,6-dihydropyrimidin-1(2*H*)-yl)phenoxy)-1-(hexylamino)butylidene)-1,3-dimethylpyrimidine-2,4,6(1*H*,3*H*,5*H*)-trione (**BA-6**): white solid, yield 90%, m.p. 201–203 °C; ^{1}H NMR (500 MHz, $CDCl_3$) δ 12.61 (s, 1H), 7.33 (d, *J* = 8.8 Hz, 1H), 6.80 (d, *J* = 6.3 Hz, 1H), 6.38 (s, 1H), 4.12 (t, *J* = 5.4 Hz, 2H), 3.59 (dd, *J* = 11.8, 6.1 Hz, 5H), 3.39–3.27 (m, 8H), 2.15 (m, 2H), 1.72 (m, 2H), 1.47–1.39 (m, 2H), 1.37–1.30 (m, 4H), 0.91 (dd, *J* = 9.2, 4.8 Hz, 3H); ^{13}C NMR (125 MHz, $CDCl_3$) δ 176.04 (s), 166.72 (s), 162.58 (s), 159.91 (s), 151.42 (d, *J* = 248.0 Hz), 151.36 (s), 151.01 (d, *J* = 2.5 Hz), 150.68 (s), 141.76 (q, *J* = 34.5 Hz), 124.45 (d, *J* = 9.3 Hz), 120.69 (d, *J* = 14.8 Hz), 119.37 (q, *J* = 275.5 Hz), 118.44 (d, *J* = 24.1 Hz), 113.49 (s), 103.09 (q, *J* = 5.4 Hz), 89.60 (s), 68.88 (s), 43.58 (s), 32.71 (q, *J* = 3.1 Hz), 31.32 (s), 29.52 (s), 27.90 (s), 27.64 (s), 27.07 (s), 26.83 (s), 26.48 (s), 22.44 (s), 13.96 (s); HRMS, *m*/*z* calcd. for $C_{28}H_{33}ClF_4N_5O_6^+$ [M + H]$^+$ 646.20500, found 646.20422.

5-(4-(2-Chloro-4-fluoro-5-(3-methyl-2,6-dioxo-4-(trifluoromethyl)-3,6-dihydropyrimidin-1(2*H*)-yl)phenoxy)-1-(cyclopropylamino)butylidene)-1,3-dimethylpyrimidine-2,4,6(1*H*,3*H*,5*H*)-trione (**BA-7**): white solid, yield 87%, m.p. 211–214 °C; ^{1}H NMR (500 MHz, $CDCl_3$) δ 12.49 (s, 1H), 7.31 (d, *J* = 8.8 Hz, 1H), 6.81 (d, *J* = 6.3 Hz, 1H), 6.38 (s, 1H), 4.16 (t, *J* = 5.5 Hz, 2H), 3.62–3.51 (m, 5H), 3.31 (s, 3H), 3.30 (s, 3H), 3.11–3.04 (m, 1H), 2.22 (m, 2H), 1.10–1.01 (m, 2H), 0.85–0.78 (m, 2H); ^{13}C NMR (125 MHz, $CDCl_3$) δ 178.48 (s), 166.60 (s), 162.31 (s), 159.92 (s), 151.38 (d, *J* = 248.1 Hz), 151.27 (s), 151.06 (d, *J* = 2.4 Hz), 150.68 (s), 141.77 (q, *J* = 34.3 Hz), 124.38 (d, *J* = 9.3 Hz), 120.69 (d, *J* = 14.9 Hz), 119.37 (q, *J* = 275.4 Hz), 118.47 (d, *J* = 24.3 Hz), 113.50 (s), 103.09 (q, *J* = 5.4 Hz), 89.94 (s), 69.07 (s), 32.73 (d, *J* = 3.5 Hz), 27.92 (s), 27.63 (s), 26.83 (s), 25.62 (s), 8.09 (s); HRMS, *m*/*z* calcd. for $C_{25}H_{25}ClF_4N_5O_6^+$ [M + H]$^+$ 602.14240, found 602.14185.

5-(4-(2-Chloro-4-fluoro-5-(3-methyl-2,6-dioxo-4-(trifluoromethyl)-3,6-dihydropyrimidin-1(2*H*)-yl)phenoxy)-1-(cyclobutylamino)butylidene)-1,3-dimethylpyrimidine-2,4,6(1*H*,3*H*,5*H*)-

trione (**BA-8**): white solid, yield 73%, m.p. 249–251 °C; ^{1}H NMR (500 MHz, $CDCl_3$) δ 12.73 (d, J = 5.9 Hz, 1H), 7.35 (d, J = 8.8 Hz, 1H), 6.80 (d, J = 6.3 Hz, 1H), 6.38 (s, 1H), 4.47 (dd, J = 15.7, 7.7 Hz, 1H), 4.12 (t, J = 5.4 Hz, 2H), 3.57 (s, 3H), 3.38–3.24 (m, 8H), 2.58–2.45 (m, 2H), 2.25–2.06 (m, 4H), 1.94–1.76 (m, 2H); ^{13}C NMR (125 MHz, $CDCl_3$) δ 174.83 (s), 166.68 (s), 162.56 (s), 159.92 (s), 151.42 (d, J = 247.8 Hz), 151.33 (s), 151.04 (d, J = 2.6 Hz), 150.69 (s), 141.79 (q, J = 34.5 Hz), 124.38 (d, J = 9.3 Hz), 120.72 (d, J = 14.9 Hz), 119.38 (q, J = 275.4 Hz), 118.50 (d, J = 24.2 Hz), 113.42 (s), 103.10 (q, J = 5.6 Hz), 89.55 (s), 68.89 (s), 47.92 (s), 32.73 (q, J = 3.5 Hz), 31.37 (s), 31.35 (s), 27.92 (s), 27.66 (s), 27.30 (s), 27.26 (s), 15.36 (s); HRMS, m/z calcd. for $C_{26}H_{27}ClF_4N_5O_6^+$ [M + H]$^+$ 616.15805, found 616.15747.

5-(4-(2-Chloro-4-fluoro-5-(3-methyl-2,6-dioxo-4-(trifluoromethyl)-3,6-dihydropyrimidin-1(2*H*)-yl)phenoxy)-1-(cyclopentylamino)butylidene)-1,3-dimethylpyrimidine-2,4,6(1*H*,3*H*,5*H*)-trione (**BA-9**): white solid, yield 29%, m.p. 264–266 °C; ^{1}H NMR (500 MHz, $CDCl_3$) δ 12.76 (d, J = 7.4 Hz, 1H), 7.33 (d, J = 8.8 Hz, 1H), 6.80 (d, J = 6.3 Hz, 1H), 6.38 (s, 1H), 4.37 (dd, J = 13.6, 6.7 Hz, 1H), 4.13 (t, J = 5.4 Hz, 2H), 3.57 (s, 3H), 3.38 (dd, J = 9.4, 6.1 Hz, 2H), 3.32 (s, 3H), 3.30 (s, 3H), 2.23–2.08 (m, 4H), 1.92–1.79 (m, 2H), 1.76–1.62 (m, 4H); ^{13}C NMR (125 MHz, $CDCl_3$) δ 174.95 (s), 166.74 (s), 162.55 (s), 159.92 (s), 151.41 (d, J = 248.1 Hz), 151.37 (s), 151.00 (d, J = 2.5 Hz), 150.68 (s), 141.78 (q, J = 34.3 Hz), 124.35 (d, J = 9.5 Hz), 120.73 (d, J = 14.8 Hz), 119.37 (q, J = 275.5 Hz), 118.45 (d, J = 24.2 Hz), 113.43 (s), 103.10 (q, J = 5.5 Hz), 89.39 (s), 68.86 (s), 54.89 (s), 34.19 (s), 32.73 (q, J = 3.1 Hz), 27.92 (s), 27.65 (s), 27.44 (s), 27.10 (s), 23.98 (s); HRMS, m/z calcd. for $C_{27}H_{29}ClF_4N_5O_6^+$ [M + H]$^+$ 630.17370, found 630.17291.

5-(4-(2-Chloro-4-fluoro-5-(3-methyl-2,6-dioxo-4-(trifluoromethyl)-3,6-dihydropyrimidin-1(2*H*)-yl)phenoxy)-1-(cyclohexylamino)butylidene)-1,3-dimethylpyrimidine-2,4,6(1*H*,3*H*,5*H*)-trione (**BA-10**): white solid, yield 23%, m.p. 264–267 °C; ^{1}H NMR (500 MHz, $CDCl_3$) δ 12.75 (d, J = 8.0 Hz, 1H), 7.33 (d, J = 8.8 Hz, 1H), 6.80 (d, J = 6.3 Hz, 1H), 6.37 (d, J = 4.3 Hz, 1H), 4.12 (t, J = 5.4 Hz, 2H), 3.93–3.83 (m, 1H), 3.57 (s, 3H), 3.38–3.28 (m, 8H), 2.16 (dt, J = 12.2, 6.3 Hz, 2H), 1.94 (d, J = 9.6 Hz, 2H), 1.79 (dd, J = 9.1, 4.0 Hz, 2H), 1.45 (m, 6H); ^{13}C NMR (125 MHz, $CDCl_3$) δ 174.54 (s), 166.80 (s), 162.57 (s), 159.92 (s), 151.43 (d, J = 248.1 Hz), 151.39 (s), 150.99 (d, J = 2.5 Hz), 150.68 (s), 141.79 (q, J = 34.4 Hz), 124.44 (d, J = 9.3 Hz), 120.73 (d, J = 14.8 Hz), 119.37 (q, J = 275.5 Hz), 118.45 (d, J = 24.1 Hz), 113.44 (s), 103.10 (q, J = 5.3 Hz), 89.31 (s), 68.82 (s), 52.14 (s), 33.58 (s), 32.74 (q, J = 3.4 Hz), 27.93 (s), 27.90 (s), 27.66 (s), 26.69 (s), 25.04 (s), 24.10 (s); HRMS, m/z calcd. for $C_{28}H_{31}ClF_4N_5O_6^+$ [M + H]$^+$ 644.18935, found 644.18866.

5-(4-(2-Chloro-4-fluoro-5-(3-methyl-2,6-dioxo-4-(trifluoromethyl)-3,6-dihydropyrimidin-1(2*H*)-yl)phenoxy)-1-(isopropylamino)butylidene)-1,3-dimethylpyrimidine-2,4,6(1*H*,3*H*,5*H*)-trione (**BA-11**): white solid, yield 48%, m.p. 264–267 °C; ^{1}H NMR (500 MHz, $CDCl_3$) δ 12.63 (d, J = 8.0 Hz, 1H), 7.33 (d, J = 8.8 Hz, 1H), 6.81 (d, J = 6.3 Hz, 1H), 6.38 (s, 1H), 4.34–4.23 (m, 1H), 4.12 (t, J = 5.4 Hz, 2H), 3.57 (s, 3H), 3.43–3.28 (m, 8H), 2.22–2.11 (m, 2H), 1.37 (s, 3H), 1.35 (s, 3H); ^{13}C NMR (125 MHz, $CDCl_3$) δ 174.59 (s), 166.76 (s), 162.58 (s), 159.92 (s), 151.44 (d, J = 248.1 Hz), 151.36 (s), 150.99 (d, J = 2.6 Hz), 150.68 (s), 141.78 (q, J = 34.6 Hz), 124.39 (d, J = 9.5 Hz), 120.73 (d, J = 14.8 Hz), 119.37 (q, J = 275.5 Hz), 118.46 (d, J = 24.1 Hz), 113.48 (s), 103.09 (q, J = 5.5 Hz), 89.26 (s), 68.84 (s), 45.57 (s), 32.73 (q, J = 3.5 Hz), 27.93 (s), 27.76 (s), 27.63 (s), 26.62 (s), 23.57 (s); HRMS, m/z calcd. for $C_{25}H_{27}ClF_4N_5O_6^+$ [M + H]$^+$ 604.15805, found 604.15765.

5-(4-(2-Chloro-4-fluoro-5-(3-methyl-2,6-dioxo-4-(trifluoromethyl)-3,6-dihydropyrimidin-1(2*H*)-yl)phenoxy)-1-(isobutylamino)butylidene)-1,3-dimethylpyrimidine-2,4,6(1*H*,3*H*,5*H*)-trione (**BA-12**): white solid, yield 76%, m.p. 241–244 °C; ^{1}H NMR (500 MHz, $CDCl_3$) δ 12.71 (s, 1H), 7.33 (d, J = 8.8 Hz, 1H), 6.80 (d, J = 6.3 Hz, 1H), 6.38 (s, 1H), 4.12 (t, J = 5.3 Hz, 2H), 3.57 (s, 3H), 3.44–3.40 (m, 2H), 3.39–3.28 (m, 8H), 2.15 (m, 2H), 2.00 (m, 1H), 1.06 (s, 3H), 1.05 (s, 3H); ^{13}C NMR (125 MHz, $CDCl_3$) δ 176.16 (s), 166.77 (s), 162.57 (s), 159.89 (s), 151.41

(d, J = 248.0 Hz), 151.34 (s), 150.97 (d, J = 2.6 Hz), 150.66 (s), 141.75 (q, J = 34.5 Hz), 124.42 (d, J = 9.5 Hz), 120.70 (d, J = 14.9 Hz), 119.37 (q, J = 275.6 Hz), 118.42 (d, J = 24.4 Hz), 113.47 (s), 103.07 (q, J = 5.4 Hz), 89.64 (s), 68.80 (s), 50.85 (s), 32.71 (q, J = 3.5 Hz), 28.71 (s), 27.90 (s), 27.65 (s), 26.99 (s), 26.79 (s), 20.12 (s); HRMS, m/z calcd. for $C_{26}H_{29}ClF_4N_5O_6^+$ [M + H]$^+$ 618.17370, found 618.17346.

5-(1-(sec-Butylamino)-4-(2-chloro-4-fluoro-5-(3-methyl-2,6-dioxo-4-(trifluoromethyl)-3,6-dihydropyrimidin-1(2*H*)-yl)phenoxy)butylidene)-1,3-dimethylpyrimidine-2,4,6(1*H*,3*H*,5*H*)-trione (**BA-13**): white solid, yield 36%, m.p. 269–271 °C; ^{1}H NMR (500 MHz, $CDCl_3$) δ 12.63 (d, J = 8.4 Hz, 1H), 7.33 (d, J = 8.8 Hz, 1H), 6.80 (d, J = 6.3 Hz, 1H), 6.38 (s, 1H), 4.18–4.06 (m, 3H), 3.57 (s, 3H), 3.45–3.28 (m, 8H), 2.26–2.07 (m, 2H), 1.74–1.62 (m, 2H), 1.32 (d, J = 6.4 Hz, 3H), 0.99 (t, J = 7.4 Hz, 3H); ^{13}C NMR (125 MHz, $CDCl_3$) δ 175.02 (s), 166.80 (s), 162.59 (s), 159.92 (s), 151.43 (d, J = 248.1 Hz), 151.38 (s), 151.01 (d, J = 2.5 Hz), 150.68 (s), 141.78 (q, J = 34.6 Hz), 124.39 (d, J = 9.3 Hz), 120.73 (d, J = 14.8 Hz), 119.37 (q, J = 275.3 Hz), 118.46 (d, J = 24.1 Hz), 113.44 (s), 103.10 (q, J = 5.1 Hz), 89.29 (s), 68.84 (s), 51.02 (s), 32.73 (q, J = 3.4 Hz), 30.27 (s), 27.92 (s), 27.70 (s), 27.64 (s), 26.64 (s), 21.49 (s), 10.35 (s); HRMS, m/z calcd. for $C_{26}H_{29}ClF_4N_5O_6^+$ [M + H]$^+$ 618.17370, found 618.17316.

5-(4-(2-Chloro-4-fluoro-5-(3-methyl-2,6-dioxo-4-(trifluoromethyl)-3,6-dihydropyrimidin-1(2*H*)-yl)phenoxy)-1-((2-hydroxyethyl)amino)butylidene)-1,3-dimethylpyrimidine-2,4,6(1*H*,3*H*,5*H*)-trione (**BA-14**): white solid, yield 82%, m.p. 214–216 °C; ^{1}H NMR (500 MHz, $CDCl_3$) δ 12.81 (s, 1H), 7.33 (d, J = 8.8 Hz, 1H), 6.80 (d, J = 6.3 Hz, 1H), 6.38 (s, 1H), 4.15 (t, J = 5.4 Hz, 2H), 3.88 (t, J = 5.1 Hz, 2H), 3.71 (dd, J = 10.4, 5.3 Hz, 2H), 3.57 (s, 3H), 3.41–3.34 (m, 2H), 3.31 (d, J = 5.5 Hz, 6H), 2.17 (m, 3H); ^{13}C NMR (125 MHz, $CDCl_3$) δ 176.53 (s), 166.65 (s), 162.52 (s), 160.02 (s), 151.43 (d, J = 248.1 Hz), 151.35 (s), 150.83 (d, J = 2.5 Hz), 150.72 (s), 141.87 (q, J = 34.7 Hz), 124.49 (d, J = 9.5 Hz), 120.67 (d, J = 14.8 Hz), 119.34 (q, J = 275.4 Hz), 118.51 (d, J = 24.1 Hz), 113.65 (s), 103.10 (q, J = 5.3 Hz), 89.92 (s), 68.69 (s), 60.66 (s), 45.45 (s), 32.78 (q, J = 3.3 Hz), 27.95 (s), 27.72 (s), 26.83 (s), 26.79 (s); HRMS, m/z calcd. for $C_{24}H_{25}ClF_4N_5O_7^+$ [M + H]$^+$ 606.13732, found 606.13708.

5-(4-(2-Chloro-4-fluoro-5-(3-methyl-2,6-dioxo-4-(trifluoromethyl)-3,6-dihydropyrimidin-1(2*H*)-yl)phenoxy)-1-((3-hydroxypropyl)amino)butylidene)-1,3-dimethylpyrimidine-2,4,6(1*H*,3*H*,5*H*)-trione (**BA-15**): white solid, yield 80%, m.p. 221–224 °C; ^{1}H NMR (500 MHz, $CDCl_3$) δ 12.66 (s, 1H), 7.33 (d, J = 8.8 Hz, 1H), 6.79 (d, J = 6.3 Hz, 1H), 6.38 (s, 1H), 4.14 (t, J = 5.4 Hz, 2H), 3.74 (t, J = 5.8 Hz, 2H), 3.70 (dd, J = 12.3, 6.4 Hz, 2H), 3.57 (s, 3H), 3.42–3.34 (m, 2H), 3.31 (s, 6H), 2.24–2.14 (m, 2H), 1.93 (p, J = 6.3 Hz, 2H), 1.74 (s, 1H); ^{13}C NMR (125 MHz, $CDCl_3$) δ 176.40 (s), 166.74 (s), 162.54 (s), 159.92 (s), 151.46 (d, J = 248.0 Hz), 151.30 (s), 151.01 (d, J = 2.3 Hz), 150.69 (s), 141.77 (q, J = 34.5 Hz), 135.64 (s), 129.22 (s), 128.27 (s), 127.30 (s), 124.51 (d, J = 9.3 Hz), 120.70 (d, J = 14.8 Hz), 119.38 (q, J = 275.2 Hz), 118.47 (d, J = 24.1 Hz), 113.56 (s), 103.09 (q, J = 5.2 Hz), 90.16 (s), 68.95 (s), 47.29 (s), 32.73 (q, J = 3.5 Hz), 27.97 (s), 27.71 (s), 27.16 (s), 26.97 (s); HRMS, m/z calcd. for $C_{25}H_{27}ClF_4N_5O_7^+$ [M + H]$^+$ 620.15297, found 620.15247.

5-(4-(2-Chloro-4-fluoro-5-(3-methyl-2,6-dioxo-4-(trifluoromethyl)-3,6-dihydropyrimidin-1(2*H*)-yl)phenoxy)-1-((2-hydroxypropyl)amino)butylidene)-1,3-dimethylpyrimidine-2,4,6(1*H*,3*H*,5*H*)-trione (**BA-16**): white solid, yield 82%, m.p. 234–237 °C; ^{1}H NMR (500 MHz, $CDCl_3$) δ 12.83 (s, 1H), 7.33 (d, J = 8.8 Hz, 1H), 6.80 (d, J = 6.3 Hz, 1H), 6.37 (d, J = 1.7 Hz, 1H), 4.14 (t, J = 5.4 Hz, 2H), 4.12–4.02 (m, 1H), 3.69–3.61 (m, 1H), 3.57 (s, 3H), 3.49–3.25 (m, 9H), 2.15 (dd, J = 12.2, 5.0 Hz, 3H), 1.27 (d, J = 6.2 Hz, 3H); ^{13}C NMR (125 MHz, $CDCl_3$) δ 176.31 (s), 166.65 (s), 162.56 (s), 160.03 (s), 159.97 (s), 151.42 (d, J = 248.2 Hz), 151.36 (s), 150.82 (d, J = 2.6 Hz), 150.74 (s), 150.69 (s), 141.86 (dd, J = 34.3, 3.7 Hz), 124.45 (d, J = 9.3 Hz), 120.68 (d, J = 14.8 Hz), 119.34 (q, J = 275.6 Hz), 118.49 (d, J = 24.3 Hz), 113.59 (s), 103.10 (p, J = 5.4 Hz), 89.89 (s), 68.57 (s), 66.07 (s), 50.28 (s), 32.77 (q, J = 3.5 Hz), 27.95 (s), 27.73 (s), 26.81 (s), 21.10 (s); HRMS, m/z calcd. for $C_{25}H_{27}ClF_4N_5O_7^+$ [M + H]$^+$ 620.15297, found 620.15240.

5-(4-(2-Chloro-4-fluoro-5-(3-methyl-2,6-dioxo-4-(trifluoromethyl)-3,6-dihydropyrimidin-1(2*H*)-yl)phenoxy)-1-((2-methoxyethyl)amino)butylidene)-1,3-dimethylpyrimidine-2,4,6(1*H*,3*H*,5*H*)-trione (**BA-17**): white solid, yield 91%, m.p. 207–209 °C; ^1H NMR (500 MHz, $CDCl_3$) δ 12.73 (s, 1H), 7.32 (d, *J* = 8.8 Hz, 1H), 6.80 (d, *J* = 6.3 Hz, 1H), 6.38 (s, 1H), 4.12 (t, *J* = 5.4 Hz, 2H), 3.80 (dd, *J* = 10.4, 5.2 Hz, 2H), 3.64 (t, *J* = 5.1 Hz, 2H), 3.57 (s, 3H), 3.44 (s, 3H), 3.37 (dd, *J* = 9.3, 6.3 Hz, 2H), 3.34 (s, 3H), 3.30 (s, 3H), 2.16 (m, 2H); ^{13}C NMR (125 MHz, $CDCl_3$) δ 176.28 (s), 166.62 (s), 162.61 (s), 159.92 (s), 151.44 (d, *J* = 248.0 Hz), 151.38 (s), 150.99 (d, *J* = 2.6 Hz), 150.68 (s), 141.78 (q, *J* = 34.5 Hz), 124.42 (d, *J* = 9.3 Hz), 120.71 (d, J = 14.9 Hz), 119.37 (q, *J* = 275.4 Hz), 118.46 (d, *J* = 24.1 Hz), 113.53 (s), 103.09 (q, *J* = 5.3 Hz), 89.94 (s), 70.25 (s), 68.85 (s), 59.22 (s), 43.38 (s), 32.73 (d, *J* = 3.4 Hz), 27.93 (s), 27.70 (s), 26.97 (s), 26.86 (s); HRMS, *m*/*z* calcd. for $C_{25}H_{27}ClF_4N_5O_7^+$ [M + H]$^+$ 620.15297, found 620.15228.

5-(4-(2-Chloro-4-fluoro-5-(3-methyl-2,6-dioxo-4-(trifluoromethyl)-3,6-dihydropyrimidin-1(2*H*)-yl)phenoxy)-1-((3-methoxypropyl)amino)butylidene)-1,3-dimethylpyrimidine-2,4,6(1*H*,3*H*,5*H*)-trione (**BA-18**): white solid, yield 79%, m.p. 197–200 °C; ^1H NMR (500 MHz, $CDCl_3$) δ 12.65 (s, 1H), 7.32 (d, *J* = 8.8 Hz, 1H), 6.80 (d, *J* = 6.3 Hz, 1H), 6.38 (s, 1H), 4.13 (t, *J* = 5.5 Hz, 2H), 3.72 (dd, *J* = 12.4, 6.6 Hz, 2H), 3.57 (s, 3H), 3.50 (t, *J* = 5.8 Hz, 2H), 3.39–3.34 (m, 5H), 3.33 (s, 3H), 3.30 (s, 3H), 2.16 (m, 2H), 2.02–1.94 (m, 2H); ^{13}C NMR (125 MHz, $CDCl_3$) δ 176.21 (s), 166.66 (s), 162.59 (s), 159.91 (s), 151.41 (d, *J* = 247.9 Hz), 151.37 (s), 151.05 (d, *J* = 2.3 Hz), 150.68 (s), 141.76 (q, *J* = 34.6 Hz), 124.53 (d, *J* = 9.3 Hz), 120.65 (d, *J* = 14.8 Hz), 119.38 (q, *J* = 275.4 Hz), 118.43 (d, *J* = 24.1 Hz), 113.50 (s), 103.09 (q, *J* = 5.4 Hz), 89.73 (s), 69.24 (s), 68.91 (s), 58.80 (s), 40.80 (s), 32.72 (q, *J* = 3.5 Hz), 29.50 (s), 27.91 (s), 27.63 (s), 27.05 (s), 26.65 (s); HRMS, *m*/*z* calcd. for $C_{26}H_{29}ClF_4N_5O_7^+$ [M + H]$^+$ 634.16862, found 634.16809.

5-(4-(2-Chloro-4-fluoro-5-(3-methyl-2,6-dioxo-4-(trifluoromethyl)-3,6-dihydropyrimidin-1(2*H*)-yl)phenoxy)-1-(phenylamino)butylidene)-1,3-dimethylpyrimidine-2,4,6(1*H*,3*H*,5*H*)-trione (**BA-19**): white solid, yield 16%, m.p. 198–200 °C; ^1H NMR (500 MHz, $CDCl_3$) δ 14.14 (s, 1H), 7.41 (t, *J* = 7.5 Hz, 2H), 7.35 (t, *J* = 7.4 Hz, 1H), 7.22 (d, *J* = 8.9 Hz, 1H), 7.17 (d, *J* = 7.6 Hz, 2H), 6.68 (d, *J* = 6.3 Hz, 1H), 6.36 (s, 1H), 3.99 (t, *J* = 5.8 Hz, 2H), 3.56 (s, 3H), 3.37 (s, 3H), 3.33 (s, 3H), 3.27–3.20 (m, 2H), 2.08 (m, 2H); ^{13}C NMR (125 MHz, $CDCl_3$) δ 176.45 (s), 167.01 (s), 162.31 (s), 159.90 (s), 151.25 (s), 151.23 (d, *J* = 247.3 Hz), 150.85 (d, *J* = 2.5 Hz), 150.67 (s), 141.73 (q, *J* = 34.1 Hz), 136.00 (s), 129.75 (s), 128.37 (s), 126.28 (s), 124.62 (d, *J* = 9.3 Hz), 120.39 (d, *J* = 14.8 Hz), 119.38 (q, *J* = 275.1 Hz), 118.30 (d, *J* = 24.2 Hz), 113.24 (s), 103.07 (q, *J* = 5.2 Hz), 90.47 (s), 68.85 (s), 32.71 (q, *J* = 3.4 Hz), 28.04 (s), 27.96 (s), 27.81 (s), 27.73 (s); HRMS, *m*/*z* calcd. for $C_{28}H_{25}ClF_4N_5O_6^+$ [M + H]$^+$ 638.14240, found 638.14160.

5-(1-(Benzylamino)-4-(2-chloro-4-fluoro-5-(3-methyl-2,6-dioxo-4-(trifluoromethyl)-3,6-dihydropyrimidin-1(2*H*)-yl)phenoxy)butylidene)-1,3-dimethylpyrimidine-2,4,6(1*H*,3*H*,5*H*)-trione (**BA-20**): white solid, yield 36%, m.p. 234–236 °C; ^1H NMR (500 MHz, $CDCl_3$) δ 12.97 (s, 1H), 7.40 (t, *J* = 7.3 Hz, 2H), 7.36–7.29 (m, 4H), 6.80 (d, *J* = 6.3 Hz, 1H), 6.38 (s, 1H), 4.81 (d, *J* = 5.8 Hz, 2H), 4.13 (t, *J* = 5.4 Hz, 2H), 3.57 (s, 3H), 3.42 (dd, *J* = 9.3, 6.0 Hz, 2H), 3.32 (s, 3H), 3.31 (s, 3H), 2.18 (m, 2H); ^{13}C NMR (125 MHz, $CDCl_3$) δ 176.40 (s), 166.75 (s), 162.54 (s), 159.88 (s), 151.50 (d, *J* = 248.0 Hz), 151.30 (s), 151.02 (d, *J* = 2.6 Hz), 150.68 (s), 141.77 (q, *J* = 34.5 Hz), 135.64 (s), 129.21 (s), 128.26 (s), 127.29 (s), 124.56 (d, *J* = 9.5 Hz), 120.72 (d, *J* = 14.8 Hz), 119.39 (q, *J* = 275.6 Hz), 118.45 (d, *J* = 24.1 Hz), 113.68 (s), 103.09 (q, *J* = 5.2 Hz), 90.17 (s), 69.02 (s), 47.30 (s), 32.70 (q, *J* = 3.5 Hz), 27.95 (s), 27.68 (s), 27.18 (s), 26.95 (s); HRMS, *m*/*z* calcd. for $C_{29}H_{27}ClF_4N_5O_6^+$ [M + H]$^+$ 652.15805, found 652.15729.

3.2. Evaluation of Herbicidal Activity

According to the methods previously reported [11], the post-emergence herbicidal activities of target compounds **BA-1**~**BA-20** against four representative plants (i.e., *B.*

campestris, A. tricolor, E. crus-galli, D. sanguinalis) were evaluated in the greenhouse. Sixteen plants, including *B. campestris, A. tricolor, L. indica, P. oleracea, T. mongolicum, C. album, B. tripartita, I. nil, E. crus-galli, D. sanguinalis, S. viridis, E. indica, S. alterniflora, P. alopecuroides, C. virgata*, and *E. dahuricus*, were chosen to investigate the herbicidal spectrum of target compound **BA-1**. Briefly, 15~20 weed seeds were uniformly sown in an 8 cm × 7 cm × 7 cm plastic pot filled with a 2:1 (w/w) mixture of sandy soil and nutrient matrix. The seedlings were cultivated in a greenhouse maintained at 28 ± 2 °C under a 16 h light–8 h dark photoperiod. The tested compounds were initially dissolved in 100% DMF and subsequently diluted with Tween-80 (concentration: 100 g/L). The resulting solutions were further diluted with distilled water (pH 7.0) to the desired concentrations prior to application. When the second true leaves had fully expanded, the seedlings were thinned to 10 plants per pot and sprayed with the evaluated compounds using a laboratory sprayer (model: 3WP-2000, Nanjing Research Institute for Agricultural Mechanization, Nanjing, Ministry of Agriculture, China), equipped with a flat-fan nozzle delivering a spray volume of 280 L ha^{-1} at 230 kPa. The initial herbicidal screening was conducted at a dosage of 150 g ha^{-1} for all target compounds. In the subsequent screening, the dosages for the selected compounds **BA-1**, **BA-2**, **BA-5**, **BA-18**, and **BA-20** were set at 75, 37.5, and 18.8 g ha^{-1}, respectively. Flumiclorac-pentyl (FP) was employed as the positive control. A control group was treated with a mixture of distilled water, DMF, and Tween-80 in equal proportions. Each treatment was replicated three times, with a one-day interval between applications. After a 14-day observation period, the herbicidal activity of each compound was evaluated. The inhibition rate was calculated using the following formula: inhibition rate (%) = ((fresh weight of control − fresh weight of treatment)/fresh weight of control) × 100%.

3.3. Crop Safety

The assay method for crop safety followed procedures previously reported in the literature [11]. Four representative crop species, i.e., *T. aestivum, Z. mays, G. hirsutum*, and *G. max*, were selected for greenhouse-based crop safety evaluation. In detail, seeds of the selected crops were planted in plastic pots and grown under controlled greenhouse conditions. When the seedlings reached the four-leaf growth stage, they were sprayed with either of the test compounds, **BA-1** or FP, at a dosage of 37.5 g ha^{-1}. The application process was conducted in accordance with the methodology described in Section 3.2. Each treatment was replicated three times, with a one-day interval between applications. Crop injury was evaluated 14 days post-treatment and expressed as the percentage of visible damage observed.

3.4. Molecular Simulation Analysis

The crystal structure of protoporphyrinogen IX oxidase (PPO, EC 1.3.3.4) from *Nicotiana tabacum* (PDB ID: 1SEZ, *Nt*PPO) was selected as the target protein for molecular docking studies. The active site was identified based on the coordinates of the co-crystallized ligand OMN using AutoDock Tools. The chemical structures of the ligands **BA-1** and FP were constructed using ChemBioDraw Ultra 14.0 and subjected to energy minimization via the MM2 force field method in ChemBio3D Ultra 14.0. The optimized structures were saved in mol2 format and subsequently converted into pdbqt format using AutoDock Tools for molecular docking analysis. Prior to docking, all water molecules and non-native ligands were removed from the protein structure. Kollman atomic charges and polar hydrogen atoms were added to ensure accurate electrostatic interactions. Molecular docking simulations between **BA-1** or FP and *Nt*PPO were performed using AutoDock Vina 4.2 [37–39]. The resulting protein-ligand complexes were visualized and analyzed using PyMOL v1.3 [40].

The molecular dynamics (MD) simulations were performed in accordance with established protocols, encompassing system preparation, force field parameter assignment, definition of initial conditions, integration of equations of motion, and data acquisition [41]. All simulations were executed using GROMACS 2023.3 on an Ubuntu 20.04.1 Linux operating system [42]. To assess the stability of the interactions over time, the complexes formed by **BA-1** or FP with *Nt*PPO were simulated separately. Each simulation system underwent a 50 ns MD simulation. Upon completion, root-mean-square deviation (RMSD) values were computed and analyzed. A lower RMSD suggests a smaller deviation from the reference structure throughout the simulation, indicating enhanced conformational stability of the complex.

3.5. Statistical Analysis

The values shown in each table are mean values ± SD of at least three repeated experiments. DPS 7.05 data processing system (DPS, Hangzhou, China) was used as a statistical software program.

4. Conclusions

In summary, twenty novel 5-(1-amino-4-phenoxybutylidene)barbituric acid derivatives incorporating an enamino diketone motif were synthesized in moderate yields and evaluated for their herbicidal activity. The bioassay results in the greenhouse demonstrated that some of the target compounds, such as **BA-1, BA-2, BA-5, BA-18**, and **BA-20**, exhibited promising herbicidal activity, and **BA-1** was confirmed as a potential herbicide lead compound due to its excellent herbicidal activity, broad herbicidal spectrum and good crop safety. The SAR study revealed that the steric effect and electronic effects of R group and the lipophilicity of target compound displayed an important effect on herbicidal activity. The molecular simulation analysis revealed that **BA-1** could bind well with *Nt*PPO, which indicated that it might be a novel ACCase inhibitor. The present work suggested that **BA-1** could represent a potential lead compound for further developing novel PPO-inhibiting herbicides. Further study on the structural optimization of **BA-1** is ongoing in our laboratory.

Supplementary Materials: The following supporting information can be downloaded at https://www.mdpi.com/article/10.3390/molecules30163445/s1, Figures S1–S60: ^{1}HNMR, ^{13}CNMR, HRMS of the target compounds **BA-1** to **BA-20**.

Author Contributions: Conceptualization, K.L. and R.L.; methodology, K.L. and R.L.; software, W.G. and J.L.; validation, K.C., S.W., S.F. and Y.Z.; formal analysis, S.W., S.F., Y.Z. and J.L.; investigation, K.C.; resources, W.G., J.L. and K.L.; data curation, K.C.; writing—original draft preparation, K.C.; writing—review and editing, K.L. and R.L.; supervision, W.G., K.L. and R.L.; project administration, K.L.; funding acquisition, W.G. and K.L. All authors have read and agreed to the published version of the manuscript.

Funding: This project was financially supported by the Natural Science Foundation of Shandong Province (No. ZR2023MC095); the National Natural Science Foundation of China (Nos. 31701827 and 32402430); the China Postdoctoral Science Foundation (No. 2020M671984).

Institutional Review Board Statement: Not applicable.

Informed Consent Statement: Not applicable.

Data Availability Statement: The data are contained within the article; further inquiries can be directed to the corresponding authors.

Conflicts of Interest: The authors declare no conflicts of interest.

References

1. Jiang, X.; Yang, F.; Jia, W.; Jiang, Y.; Wu, X.; Song, S.; Shen, H.; Shen, J. Nanomaterials and nanotechnology in agricultural pesticide delivery: A review. *Langmuir* **2024**, *40*, 18806–18820. [CrossRef] [PubMed]
2. Zhang, B.; Lv, F.; Yang, J. Pesticides toxicity, removal and detoxification in plants: A Review. *Agronomy* **2024**, *14*, 1260. [CrossRef]
3. Giugliano, R.; Armenio, V.; Savio, V.; Vaccaro, E.; Ciccotelli, V.; Vivaldi, B. Monitoring of non-maximum-residue-level pesticides in animal feed: A study from 2019 to 2023. *Toxics* **2024**, *12*, 680. [CrossRef] [PubMed]
4. Oerke, E.C. Crop losses to pests. *J. Agric. Sci.* **2005**, *144*, 31–34. [CrossRef]
5. Peterson, M.A.; Collavo, A.; Ovejero, R.; Shivrain, V.; Walsh, M.J. The challenge of herbicide resistance around the world: A current summary. *Pest Manag. Sci.* **2018**, *74*, 2246–2259. [CrossRef]
6. Yang, R.; Lv, M.; Xu, H. Synthesis of piperine analogs containing isoxazoline/pyrazoline scaffold and their pesticidal bioactivities. *J. Agric. Food Chem.* **2018**, *66*, 11254–11264. [CrossRef]
7. Fang, J.P.; He, Z.Z.; Liu, T.T.; Li, J.; Dong, L.Y. A novel mutation Asp-2078-Glu in ACCase confers resistance to ACCase herbicides in barnyardgrass (*Echinochloa crus-galli*). *Pestic. Biochem. Physiol.* **2020**, *168*, 104634. [CrossRef]
8. Wang, J.Z.; Peng, Y.J.; Chen, W.; Yu, Q.; Bai, L.Y.; Pan, L. The Ile-2041-Val mutation in the ACCase gene confers resistance to clodinafop-propargyl in American sloughgrass (*Beckmannia syzigachne Steud*). *Pest Manag. Sci.* **2021**, *77*, 2425–2432. [CrossRef]
9. Darmency, H.; Colbach, N.; Corre, V.L. Relationship between weed dormancy and herbicide rotations: Implications in resistance evolution. *Pest Manag. Sci.* **2017**, *73*, 1994–1999. [CrossRef]
10. Chio, E.H.; Li, Q.X. Pesticide research and development: General discussion and Spinosad case. *J. Agric. Food Chem.* **2022**, *70*, 8913–8919. [CrossRef]
11. Han, S.B.; Wang, S.M.; Fu, S.Y.; Chen, K.; Gao, G.; Cheng, Y.N.; Liu, M.; Zhang, X.M.; Lei, K. Design, synthesis, and herbicidal activity of novel 5-acylbarbituric acid derivatives containing maleimide moieties and evaluation of their mode of action. *J. Agric. Food Chem.* **2025**, *73*, 11386–11398. [CrossRef]
12. Sun, S.S.; Kou, S.; Wang, W.F.; Li, Y.Z.; Wang, Z.R.; Huo, J.Q.; An, Z.X.; Zhu, L.; Chen, L.; Zhang, J.L. Synthesis of novel propionamide-methylpyrazole carboxylates as herbicidal candidates. *J. Agric. Food Chem.* **2024**, *72*, 21401–21409. [CrossRef]
13. Feng, T.; Liu, Q.; Xu, Z.Y.; Li, H.T.; Wei, W.; Shi, R.C.; Zhang, L.; Cao, Y.M.; Liu, S.Z. Design, synthesis, herbicidal activity, and structure-activity relationship study of novel 6-(5-aryl-substituted-1-pyrazolyl)-2-picolinic acid as potential herbicides. *Molecules* **2023**, *28*, 1431. [CrossRef] [PubMed]
14. Wang, D.W.; Zhang, R.B.; Yu, S.Y.; Liang, L.; Ismail, I.; Li, Y.H.; Xu, H.; Wen, X.; Xi, Z. Discovery of novel N-isoxazolinylphenyltriazinones as promising protoporphyrinogen IX oxidase inhibitors. *J. Agric. Food Chem.* **2019**, *67*, 12382–12392. [CrossRef] [PubMed]
15. Gross, E.M.; Wolk, C.P.; Jüttner, F. Fischerellin, a new allelochemical from the freshwater cyanobacterium *Fischerella musicola*. *J. Phycol.* **1991**, *27*, 686–692. [CrossRef]
16. Ding, L.; Dahse, H.-M.; Hertweck, C. Cytotoxic alkaloids from *Fusarium incarnatum* associated with the mangrove tree *Aegiceras corniculatum*. *J. Nat. Prod.* **2012**, *75*, 617–621. [CrossRef]
17. Avdović, E.H.; Stojković, D.L.; Jevtić, V.V.; Milenković, D.; Marković, Z.S.; Vuković, N.; Potočňák, I.; Radojević, I.D.; Čomić, L.R.; Trifunović, S.R. Preparation and antimicrobial activity of a new palladium(II) complexes with a coumarin-derived ligands. crystal structures of the 3-(1-(o-toluidino)ethylidene)-chroman-2,4-dione and 3-(1-(m-toluidino) ethylidene)-chroman-2,4-dione. *Inorg. Chim. Acta* **2019**, *484*, 52–59. [CrossRef]
18. Mladenović, M.; Vuković, N.; Nićiforović, N.; Sukdolak, S.; Solujić, S. Synthesis and molecular descriptor characterization of novel 4-hydroxy-chromene-2-one derivatives as antimicrobial agents. *Molecules* **2009**, *14*, 1495–1512. [CrossRef]
19. Baldwin, A.G.; Bevan, J.; Brough, D.; Ledder, R.; Freeman, S. Synthesis and antibacterial activities of enamine derivatives of dehydroacetic acid. *Med. Chem. Res.* **2018**, *27*, 884–889. [CrossRef]
20. Garmaise, D.L.; Chu, D.T.W.; Bernstein, E.; Inaba, M. Synthesis and antibacterial activity of 2′-substituted chelocardin analogues. *J. Med. Chem.* **1979**, *22*, 559–564. [CrossRef]
21. Bangalore, P.K.; Vagolu, S.K.; Bollikanda, R.K.; Veeragoni, D.K.; Choudante, P.C.; Misra, S.; Sriram, D.; Sridhar, B.; Kantevari, S. Usnic acid enaminone-coupled 1,2,3-triazoles as antibacterial and antitubercular agents. *J. Nat. Prod.* **2020**, *83*, 26–35. [CrossRef] [PubMed]
22. Canela, M.D.; Pérez-Pérez, M.J.; Noppen, S.; Sáez-Calvo, G.; Díaz, J.F.; Camarasa, M.J.; Liekens, S.; Priego, E.M. Novel colchicine-site binders with a cyclohexanedione scaffold identified through a ligand-based virtual screening approach. *J. Med. Chem.* **2014**, *57*, 3924–3938. [CrossRef] [PubMed]
23. Ilić, D.R.; Jevtić, V.V.; Radić, G.P.; Arsikin, K.; Ristić, B.; Harhaji-Trajković, L.; Vuković, N.; Sukdolak, S.; Klisurić, O.; Trajković, V.; et al. Synthesis, characterization and cytotoxicity of a new palladium(II) complex with a coumarine-derived ligand. *Eur. J. Med. Chem.* **2014**, *74*, 502–508. [CrossRef] [PubMed]

24. Budzisz, E.; Keppler, B.K.; Giester, G.; Wozniczka, M.; Kufelnicki, A.; Nawrot, B. Synthesis, crystal structure and biological characterization of a novel Palladium(II) complex with a coumarin-derived ligand. *Eur. J. Inorg. Chem.* **2004**, 22, 4412–4419. [CrossRef]
25. Budzisz, E.; Małecka, M.; Lorenz, I.P.; Mayer, P.; Kwiecien, R.A.; Paneth, P.; Krajewska, U.; Rozalski, M. Synthesis, cytotoxic effect, and structure–activity relationship of Pd(II) complexes with coumarin derivatives. *Inorg. Chem.* **2006**, *45*, 9688–9695. [CrossRef]
26. Budzisz, E.; Brzezinska, E.; Krajewska, U.; Rozalski, M. Cytotoxic effects, alkylating properties and molecular modelling of coumarin derivatives and their phosphonic analogues. *Eur. J. Med. Chem.* **2003**, *38*, 597–603. [CrossRef]
27. Dias, L.C.; Demuner, A.J.; Valente, V.V.M.; Barbosa, L.C.A.; Martins, F.T.; Doriguetto, A.C.; Ellena, J. Preparation of achiral and chiral (E)-enaminopyran-2,4-diones and their phytotoxic activity. *J. Agric. Food Chem.* **2009**, *57*, 1399–1405. [CrossRef]
28. Serban, A.; Watson, K.G.; Bird, G.J.; Farquharson, G.J.; Cross, L.E. Preparation of 2-[1-(Ethoxyimino)Propyl]-5-Indanylcyclohexene-1,3-Diones and Analogs as Herbicides and Plant Growth Regulators. US 4952722A, 28 August 1990.
29. Liu, Y.X.; Zhao, H.P.; Wang, Z.W.; ·Li, Y.H.; Song, H.B.; Riches, H.; Beattie, D.; Gu, Y.C.; Wang, Q.M. The discovery of 3-(1-aminoethylidene)quinoline-2,4(1*H*,3*H*)-dione derivatives as novel PSII electron transport inhibitors. *Mol. Divers.* **2013**, *17*, 701–710. [CrossRef]
30. Batran, R.Z.; Khedr, M.A.; Abdel Latif, N.A.; Abd El Aty, A.A.; Shehata, A.N. Synthesis, homology modeling, molecular docking, dynamics, and antifungal screening of new 4-hydroxycoumarin derivatives as potential chitinase inhibitors. *J. Mol. Struct.* **2019**, *1180*, 260–271. [CrossRef]
31. Lv, P.; Chen, Y.L.; Zhao, Z.; Shi, T.Z.; Wu, X.W.; Xue, J.Y.; Li, Q.X.; Hua, R.M. Design, synthesis, and antifungal activities of 3-acyl thiotetronic acid derivatives: New fatty acid synthase inhibitors. *J. Agric. Food Chem.* **2018**, *66*, 1023–1032. [CrossRef]
32. Neumann, D.M.; Cammarata, A.; Backes, G.; Palmer, G.E.; Jursic, B.S. Synthesis and antifungal activity of substituted 2,4,6-pyrimidinetrione carbaldehyde hydrazones. *Bioorg. Med. Chem.* **2014**, *22*, 813–826. [CrossRef] [PubMed]
33. Guo, H.Y.; Jin, C.M.; Zhang, H.M.; Jin, C.-M.; Shen, Q.K.; Quan, Z.S. Synthesis and biological evaluation of (+)-usnic acid derivatives as potential anti-toxoplasma gondii agents. *J. Agric. Food Chem.* **2019**, *67*, 9630–9642. [CrossRef] [PubMed]
34. Wang, C.C.; Chen, K.; Li, N.; Wang, X.K.; Wang, S.B.; Li, P.; Hua, X.W.; Lei, K.; Ji, L.S. Discovery of 3-(1-amino-2-phenoxyethylidene)-6-methyl-2*H*-pyran-2,4(3*H*)-dione derivatives as novel herbicidal leads. *Agronomy* **2022**, *12*, 202. [CrossRef]
35. Wang, C.C.; Liu, H.; Zhao, W.; Li, P.; Ji, L.S.; Liu, R.M.; Lei, K.; Xu, X.H. Synthesis and herbicidal activity of 5-(1-amino-2-phenoxyethylidene)barbituric acid derivatives. *Chin. J. Org. Chem.* **2021**, *41*, 2063–2073. [CrossRef]
36. Hwang, J.-I.; Norsworthy, J.K.; Gonzalez-Torralva, F.; Piveta, L.B.; Tom Barber, L.; Butts, T.R. Cross-resistance of Barnyardgrass [*Echinochloa crus-galli* (L.) P. Beauv.] to aryloxyphenoxypropionate herbicides. *Pest. Biochem. Physiol.* **2022**, *184*, 105089. [CrossRef]
37. Trott, O.; Olson, A.J. Autodock vina: Improving the speed and accuracy of docking with a new scoring function, efficient optimization, and multithreading. *J. Comput. Chem.* **2010**, *31*, 455–461. [CrossRef]
38. Tanchuk, V.Y.; Tanin, V.O.; Vovk, I.; Poda, G. A new improved hybrid scoring function for molecular docking and scoring based on autodock and autodock vina. *Chem. Biol. Drug Des.* **2016**, *87*, 618–625. [CrossRef]
39. Di, M.E.; Toti, D.; Polticelli, F. Dockingapp: A user friendly interface for facilitated docking simulations with autodock vina. *J. Comput. Aid. Mol. Des.* **2017**, *31*, 213–218.
40. Chaudhari, R.; Li, Z. Pymine: A pymol plugin to integrate and visualize data for drug discovery. *BMC Res. Notes* **2015**, *8*, 517. [CrossRef]
41. Lv, Y.; Li, K.; Lei, L.; Yu, Z.W.; Wu, R.Z.; Chen, A.K.; Tian, R.X.; Deng, Y.X.; Tang, L.F.; Fan, Z.J. Design, synthesis, and assessment of fungicidal activity of active substructure 1,2,4-triazole containing coumarin. *J. Agric. Food Chem.* **2024**, *72*, 27075–27083. [CrossRef]
42. Abraham, M.J.; Murtola, T.; Schulz, R.; Páll, S.; Smith, J.C.; Hess, B.; Lindahl, E. GROMACS: High performance molecular simulations through multi-level parallelism from laptops to supercomputers. *SoftwareX* **2015**, *1–2*, 19–25. [CrossRef]

molecules

MDPI

Article

Disubstituted Meldrum's Acid: Another Scaffold with SuFEx-like Reactivity

Baoqi Chen, Zhenguo Wang, Xiaole Peng, Jijun Xie, Zhixiu Sun and Le Li *

PCFM Lab and GDHPRC Lab, School of Chemistry, Sun Yat-sen University, Guangzhou 510275, China; benchan93@163.com (B.C.); wangzhg28@mail2.sysu.edu.cn (Z.W.); pengxle@mail2.sysu.edu.cn (X.P.); xiejj35@mail2.sysu.edu.cn (J.X.); sunzx1996@163.com (Z.S.)

* Correspondence: lile26@mail.sysu.edu.cn

Abstract

Sulfur Fluoride Exchange (SuFEx) chemistry represents an emerging class of click reactions that has found broad applications in drug discovery and materials science. Traditionally, SuFEx reactivity has been regarded as the exclusive privilege of sulfur and fluorine. Accordingly, the scaffolds exhibiting SuFEx-like reactivity without sulfur or fluorine have remained underdeveloped. Indeed, SuFEx reactions may represent a more generalizable mode of chemical reactivity. By enhancing the electrophilicity of the carbonyl group and increasing the steric hindrance around the carbon center, we identified disubstituted Meldrum's acid as a novel carbon-based scaffold with SuFEx-like reactivity. Various O-, S-, and N-nucleophiles are viable exchange partners in the presence of Barton's base or DBU. In addition to the original method, a catalytic protocol was developed and successfully applied to drug derivatization, including the gram-scale modification of acetaminophen.

Keywords: disubstituted Meldrum's acid; esterification; amidation; decarboxylation; SuFEx

1. Introduction

The concept of Sulfur Fluoride Exchange (SuFEx) [1–6], first introduced by Sharpless and coworkers, represents a unique class of nucleophilic exchange reactions in which stable sulfur(VI) fluoride compounds can be selectively activated under specific environments [7–12], in the presence of promoters [13,14], or under catalytic conditions [15–20] to form covalent linkages. This "dormant awakening reactivity" has enabled broad applications across chemical biology [21–27], drug discovery [28–38], and materials science [39–52]. Initially, SuFEx reactivity was attributed to the distinctive characteristics of the S(VI)–F bond (Scheme 1a). Following this paradigm, a variety of building blocks containing an S–F bond have been developed, greatly expanding the SuFEx toolbox [53–65]. However, the reliance on either sulfur or fluorine elements in SuFEx chemistry has been challenged by recent discoveries. For instance, Zuilhof and coworkers introduced the concept of sulfur-phenolate exchange (SuPhenEx) in their latest work, demonstrating that S(VI) centers can undergo efficient exchange reactions without the involvement of fluorine (Scheme 1b) [66–69]. In 2023, Moses and coworkers discovered a set of phosphorus-based exchange reactions, termed Phosphorus Fluoride Exchange (PFEx), wherein P(V) fluorides exhibit similar latent reactivity with nucleophiles (Scheme 1c) [70–73]. These findings suggest that SuFEx-like reactivity may not be limited to S- or F-based systems, but rather represent a more general reactivity mode for robust covalent bond formation. Therefore, it is highly desirable to discover new scaffolds capable of mimicking SuFEx-type reactivity. Herein, we report a carbon-based scaffold, disubstituted Meldrum's acid, that exhibits SuFEx-like reactivity under mild conditions (Scheme 1d).

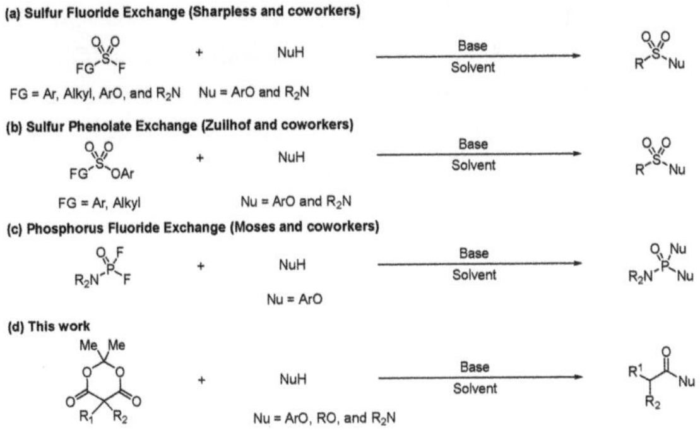

Scheme 1. Development of novel scaffolds with SuFEx reactivity.

Acyl fluorides were the original candidates for this project. However, due to the relatively low steric hindrance around the acyl carbon, acyl fluorides, despite their high exchange reactivity, exhibited significantly lower hydrolytic stability compared to S(VI)–fluorides. This limitation led us to shift our focus to other carbonyl compounds with high intrinsic reactivity. Ultimately, disubstituted Meldrum's acid was identified as a promising candidate. Although Meldrum's acid may seem unrelated to SuFEx-like reactivity at first glance, its cyclic ester structure [74–78] endows it with both high electrophilicity and hydrolytic stability. This pairing of electrophilicity and stability strongly resonates with the design principles of conventional SuFEx reagents. (Figure 1). In addition, disubstituted Meldrum's acids are highly tunable building blocks and can be readily prepared from Meldrum's acid via alkylations, Michael additions, and reductive Knoevenagel condensations [79,80]. This ease of double substitution imparts remarkable structural diversity to disubstituted Meldrum's acids, which in turn facilitates multidimensional connectivity via nucleophilic ring-opening reactions. Meanwhile, disubstituted Meldrum's acids possess markedly enhanced stability relative to their less substituted counterparts. However, several challenges persist in the proposed decarboxylative nucleophilic ring-opening reaction. Notably, while the nucleophilic ring-opening of disubstituted Meldrum's acids occurs readily [79,81–89], only a very limited number of them undergo decarboxylation under mild conditions [90–92]. In many cases, decarboxylation still requires elevated temperatures or the use of excess reagents to achieve efficient conversion [93–101]. These existing conditions fail to meet the standards of SuFEx chemistry. Therefore, a facile protocol compatible with more complex synthetic settings is highly desirable.

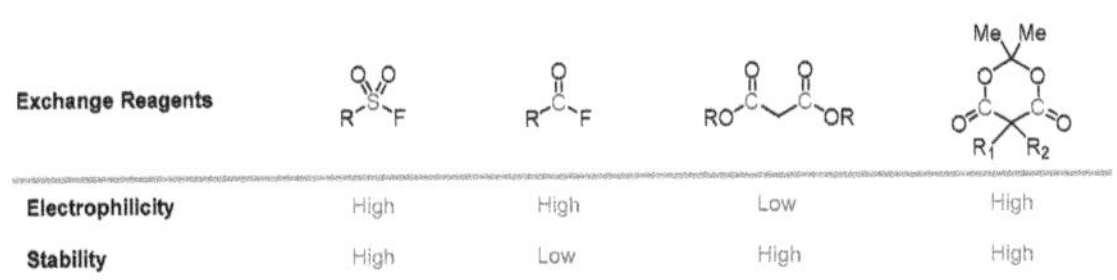

Figure 1. The design of carbon exchange reagents.

2. Results

Initially, we chose **2a** as a nucleophile to investigate the nucleophilic exchange reactions of **1a**. A control experiment conducted in the absence of any base showed no formation of the expected product, and **1a** remained intact (Table 1, entry 1). In addition, either inorganic bases or weaker organic bases resulted in negligible formation of **3a** (Table 1, entries 2–8). Further investigation revealed that **1a** was completely consumed when a strong inorganic base, such as cesium carbonate, potassium carbonate, or potassium phosphate, was used. In these cases, the nucleophilic ring-opening product, malonate half ester **3a'** was obtained instead of **3a**. In the other cases using sodium carbonate, 4-dimethylaminopyridine (DMAP), triethylamine (TEA), and *N*,*N*-diisopropylethylamine (DIPEA), most of 1a remained unchanged. Gratifyingly, both nucleophilic substitution and decarboxylation proceeded smoothly at room temperature in the presence of 1,8-diazabicyclo[5.4.0]undec-7-ene (DBU) or Barton's base (2-tert-Butyl-1,1,3,3-tetramethylguanidine, BTMG) (Table 1, entry 9–10). These results were somewhat unexpected, as the decarboxylation of malonate half-esters typically requires elevated temperatures. Next, we extended the reaction time from 4 h to 12 h and evaluated the compatibility of this reaction with a variety of common solvents (Table 1, entries 11–16). To our delight, nearly quantitative yields were obtained in acetonitrile, toluene, tetrahydrofuran (THF), *N*-methyl-pyrrolidinone (NMP), and dimethyl sulfoxide (DMSO), while a slightly lower yield (87%) was observed in dichloromethane. To evaluate the potential applicability of this transformation in biological settings, aqueous DMSO solutions were tested, and satisfactory yields were obtained (Table 1, entries 17–18). The high efficiency of this transformation across various solvents aligned well with the principles of click chemistry.

Table 1. Optimization of reaction conditions[a].

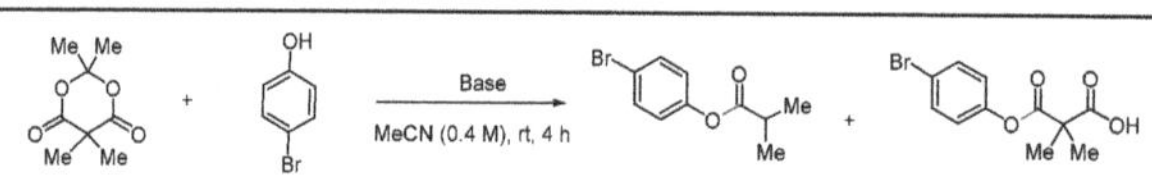

1a 2a 3a 3a'

Entry	Base	Solvent	Time(h)	3a[b](%)
1	none	MeCN	4	0
2	Cs_2CO_3	MeCN	4	2
3	K_2CO_3	MeCN	4	0
4	K_3PO_4	MeCN	4	0
5	Na_2CO_3	MeCN	4	0
6	DMAP	MeCN	4	0
7	TEA	MeCN	4	0
8	DIPEA	MeCN	4	2
9	DBU	MeCN	4	65
10	BTMG	MeCN	4	82
11	BTMG	MeCN	12	100
12	BTMG	Dichloromethane	12	87
13	BTMG	Toluene	12	100
14	BTMG	Tetrahydrofuran	12	100
15	BTMG	*N*-methyl-pyrrolidinone	12	100
16	BTMG	Dimethyl sulfoxide	12	99
17[c]	BTMG	Dimethyl sulfoxide	1	87
18[d]	BTMG	Dimethyl sulfoxide	1	80

[a] Reactions were run with **1a** (0.10 mmol), *p*-bromophenol (1.10 equiv), and base (1.10 equiv) in anhydrous acetonitrile (250.0 μL) at rt for 4 h. [b] Yields were determined by ^1H NMR with 1,3,5-trimethoxybenzene as an internal standard. [c] Reactions were run in 5% H_2O–DMSO at 60 °C for 1 h. [d] Reactions were run in 20% H_2O–DMSO at 60 °C for 1 h.

With the optimal protocol in hand, the substrate scope was acid and phenolic nucleophiles were well tolerated and α,α-disubstituted phenyl acetates were obtained in excellent isolated yields (**3a–3y**) (Figure 2). For the Meldrum's acid component, we focus on evaluating the substrates with a larger alkyl group. The results indicated that a variety of benzyl-substituted substrates afforded excellent yields (**3f–3j**). Notably, more sterically hindered alkyl substrates (**1b–1e**) also provided satisfactory results. For phenolic nucleophiles, we examined the influence of functional group tolerance, electronic properties, and steric hindrance. The method demonstrated excellent tolerance toward diverse functional groups. A wide array of α,α-disubstituted phenylacetates bearing diverse functional groups such as halogens (**3t**, **3x**, and **3y**), trifluoromethyl (**3l**), amino (**3n**), alkoxy (**3o** and **3w**), nitro (**3k**), ester (**3p**), aldehyde (**3q**), alkenyl (**3w**), and various heterocycles (**3m**, **3x**, and **3y**), were obtained in excellent yields. Although the method was generally insensitive to electronic effects, the most electron-deficient phenol, 4-nitrophenol (**2k**), and the most electron-rich one, 4-dimethylaminophenol (**2n**), required a more polar solvent, NMP, and a more concentrated condition (0.8 M) to complete the reaction at room temperature. In terms of steric effects, *ortho*-substituted substrates (**2s**, **2t**, and **2u**) and 1-naphthol (**2r**) reacted smoothly under standard conditions. The only exception was the highly sterically hindered 2,6-dimethylphenol (**2v**), which required heating at 60 °C to achieve full conversion.

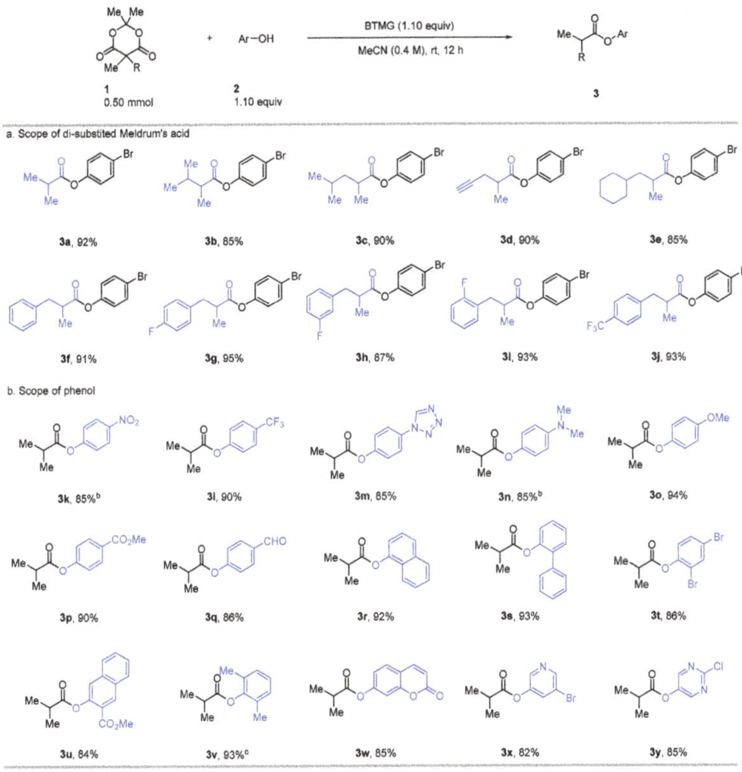

Figure 2. The scope of disubstituted Meldrum's acids and phenolic nucleophiles[a]. [a]Reactions were run with **1** (0.50 mmol, 1.00 equiv), **2** (0.55 mmol, 1.10 equiv), and BTMG (0.55 mmol, 1.10 equiv) in anhydrous acetonitrile (1.25 mL) at rt for 12 h. All yields were isolated yields. [b]Reactions were run in NMP (625.0 μL). [c]Reaction was run at 60 °C.

Next, we turned our attention to the use of alcohols, thiols, and amines as nucleophilic partners. Several representative nucleophiles were selected for evaluation. Not surprisingly, no desired α,α-disubstituted acetate products were obtained when alcohols were used as nucleophiles under the standard conditions developed for phenols, even at 40 °C. However, small amounts of the desired products could be detected upon raising the reaction temperature to 60 °C in acetonitrile. Analysis of the reaction mixtures revealed that the major products under these conditions were the non-decarboxylated malonate half-esters. To improve the yield of the expected ester product, we employed NMP as the solvent to promote decarboxylation. Gratifyingly, this subtle adjustment successfully led to the formation of the desired esters (**4a, 4b, 4c**, and **4d**) in high yields from alcohol nucleophiles (Figure 3). Indeed, primary alcohols such as (4-bromophenyl)methanol and 3-phenylpropan-1-ol, as well as secondary diphenylmethanol, reacted smoothly at 60 °C. Furthermore, cyclohexanol, due to its increased steric hindrance, required the use of a less hindered base (DBU) in place of BTMG, along with a slightly higher temperature (80 °C) to afford the product **4d**. Interestingly, the reactivity of thiol and thiophenol more closely resembles that of phenols rather than alcohols. Thioesters (**4e** and **4f**) were delivered in excellent yields at room temperature. Encouraged by these results, we further increased the reaction temperature to 100 °C for amidations and confirmed that primary amines were viable nucleophiles under elevated temperature (Figure 3). The corresponding amide products (**4g, 4h, 4i**, and **4j**) were obtained at 100 °C in satisfactory yields. We also investigated a secondary amine (morpholine) as the nucleophile. As a result, **4k** was obtained in 62% isolated yield using the conditions for primary amines. As anticipated, the sterically hindered tert-butanol and tert-butylamine did not undergo nucleophilic exchange reactions and failed to yield the desired products **4l** and **4m** even at 100 °C.

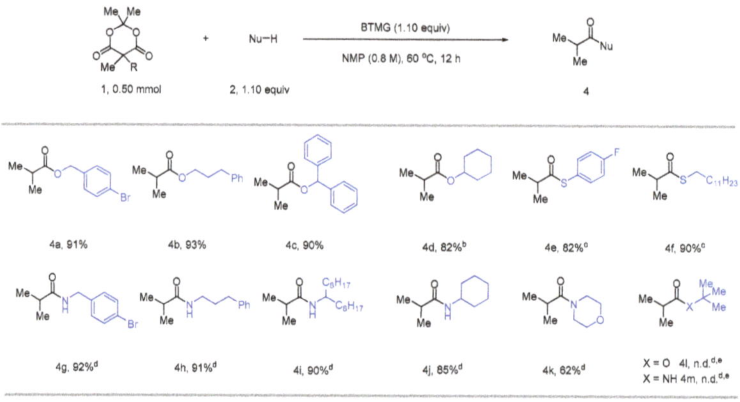

Figure 3. The scope of alcohol, thiols, and amine nucleophiles[a]. [a]Reactions were run with **1a** (0.50 mmol, 1.00 equiv), **2** (0.55 mmol, 1.10 equiv), and BTMG (0.55 mmol, 1.10 equiv) in NMP (625.0 µL) at 60 °C for 12 h. All yields were isolated yields. [b]Reaction was run with using DBU instead of BTMG at 80 °C for 12 h. [c]Reaction was run in anhydrous acetonitrile (1.25 mL) at rt for 12 h. [d]Reactions were run at 100 °C in NMP (1.25 mL). [e]n.d. = not detected.

After evaluating the scope of nucleophilic exchange partners, we sought to improve the practicality of the current methodology in scalable synthesis. To avoid the use of stoichiometric amounts of BTMG, we aimed to develop a catalytic protocol for this transformation. Acetaminophen, a widely used over-the-counter (OTC) fever and pain reliever, was selected as the model substrate. Gratifyingly, using a catalytic amount of BTMG in NMP at 60 °C for 12 h, the desired acylated product was obtained in 96% yield on a 2.12 g scale (Scheme 2a). In addition, we are able to isolate the malonate half-ester **5** by using a modified protocol (Scheme 2b). Subsequently, the Curtius rearrangement of **5** successfully delivered the valuable α-amino acid derivatives **6** in 76% yield (Scheme 2c). Further investigation revealed that the isolation of the malonate half-ester **5** was not required. Accordingly, a one-pot synthesis of malonyl monoester amide **7** from **1a** and **2** was successfully achieved (Scheme 2d).

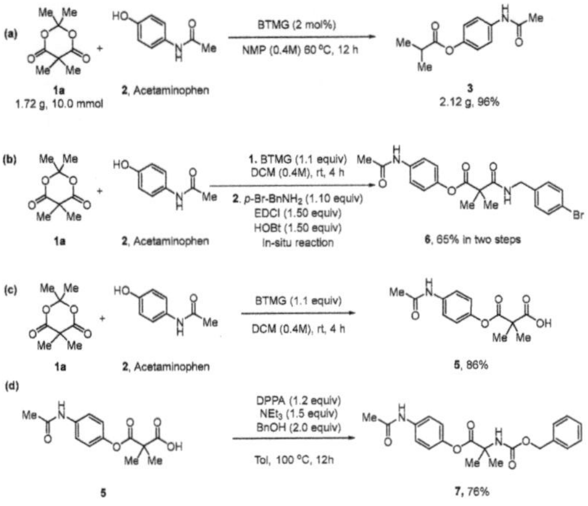

Scheme 2. Preparation-scale derivatization of Acetaminophen.

Based on the experimental data we obtained, a plausible catalytic cycle is proposed. The reaction proceeds via decarboxylation of the malonate half-ester followed by reprotonation (Scheme 3) [102,103]. The superior results obtained with BTMG, in contrast to inorganic bases, are likely due to its excellent solubility in various organic solvents, which is particularly important for facilitating the decarboxylation. This pathway is distinct from the ketene mechanism observed under thermal conditions (>150 °C) [104–107]. To further support this mechanistic proposal, the malonate half-ester **3a′** was treated with a stoichiometric amount of BTMG at room temperature. The decarboxylation of **3a′** occurred readily, affording the product **3a** (see Supplementary Materials).

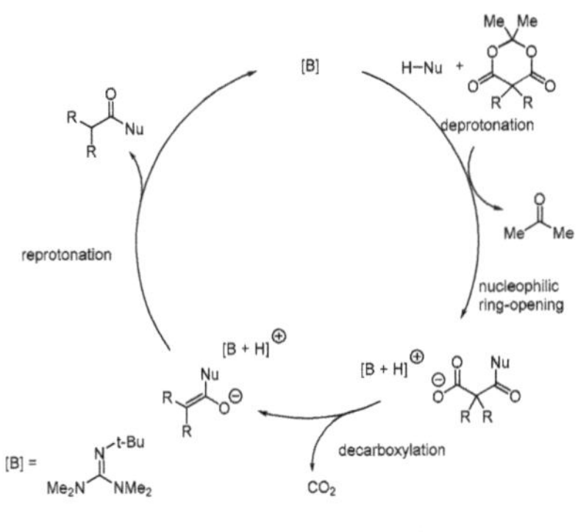

Scheme 3. Proposed Catalytic Cycle.

3. Materials and Methods

3.1. Reagents and General Methods

All reagents were purchased from commercial sources(Energy Chemical, Shanghai, China) and used without further purification unless otherwise noted. Acetonitrile, *N*-methyl-pyrrolidinone and dimethyl sulfoxide used in the reactions were anhydrous solvents purchased from commercial suppliers (Energy Chemical, Shanghai, China) and used without further drying (≥99.9%, LC-MS, Energy Chemical, China). The petroleum ether (Energy Chemical, Shanghai, China) used was in a boiling range of 60–90 °C. Other solvents were purified according to standard procedures [108]. All reactions were carried out with oven-dried glassware and monitored by thin-layer chromatography (0.20 mm

HP-TLC silica gel 60 GF-254 plates, Leyan, Shanghai, China). Visualization was accomplished with UV light, and/or potassium permanganate, or 2% ninhydrin in ethanol stain followed by heating. Flash column chromatography was performed on 200–300 mesh silica gel (Leyan, Shanghai, China). Meldrum's acid (2,2-dimethyl-1,3-dioxane-4,6-dione) and 5-methyl Meldrum's acid (2,2,5-trimethyl-1,3-dioxane-4,6-dione) were purchased from Bide Pharm, Shanghai, China, and used without further purification. The deuterated chloroform ($CDCl_3$) (Energy Chemical, Shanghai, China) used contains 0.03% (*v*/*v*) of tetramethylsilane (TMS).

^{1}H, ^{19}F, and ^{13}C NMR spectra were recorded on a Bruker AVANCE III 400 MHz spectrometer (Bruker, Billerica, MA, USA) at 298 K and referenced to residual protium in the NMR solvent ($CDCl_3$, δ 7.26, DMSO-d_6, 2.50 in ^{1}H NMR) and the carbon resonances of the solvent ($CDCl_3$, δ 77.16, DMSO-d_6, 39.52 in ^{13}C NMR). Chemical shifts were reported in parts per million (ppm, δ) downfield from tetramethylsilane. NMR peaks are described as singlet (s), doublet (d), triplet (t), quartet (q), multiplet (m), heptet (hept), complex (comp), and approximate (app). High-resolution mass spectra (HRMS) were recorded on a Thermo Fisher Scientific's Q Exactive UHMR Hybrid Quadrupole-Orbitrap Mass Spectrometer LC/MS (ESI/APCI) (Thermo Fisher, Waltham, MA, USA).

TEAF = triethylammonium formate, TEA = triethylamine, DIPEA = *N*,*N*-diisopropylethylamine, DBU = 1,8-diazabicyclo[5.4.0]undec-7-ene, DMAP = 4-dimethylaminopyridine, BTMG = 2-*tert*-butyl-1,1,3,3-tetramethylguanidine, NMI = *N*-methylimidazole, DPPA = diphenyl azidophosphate, HOBt = 1-hydroxybenzotriazole, EDC = 1-ethyl-3-(3-dimethylaminopropyl) carbodiimide, EA = ethyl acetate, DMF = *N*,*N*-dimethylformamide, DCM = dichloromethane, DCE = dichloroethane, DMSO = dimethyl sulfoxide, THF = tetrahydrofuran, NMP = *N*-methylpyrrolidinone, TLC = thin-layer chromatography, *v*/*v* = volume per volume, equiv = equivalent, w/o = without, rt = room temperature.

3.2. Synthetic Procedures

3.2.1. A General Procedure for the 5-Substituted-5-methyl-1,3-dioxane-4,6-dione

General Procedure: Substituted-Meldrum's acids were prepared according to the literature procedure [109]. 5-methyl Meldrum's acid (1.00 equiv) and K_2CO_3 (1.30 equiv) were dissolved in anhydrous DMF, followed by the addition of alkyl bromide (1.20 equiv). The mixture was then heated to 60 °C for 12 h. After reaction completion, the mixture was diluted with 50 mL of EA and 50 mL of water. The organic phase was separated. The aqueous phase was further extracted with 2 × 50 mL of EA. The combined organic layer was separated, washed with saturated aqueous $NaHCO_3$ solution and saturated aqueous NaCl solution, dried over anhydrous sodium sulfate, and concentrated in vacuo to afford the crude product. The crude product was purified by flash column chromatography to afford the purified product.

3.2.2. A General Procedure for the Preparation of the Esters **3**

In a 4.0-mL vial, 5,5-substituted-Meldrum's acid **1** (0.50 mmol, 1.00 equiv), BTMG (94.2 mg, 0.55 mmol, 1.10 equiv) were dissolved in anhydrous MeCN (1.25 mL). The phenol (0.55 mmol, 1.10 equiv) was added and stirred at rt for 12 h. After the reaction was completed, the mixture was diluted with EA (20 mL), washed with 2 M aqueous HCl solution (15 mL). The organic layer was separated, washed with saturated brine (20 mL), dried over anhydrous sodium sulfate, filtered, and concentrated in vacuo. The crude product was then purified by silica gel column chromatography.

4-Bromophenyl isobutyrate (**3a**): Compound **3a** was prepared according to the general procedure using **1a** (86.0 mg, 0.50 mmol, 1.00 equiv) and *p*-bromophenol (95.2 mg, 0.55 mmol, 1.10 equiv) at rt for 12 h. Purification by flash column chromatography (petroleum ether/ethyl acetate = 20/1, *v*/*v*) afforded 4-bromophenyl isobutyrate (**3a**) as a colorless oil (111.8 mg, 92%). R_f = 0.40 (petroleum ether/ethyl acetate = 40/1, *v*/*v*). **^{1}H NMR** (400 MHz, $CDCl_3$) δ 7.48 (d, *J* = 7.5 Hz, 2H), 6.97 (d, *J* = 7.5 Hz, 2H), 2.79 (hept, *J* = 6.9 Hz, 1H), 1.31 (d, *J* = 6.9 Hz, 6H). **^{13}C NMR** (101 MHz, $CDCl_3$) δ 175.3, 149.9, 132.4 (2C), 123.4 (2C), 118.7, 34.2, 18.9 (2C). **HRMS−ESI** (*m*/*z*) for $C_{10}H_{11}BrO_2$ $[M + Na]^+$: calcd 264.9834 (^{79}Br), 266.9814 (^{81}Br), found 264.9835 (^{79}Br), 266.9814 (^{81}Br).

4-Bromophenyl 2,3-dimethylbutanoate (**3b**): Compound **3b** was prepared according to the general procedure using **1b** (100.0 mg, 0.50 mmol, 1.00 equiv) and *p*-bromophenol (95.2 mg, 0.55 mmol, 1.10 equiv) at rt for 12 h. Purification by flash column chromatography (petroleum ether/ethyl acetate = 20/1, *v*/*v*) afforded 4-bromophenyl 2,3-dimethylbutanoate (**3b**) as a colorless oil (115.2 mg, 85%). **R_f** = 0.40 (petroleum ether/ethyl acetate = 40/1, *v*/*v*). **^{1}H NMR** (400 MHz, $CDCl_3$) δ 7.5 (d, *J* = 8.8 Hz, 2H), 7.0 (d, *J* = 8.9 Hz, 2H), 2.5 (m, 1H), 2.1 (m, 1H), 1.3 (d, *J* = 7.1 Hz, 3H), 1.04 (d, *J* = 6.8 Hz, 1H), 1.00 (d, *J* = 6.7 Hz, 1H). **^{13}C NMR** (101 MHz, $CDCl_3$) δ 174.5, 149.9, 132.4 (2C), 123.4 (2C), 118.7, 46.2, 31.2, 20.7, 19.2, 13.7. **HRMS−ESI** (*m*/*z*) for $C_{12}H_{15}BrO_2$ $[M + Na]^+$: calcd 293.0147 (^{79}Br), 295.0127 (^{81}Br), found 293.0149 (^{79}Br), 295.0127 (^{81}Br).

4-Bromophenyl 2,4-dimethylpentanoate (**3c**): Compound **3c** was prepared according to the general procedure using **1c** (107.0 mg, 0.50 mmol, 1.00 equiv) and *p*-bromophenol (95.2 mg, 0.55 mmol, 1.10 equiv) at rt for 12 h. Purification by flash column chromatography (petroleum ether/ethyl acetate = 20/1, *v*/*v*) afforded 4-bromophenyl 2,4-dimethylpentanoate (**3c**) as a colorless oil (126.4 mg, 90%). **R_f** = 0.40 (petroleum ether/ethyl acetate = 40/1, *v*/*v*). **^{1}H NMR** (400 MHz, $CDCl_3$) δ 7.48 (d, *J* = 8.8 Hz, 2H), 6.96 (d, *J* = 8.7 Hz, 2H), 2.84–2.64 (m, 1H), 1.83–1.64 (comp, 2H), 1.42–1.31 (m, 1H), 1.28 (d, *J* = 6.9 Hz, 3H), 0.97 (d, *J* = 6.2 Hz, 1H), 0.94 (d, *J* = 6.1 Hz, 1H). **^{13}C NMR** (101 MHz, $CDCl_3$) δ 175.4, 150.0, 132.5 (2C), 123.5 (2C), 118.9, 43.0, 37.9, 26.2, 22.7, 22.6, 17.5. **HRMS−ESI** (*m*/*z*) for $C_{13}H_{17}BrO_2$ $[M + Na]^+$: calcd 307.0304 (^{79}Br), 309.0283 (^{81}Br), found 307.0304 (^{79}Br), 309.0288 (^{81}Br).

4-Bromophenyl 2-methylpent-4-ynoate (**3d**): Compound **3d** was prepared according to the general procedure using **1d** (98.0 mg, 0.50 mmol, 1.00 equiv) and *p*-bromophenol (95.2 mg, 0.55 mmol, 1.10 equiv) at rt for 12 h. Purification by flash column chromatography (petroleum ether/ethyl acetate = 20/1, *v*/*v*) afforded 4-bromophenyl 2-methylpent-4-ynoate (**3d**) as a colorless oil (121.9 mg, 90%). **R_f** = 0.40 (petroleum ether/ethyl acetate = 40/1, *v*/*v*). **^{1}H NMR** (400 MHz, $CDCl_3$) δ 7.49 (d, *J* = 8.9 Hz, 2H), 6.99 (d, *J* = 8.8 Hz, 2H), 2.91 (m, 1H), 2.59 (comp, 2H), 2.06 (s, 1H), 1.41 (d, *J* = 7.1 Hz, 3H). **^{13}C NMR** (101 MHz, $CDCl_3$) δ 173.1, 149.9, 132.6 (2C), 123.5 (2C), 119.1, 81.0, 70.5, 39.0, 22.9, 16.4. **HRMS−ESI** (*m*/*z*) for $C_{12}H_{11}BrO_2$ $[M + Na]^+$: calcd 288.9835 (^{79}Br), 290.9815 (^{81}Br), found 288.9831 (^{79}Br), 290.9815 (^{81}Br).

4-Bromophenyl 3-cyclohexyl-2-methylpropanoate (**3e**): Compound **3e** was prepared according to the general procedure using **1e** (127.0 mg, 0.50 mmol, 1.00 equiv) and *p*-bromophenol (95.2 mg, 0.55 mmol, 1.10 equiv) at rt for 12 h. Purification by flash column chromatography (petroleum ether/ethyl acetate = 20/1, *v*/*v*) afforded 4-bromophenyl 3-cyclohexyl-2-methylpropanoate (**3e**) as a colorless oil (137.7 mg, 85%). **R_f** = 0.40 (petroleum ether/ethyl acetate = 40/1, *v*/*v*). **^{1}H NMR** (400 MHz, $CDCl_3$) δ 7.48 (d, *J* = 8.8 Hz, 2H), 6.96 (d, *J* = 8.8 Hz, 2H), 2.84–2.71 (m, 1H), 1.84–1.62 (comp, 6H), 1.37 (comp, 2H), 1.27 (d, *J* = 6.9 Hz, 3H), 1.23–1.10 (comp, 3H), 0.93 (comp, 2H). **^{13}C NMR** (101 MHz, $CDCl_3$) δ 175.5, 150.1, 132.6 (2C), 123.5 (2C), 118.8, 41.6, 37.2, 35.7, 33.5, 33.3, 26.7, 26.4, 26.4, 17.6. **HRMS−ESI** (*m*/*z*) for $C_{16}H_{21}BrO_2$ $[M + Na]^+$: calcd 347.0617 (^{79}Br), 349.0596 (^{81}Br), found 347.0617 (^{79}Br), 349.0598 (^{81}Br).

4-Bromophenyl 2-methyl-3-phenylpropanoate (**3f**): Compound **3f** was prepared according to the general procedure using **1f** (124.0 mg, 0.50 mmol, 1.00 equiv) and *p*-bromophenol

(95.2 mg, 0.55 mmol, 1.10 equiv) at rt for 12 h. Purification by flash column chromatography (petroleum ether/ethyl acetate = 20/1, *v*/*v*) afforded 4-bromophenyl 2-methyl-3-phenylpropanoate (**3f**) as a colorless oil (145.2 mg, 91%). $\mathbf{R}_f$ = 0.40 (petroleum ether/ethyl acetate = 40/1, *v*/*v*). ^{1}**H NMR** (400 MHz, $CDCl_3$) δ 7.44 (d, *J* = 8.4 Hz, 2H), 7.31 (m, 2H), 7.23 (comp, 3H), 6.79 (d, *J* = 8.3 Hz, 2H), 3.09 (dd, *J* = 13.3, 7.7 Hz, 1H), 2.99 (m, 1H), 2.83 (dd, *J* = 13.3, 6.6 Hz, 1H), 1.32 (d, *J* = 6.6 Hz, 3H). ^{13}**C NMR** (101 MHz, $CDCl_3$) δ 174.4, 149.8, 139.0, 132.5 (2C), 129.2 (2C), 128.6 (2C), 126.7, 123.4 (2C), 118.9, 41.8, 40.0, 17.1. **HRMS—ESI** (*m*/*z*) for $C_{16}H_{15}BrO_2$ $[M + Na]^+$: calcd 341.0148 (^{79}Br), 343.0128 (^{81}Br), found 341.0149 (^{79}Br), 343.0132 (^{81}Br).

4-Bromophenyl 3-(4-fluorophenyl)-2-methylpropanoate (**3g**): Compound **3g** was prepared according to the general procedure using **1g** (133.0 mg, 0.50 mmol, 1.00 equiv) and *p*-bromophenol (95.2 mg, 0.55 mmol, 1.10 equiv) at rt for 12 h. Purification by flash column chromatography (petroleum ether/ethyl acetate = 20/1, *v*/*v*) afforded 4-bromophenyl 3-(4-fluorophenyl)-2-methylpropanoate (**3g**) as a colorless oil (151.7 mg, 95%). $\mathbf{R}_f$ = 0.40 (petroleum ether/ethyl acetate = 40/1, *v*/*v*). ^{1}**H NMR** (400 MHz, $CDCl_3$) δ 7.46 (d, *J* = 8.8 Hz, 2H), 7.19 (dd, *J* = 8.3, 5.4 Hz, 2H), 7.00 (t, *J* = 8.5 Hz, 2H), 6.81 (d, *J* = 8.8 Hz, 2H), 3.07 (dd, *J* = 13.4, 7.7 Hz, 1H), 2.94 (m, 1H), 2.81 (dd, *J* = 13.4, 6.8 Hz, 1H), 1.31 (d, *J* = 6.9 Hz, 3H). ^{19}**F NMR** (377 MHz, $CDCl_3$) δ −116.4. ^{13}**C NMR** (101 MHz, $CDCl_3$) δ 174.2, 161.9 (d, J_{C-F} = 244.7 Hz), 149.8, 134.7 (d, J_{C-F} = 3.2 Hz), 132.6 (2C), 130.6 (d, J_{C-F} = 7.8 Hz, 2C), 123.4 (2C), 119.0, 115.5 (d, J_{C-F} = 21.2 Hz, 2C), 41.9, 39.1, 17.0. **HRMS—ESI** (*m*/*z*) for $C_{16}H_{14}BrFO_2$ $[M + Na]^+$: calcd 359.0053 (^{79}Br), 361.0033 (^{81}Br), found 359.0052 (^{79}Br), 361.0035 (^{81}Br).

4-Bromophenyl 3-(3-fluorophenyl)-2-methylpropanoate (**3h**): Compound **3h** was prepared according to the general procedure using **1h** (133.0 mg, 0.50 mmol, 1.00 equiv) and *p*-bromophenol (95.2 mg, 0.55 mmol, 1.10 equiv) at rt for 12 h. Purification by flash column chromatography (petroleum ether/ethyl acetate = 20/1, *v*/*v*) afforded 4-bromophenyl 3-(3-fluorophenyl)-2-methylpropanoate (**3h**) as a colorless oil (146.7 mg, 87%). $\mathbf{R}_f$ = 0.40 (petroleum ether/ethyl acetate = 40/1, *v*/*v*). ^{1}**H NMR** (400 MHz, $CDCl_3$) δ 7.46 (d, *J* = 8.8 Hz, 2H), 7.26 (m, 1H), 7.00 (m, 1H), 6.95 (comp, 2H), 6.83 (d, *J* = 8.4 Hz, 2H), 3.10 (dd, *J* = 13.4, 7.7 Hz, 1H), 2.98 (m, 1H), 2.82 (dd, *J* = 13.4, 6.9 Hz, 1H), 1.32 (d, *J* = 6.9 Hz, 3H). ^{19}**F NMR** (377 MHz, $CDCl_3$) δ −113.3. ^{13}**C NMR** (101 MHz, $CDCl_3$) δ 174.0, 162.9 (d, J_{C-F} = 246.0 Hz), 149.6, 141.4 (d, J_{C-F} = 7.2 Hz), 132.4 (2C), 130.0 (d, J_{C-F} = 8.3 Hz), 124.7 (d, J_{C-F} = 2.9 Hz), 123.2 (2C), 118.9, 115.9 (d, J_{C-F} = 21.1 Hz), 113.6 (d, J_{C-F} = 21.1 Hz), 41.4, 39.4, 17.0. **HRMS—ESI** (*m*/*z*) for $C_{16}H_{14}BrFO_2$ $[M + Na]^+$: calcd 359.0053 (^{79}Br), 361.0033 (^{81}Br), found 359.0052 (^{79}Br), 361.0032 (^{81}Br).

4-Bromophenyl 3-(2fluorophenyl)-2-methylpropanoate (**3i**): Compound **3i** was prepared according to the general procedure using **1i** (133.0 mg, 0.50 mmol, 1.00 equiv) and *p*-bromophenol (95.2 mg, 0.55 mmol, 1.10 equiv) at rt for 12 h. Purification by flash column chromatography (petroleum ether/ethyl acetate = 20/1, *v*/*v*) afforded 4-bromophenyl 3-(2-fluorophenyl)-2-methylpropanoate (**3i**) as a colorless oil (143.3 mg, 93%). $\mathbf{R}_f$ = 0.40 (petroleum ether/ethyl acetate = 40/1, *v*/*v*). ^{1}**H NMR** (400 MHz, $CDCl_3$) δ 7.45 (d, *J* = 8.8 Hz, 2H), 7.25–7.17 (comp, 2H), 7.11–7.00 (comp, 2H), 6.82 (d, *J* = 8.8 Hz, 2H), 3.14–2.99 (comp, 2H), 2.97–2.85 (m, 1H), 1.33 (d, *J* = 6.6 Hz, 3H). ^{19}**F NMR** (377 MHz, $CDCl_3$) δ −117.6. ^{13}**C NMR** (101 MHz, $CDCl_3$) δ 174.1, 161.4 (d, J_{C-F} = 245.3 Hz), 149.7, 132.4 (2C), 131.5 (d, J_{C-F} = 4.7 Hz), 128.5 (d, J_{C-F} = 8.2 Hz), 125.8 (d, J_{C-F} = 15.7 Hz), 124.1 (d, J_{C-F} = 3.6 Hz), 123.3 (2C), 118.8, 115.4 (d, J_{C-F} = 22.1 Hz), 40.2, 33.2 (d, J_{C-F} = 2.1 Hz), 17.0. **HRMS—ESI** (*m*/*z*) for $C_{16}H_{14}BrFO_2$ $[M + Na]^+$: 359.0053 (^{79}Br), 361.0033 (^{81}Br), found 359.0054 (^{79}Br), 361.0033 (^{81}Br).

4-Bromophenyl 3-cyclohexyl-2-methylpropanoate (**3j**): Compound **3j** was prepared according to the general procedure using **1j** (158.0 mg, 0.50 mmol, 1.00 equiv) and *p*-bromophenol

(95.2 mg, 0.55 mmol, 1.10 equiv) at rt for 12 h. Purification by flash column chromatography (petroleum ether/ethyl acetate = 20/1, v/v) afforded 4-bromophenyl 3-cyclohexyl-2-methylpropanoate (**3j**) as a colorless oil (168.0 mg, 93%). $\mathbf{R}_f$ = 0.40 (petroleum ether/ethyl acetate = 40/1, v/v). **^{1}H NMR** (400 MHz, $CDCl_3$) δ 7.57 (d, J = 7.9 Hz, 2H), 7.46 (d, J = 8.8 Hz, 2H), 7.35 (d, J = 7.9 Hz, 2H), 6.80 (d, J = 8.9 Hz, 2H), 3.16 (dd, J = 13.4, 7.7 Hz, 1H), 3.01 (m, 1H), 2.88 (dd, J = 13.4, 7.0 Hz, 1H), 1.34 (d, J = 6.8 Hz, 3H). **^{19}F NMR** (377 MHz, $CDCl_3$) δ –62.8. **^{13}C NMR** (101 MHz, $CDCl_3$) δ 173.9, 149.7, 143.1, 132.6 (2C), 129.5 (2C), 129.1 (q, J_{C-F} = 32.1 Hz), 125.6 (q, J_{C-F} = 3.8 Hz, 2C), 124.3 (q, J_{C-F} = 272.0 Hz), 123.3 (2C), 119.1, 41.5, 39.5, 17.1. **HRMS—ESI** (m/z) for $C_{17}H_{14}BrF_3O_2$ $[M + Na]^+$: calcd 409.0021 (^{79}Br), 411.0001 (^{81}Br), found 409.0025 (^{79}Br), 411.0014 (^{81}Br).

4-Nitrophenyl isobutyrate (**3k**): Compound **3k** was prepared according to the general procedure using **1a** (86.0 mg, 0.50 mmol, 1.00 equiv) and *p*-nitrophenol (76.5 mg, 0.55 mmol, 1.10 equiv) at rt for 12 h. Purification by flash column chromatography (petroleum ether/ethyl acetate = 10/1, v/v) afforded 4-nitrophenyl isobutyrate (**3k**) as a white solid (88.8 mg, 85%). The NMR data of **3k** were in agreement with the literature data [109]. $\mathbf{R}_f$ = 0.50 (petroleum ether/ethyl acetate = 10/1, v/v). **HRMS—ESI** (m/z) for $C_{10}H_{11}NO_4$ $[M + Na]^+$: calcd 232.0581, found 232.0580.

4-(Trifluoromethyl)phenyl isobutyrate (**3l**): Compound **3l** was prepared according to the general procedure using **1a** (86.0 mg, 0.50 mmol, 1.00 equiv) and 4-(trifluoromethyl)phenol (89.2 mg, 0.55 mmol, 1.10 equiv) at rt for 12 h. Purification by flash column chromatography (petroleum ether/ethyl acetate = 40/1, v/v) afforded 4-(trifluoromethyl)phenyl isobutyrate (**3l**) as a colorless oil (104.4 mg, 90%). $\mathbf{R}_f$ = 0.40 (petroleum ether/ethyl acetate = 40/1, v/v). **^{1}H NMR** (400 MHz, $CDCl_3$) δ 7.64 (d, J = 8.6 Hz, 2H), 7.20 (d, J = 8.6 Hz, 2H), 2.82 (hept, J = 7.0 Hz, 1H), 1.33 (d, J = 7.0 Hz, 6H). **^{19}F NMR** (377 MHz, $CDCl_3$) δ –62.2. **^{13}C NMR** (101 MHz, $CDCl_3$) δ175.1, 153.4, 128.1 (q, J_{C-F} = 31.2 Hz), 126.7 (q, J_{C-F} = 3.8 Hz, 2C), 126.2 (q, J_{C-F} = 271.3 Hz), 122.0 (2C), 34.2, 18.8 (2C). **HRMS—ESI** (m/z) for $C_{11}H_{11}F_3O_2$ $[M + Na]^+$: calcd 255.0603, found 255.0607.

4-(1H-Tetrazol-1-yl)phenyl isobutyrate (**3m**): Compound **3m** was prepared according to the general procedure using **1a** (86.0 mg, 0.50 mmol, 1.00 equiv) and 4-(1H-tetrazol-1-yl)phenol (89.2 mg, 0.55 mmol, 1.10 equiv) at rt for 12 h. Purification by flash column chromatography (petroleum ether/ethyl acetate = 10/1, v/v) afforded 4-(1H-tetrazol-1-yl)phenyl isobutyrate (**3m**) as a colorless oil (98.7 mg, 85%). $\mathbf{R}_f$ = 0.35 (petroleum ether/ethyl acetate = 10/1, v/v). **^{1}H NMR** (400 MHz, $CDCl_3$) δ 8.97 (s, 1H), 7.72 (d, J = 8.6 Hz, 2H), 7.33 (d, J = 8.6 Hz, 2H), 2.85 (hept, J = 7.0 Hz, 1H), 1.35 (d, J = 7.0 Hz, 6H). **^{13}C NMR** (101 MHz, $CDCl_3$) δ 175.1, 151.9, 140.6, 131.1, 123.5 (2C), 122.5 (2C), 34.2, 18.8 (2C). **HRMS—ESI** (m/z) for $C_{11}H_{12}N_4O_2$ $[M + Na]^+$: calcd 255.0852, found 255.0854.

4-(Dimethylamino)phenyl isobutyrate (**3n**): Compound **3n** was prepared according to the general procedure using **1a** (86.0 mg, 0.50 mmol, 1.00 equiv) and 4-(dimethylamino)phenol (75.4 mg, 0.55 mmol, 1.10 equiv) at rt for 12 h. Purification by flash column chromatography (petroleum ether/ethyl acetate = 20/1, v/v) afforded 4-(dimethylamino)phenyl isobutyrate (**3n**) as a white solid (88.0 mg, 85%). $\mathbf{R}_f$ = 0.40 (petroleum ether/ethyl acetate = 40/1, v/v). **mp** 59–60 °C (petroleum ether). **^{1}H NMR** (400 MHz, $CDCl_3$) δ 6.93 (d, J = 9.1 Hz, 2H), 6.70 (d, J = 9.0 Hz, 2H), 2.92 (s, 6H), 2.76 (hept, J = 7.0 Hz, 1H), 1.30 (d, J = 7.0 Hz, 6H). **^{13}C NMR** (101 MHz, $CDCl_3$) δ 176.2, 148.7, 141.8, 121.7 (2C), 113.2 (2C), 41.0 (2C), 34.1, 19.0 (2C). **HRMS—ESI** (m/z) for $C_{12}H_{17}NO_2$ $[M + H]^+$: calcd 208.1332, found 208.1334.

4-Methoxyphenyl isobutyrate (**3o**): Compound **3o** was prepared according to the general procedure using **1a** (86.0 mg, 0.50 mmol, 1.00 equiv) and 4-methoxyphenol (68.3 mg, 0.55 mmol, 1.10 equiv) at rt for 12 h. Purification by flash column chromatography (petroleum ether/ethyl acetate = 20/1, v/v) afforded 4-methoxyphenyl isobutyrate (**3o**) as a colorless oil (91.2 mg, 94%). The NMR data of **3o** were in agreement with the literature data [110]. $\mathbf{R}_f$ = 0.40 (petroleum ether/ethyl acetate = 20/1, *v*/*v*). **HRMS—ESI** (*m*/*z*) for $C_{11}H_{14}O_3$ [M + Na]$^+$: calcd 217.0835, found 217.0837.

Methyl 4-(isobutyryloxy)benzoate (**3p**): Compound **3p** was prepared according to the general procedure using **1a** (86.0 mg, 0.50 mmol, 1.00 equiv) and methyl 4-hydroxybenzoate (83.7 mg, 0.55 mmol, 1.10 equiv) at rt for 4 h. Purification by flash column chromatography (petroleum ether/ethyl acetate = 20/1, *v*/*v*) afforded methyl 4-(isobutyryloxy)benzoate (**3p**) as a colorless oil (100.0 mg, 90%). $\mathbf{R}_f$ = 0.40 (petroleum ether/ethyl acetate = 40/1, *v*/*v*). ^{1}**H NMR** (400 MHz, $CDCl_3$) δ 8.07 (d, *J* = 9.1 Hz, 2H), 7.15 (d, *J* = 9.1 Hz, 2H), 3.91 (s, 3H), 2.81 (hept, *J* = 7.0 Hz, 1H), 1.32 (d, *J* = 6.9 Hz, 6H). ^{13}**C NMR** (101 MHz, $CDCl_3$) δ 175.1, 166.4, 154.6, 131.1 (2C), 127.6, 121.6 (2C), 52.2, 34.2, 18.9 (2C). **HRMS—ESI** (*m*/*z*) for $C_{12}H_{14}O_4$ [M + Na]$^+$: calcd 245.0785, found 245.0787.

4-Formylphenyl isobutyrate (**3q**): Compound **3q** was prepared according to the general procedure using **1a** (86.0 mg, 0.50 mmol, 1.00 equiv) and 4-hydroxybenzaldehyde (67.2 mg, 0.55 mmol, 1.10 equiv) at rt for 12 h. Purification by flash column chromatography (petroleum ether/ethyl acetate = 20/1, *v*/*v*) afforded 4-formylphenyl isobutyrate (**3q**) as a colorless oil (82.6 mg, 86%). $\mathbf{R}_f$ = 0.40 (petroleum ether/ethyl acetate = 40/1, *v*/*v*). ^{1}**H NMR** (400 MHz, $CDCl_3$) δ 9.99 (s, 1H), 7.92 (d, *J* = 8.5 Hz, 2H), 7.27 (d, *J* = 8.4 Hz, 2H), 2.83 (hept, *J* = 6.9 Hz, 1H), 1.35 (d, *J* = 6.9 Hz, 6H). ^{13}**C NMR** (101 MHz, $CDCl_3$) δ 190.9, 174.9, 155.7, 133.9, 131.2 (2C), 122.3 (2C), 34.3, 18.8 (2C). **HRMS—ESI** (*m*/*z*) for $C_{11}H_{12}O_3$ [M + Na]$^+$: calcd 215.0679, found 215.0681.

Naphthalen-1-yl isobutyrate (**3r**): Compound **3r** was prepared according to the general procedure using **1a** (86.0 mg, 0.50 mmol, 1.00 equiv) and naphthalen-1-ol (79.3 mg, 0.55 mmol, 1.10 equiv) at rt for 12 h. Purification by flash column chromatography (petroleum ether/ethyl acetate = 20/1, *v*/*v*) afforded naphthalen-1-yl isobutyrate (**3r**) as a colorless oil (98.6mg, 92%). $\mathbf{R}_f$ = 0.40 (petroleum ether/ethyl acetate = 40/1, *v*/*v*). ^{1}**H NMR** (400 MHz, $CDCl_3$) δ 8.00–7.86 (comp, 2H), 7.77 (d, *J* = 8.3 Hz, 1H), 7.60–7.46 (comp, 3H), 7.28 (d, *J* = 7.4 Hz, 1H), 3.04 (hept, *J* = 7.0 Hz, 1H), 1.49 (d, *J* = 7.0 Hz, 6H). ^{13}**C NMR** (101 MHz, $CDCl_3$) δ 175.6, 146.7, 134.7, 128.1, 127.0, 126.4, 126.4, 125.9, 125.4, 121.1, 118.0, 34.5, 19.2 (2C). **HRMS—ESI** (*m*/*z*) for $C_{14}H_{14}O_2$ [M + Na]$^+$: calcd 237.0886, found 237.0887.

[1,1′-Biphenyl]-2-yl isobutyrate (**3s**): Compound **3s** was prepared according to the general procedure using **1a** (86.0 mg, 0.50 mmol, 1.00 equiv) and [1,1′-biphenyl]-2-ol (93.6 mg, 0.55 mmol, 1.10 equiv) at rt for 12 h. Purification by flash column chromatography (petroleum ether/ethyl acetate = 20/1, *v*/*v*) afforded [1,1′-biphenyl]-2-yl isobutyrate (**3s**) as a colorless oil (111.7 mg, 93%). $\mathbf{R}_f$ = 0.40 (petroleum ether/ethyl acetate = 40/1, *v*/*v*). ^{1}**H NMR** (400 MHz, $CDCl_3$) δ 7.45–7.29 (comp, 8H), 7.13 (d, *J* = 7.9 Hz, 1H), 2.62 (hept, *J* = 6.9 Hz, 1H), 1.10 (d, *J* = 6.8 Hz, 6H). ^{13}**C NMR** (101 MHz, $CDCl_3$) δ 175.4, 147.9, 137.6, 135.2, 130.9, 129.1 (2C), 128.5, 128.1 (2C), 127.4, 126.1, 122.8, 34.1, 18.7 (2C). **HRMS—ESI** (*m*/*z*) for $C_{16}H_{16}O_2$ [M + Na]$^+$: calcd 263.1042, found 263.1044.

2,4-Dibromophenyl isobutyrate (**3t**): Compound **3t** was prepared according to the general procedure using **1a** (86.0 mg, 0.50 mmol, 1.00 equiv) and 2,4-dibromophenol (138.5 mg, 0.55 mmol, 1.10 equiv) at rt for 12 h. Purification by flash column chromatography (petroleum ether/ethyl acetate = 20/1, *v*/*v*) afforded methyl 2,4-dibromophenyl isobutyrate (**3t**) as a colorless oil (137.2 mg, 86%). $\mathbf{R}_f$ = 0.40 (petroleum ether/ethyl acetate = 40/1, *v*/*v*). ^{1}**H NMR** (400 MHz, $CDCl_3$) δ 7.46 (d, *J* = 8.7 Hz, 1H), 7.33–7.22 (comp, 2H), 2.86 (hept, *J* = 7.0 Hz, 1H), 1.36 (d, *J* = 7.0 Hz, 6H). ^{13}**C NMR** (101 MHz, $CDCl_3$) δ 174.2, 148.9, 134.2, 130.3, 127.1, 121.1, 115.3, 34.2, 18.9 (2C). **HRMS—ESI** (*m*/*z*) for $C_{10}H_{10}{}^{79}Br_2O_2$ [M + Na]$^+$: calcd 342.8940, found 342.8944; $C_{10}H_{10}{}^{79}Br^{81}Br\ O_2$ [M + Na]$^+$: calcd 344.8920, found 344.8919.

Methyl 3-(isobutyryloxy)-2-naphthoate (**3u**): Compound **3u** was prepared according to the general procedure using **1a** (86.0 mg, 0.50 mmol, 1.00 equiv) and methyl 3-hydroxy-

2-naphthoate (111.2 mg, 0.55 mmol, 1.10 equiv) at rt for 12 h. Purification by flash column chromatography (petroleum ether/ethyl acetate = 20/1, *v*/*v*) afforded methyl 3-(isobutyryloxy)-2-naphthoate (**3u**) as a white solid (114.7 mg, 84%). **R**$_f$ = 0.40 (petroleum ether/ethyl acetate = 20/1, *v*/*v*). **mp** 58–59 °C (petroleum ether). ^{1}**H NMR** (400 MHz, $CDCl_3$) δ 8.58 (s, 1H), 7.93 (d, *J* = 8.2 Hz, 1H), 7.80 (d, *J* = 8.2 Hz, 1H), 7.63–7.48 (comp, 3H), 3.92 (s, 3H), 2.93 (hept, *J* = 7.0 Hz, 1H), 1.39 (d, *J* = 7.1 Hz, 6H). ^{13}**C NMR** (101 MHz, $CDCl_3$) δ176.1, 165.3, 147.0, 135.7, 133.7, 130.7, 129.1, 128.9, 127.3, 126.6, 122.5, 121.1, 52.3, 34.3, 19.0 (2C). **HRMS—ESI** (*m*/*z*) for $C_{16}H_{16}O_4$ $[M + Na]^+$: calcd 295.0941, found 295.0943.

2,6-Dimethylphenyl isobutyrate (**3v**): Compound **3v** was prepared according to the general procedure using **1a** (86.0 mg, 0.50 mmol, 1.00 equiv) and 2,6-dimethylphenol (68.2 mg, 0.55 mmol, 1.10 equiv) at 60 °C for 12 h. Purification by flash column chromatography (petroleum ether/ethyl acetate = 20/1, *v*/*v*) afforded 2,6-dimethylphenyl isobutyrate (**3v**) as a colorless oil (89.4 mg, 93%). **R**$_f$ = 0.40 (petroleum ether/ethyl acetate = 40/1, *v*/*v*). ^{1}**H NMR** (400 MHz, $CDCl_3$) δ 7.15–6.93 (comp, 3H), 2.87 (hept, *J* = 7.0 Hz, 1H), 2.13 (s, 6H), 1.36 (d, *J* = 7.0 Hz, 6H). ^{13}**C NMR** (101 MHz, $CDCl_3$) δ 174.7, 148.1, 130.1, 128.6 (2C), 125.7 (2C), 34.3, 19.2 (2C), 16.3 (2C). **HRMS—ESI** (*m*/*z*) for $C_{12}H_{16}O_2$ $[M + Na]^+$: calcd 215.1042, found 215.1041.

2-Oxo-2H-chromen-7-yl isobutyrate (**3w**): Compound **3w** was prepared according to the general procedure using **1a** (86.0 mg, 0.50 mmol, 1.00 equiv) and 7-hydroxy-2H-chromen-2-one (89.2 mg, 0.55 mmol, 1.10 equiv) at rt for 12 h. Purification by flash column chromatography (petroleum ether/ethyl acetate = 20/1, *v*/*v*) afforded 2-oxo-2H-chromen-7-yl isobutyrate (**3w**) as a white solid (98.7 mg, 85%). **R**$_f$ = 0.45 (petroleum ether/ethyl acetate = 20/1, *v*/*v*). **mp** 104–105 °C (petroleum ether). ^{1}**H NMR** (400 MHz, $CDCl_3$) δ 7.69 (d, *J* = 9.5 Hz, 1H), 7.49 (d, *J* = 8.4 Hz, 1H), 7.10 (s, 1H), 7.04 (d, *J* = 8.4 Hz, 1H), 6.39 (d, *J* = 9.5 Hz, 1H), 2.84 (hept, *J* = 7.0 Hz, 1H), 1.34 (d, *J* = 6.9 Hz, 6H). ^{13}**C NMR** (101 MHz, $CDCl_3$) δ 174.9, 160.4, 154.7, 153.5, 142.9, 128.5, 118.4, 116.6, 116.0, 110.4, 34.2, 18.8 (2C). **HRMS—ESI** (*m*/*z*) for $C_{13}H_{12}O_4$ $[M + Na]^+$: calcd 255.0628, found 255.0628.

5-Bromopyridin-3-yl isobutyrate (**3x**): Compound **3x** was prepared according to the general procedure using **1a** (86.0 mg, 0.50 mmol, 1.00 equiv) and 5-bromopyridin-3-ol (95.7 mg, 0.55 mmol, 1.10 equiv) at rt for 12 h. Purification by flash column chromatography (petroleum ether/ethyl acetate = 20/1, *v*/*v*) afforded 5-bromopyridin-3-yl isobutyrate (**3x**) as a colorless oil (100.1 mg, 82%). **R**$_f$ = 0.45 (petroleum ether/ethyl acetate = 20/1, *v*/*v*). ^{1}**H NMR** (400 MHz, $CDCl_3$) δ 8.57 (s, 1H), 8.38 (s, 1H), 7.71 (s, 1H), 2.86 (hept, *J* = 7.0 Hz, 1H), 1.35 (d, *J* = 7.0 Hz, 6H). ^{13}**C NMR** (101 MHz, $CDCl_3$) δ 174.6, 147.9, 147.5, 141.6, 132.1, 119.9, 34.1, 18.8 (2C). **HRMS—ESI** (*m*/*z*) for $C_9H_{10}BrNO_2$ $[M + H]^+$: calcd 243.9968 (^{79}Br), 245.9947 (^{81}Br), found 243.9970 (^{79}Br), 245.9948 (^{81}Br).

2-Chloropyrimidin-5-yl isobutyrate (**3y**): Compound **3y** was prepared according to the general procedure using **1a** (86.0 mg, 0.50 mmol, 1.00 equiv) and 2-chloropyrimidin-5-ol (71.8 mg, 0.55 mmol, 1.10 equiv) at rt for 12 h. Purification by flash column chromatography (petroleum ether/ethyl acetate = 20/1, *v*/*v*) afforded 2-chloropyrimidin-5-yl isobutyrate (**3y**) as a colorless oil (85.3 mg, 85%). **R**$_f$ = 0.45 (petroleum ether/ethyl acetate = 20/1, *v*/*v*). ^{1}**H NMR** (400 MHz, $CDCl_3$) δ 8.50 (s, 2H), 2.87 (hept, *J* = 7.0 Hz, 1H), 1.34 (d, *J* = 7.0 Hz, 6H). ^{13}**C NMR** (101 MHz, $CDCl_3$) δ 174.1, 157.1, 152.6 (2C), 145.1, 34.1, 18.7 (2C). **HRMS—ESI** (*m*/*z*) for $C_8H_9ClN_2O_2$ $[M + H]^+$: calcd 201.0426, found 201.0426.

3.2.3. A General Procedure for Alcohols, Thiol, Thiophenol, and Amines

In a 4.0-mL vial, 2,2,5,5-tetramethyl-1,3-dioxane-4,6-dione (**1a**) (86.0 mg, 0.50 mmol, 1.00 equiv), BTMG (94.2 mg, 0.55 mmol, 1.10 equiv) were dissolved in anhydrous NMP (625.0 μL). Then, the nucleophile (0.55 mmol, 1.10 equiv) was added, and the mixture was stirred at 60 °C for 12 h. After the reaction was completed, the mixture was diluted with

EA (20 mL) and washed with 2 M aqueous HCl solution (15 mL). The organic layer was separated, washed with saturated brine (20 mL), dried over anhydrous sodium sulfate, filtered, and concentrated in vacuo. The crude product was then purified by silica gel column chromatography.

4-Bromobenzyl isobutyrate (**4a**): Compound **4a** was prepared according to the general procedure using **1a** (86.0 mg, 0.50 mmol, 1.00 equiv) and (4-bromophenyl)methanol (102.9 mg, 0.55 mmol, 1.10 equiv) at 60 °C for 12 h. Purification by flash column chromatography (petroleum ether/ethyl acetate = 20/1, v/v) afforded 4-bromobenzyl isobutyrate (**4a**) as a colorless oil (117.0 mg, 91%). $\mathbf{R_f}$ = 0.55 (petroleum ether/ethyl acetate = 20/1, v/v). **^{1}H NMR** (400 MHz, $CDCl_3$) δ 7.49 (d, J = 8.3 Hz, 2H), 7.22 (d, J = 8.3 Hz, 2H), 5.06 (s, 2H), 2.59 (hept, J = 7.0 Hz, 1H), 1.18 (d, J = 7.1 Hz, 6H). **^{13}C NMR** (101 MHz, $CDCl_3$) δ 176.8, 135.3, 131.7 (2C), 129.7 (2C), 122.1, 65.2, 34.0, 19.0 (2C). **HRMS—ESI** (m/z) for $C_{11}H_{13}BrO_2$ $[M + Na]^+$: calcd 278.9992 (^{79}Br), 280.9971 (^{81}Br), found 278.9991 (^{79}Br), 280.9977 (^{81}Br).

3-Phenylpropyl isobutyrate (**4b**): Compound **4b** was prepared according to the general procedure using **1a** (86.0 mg, 0.50 mmol, 1.00 equiv) and 3-phenylpropanol (74.9 mg, 0.55 mmol, 1.10 equiv) at 60 °C for 12 h. Purification by flash column chromatography (petroleum ether/ethyl acetate = 20/1, v/v) afforded 3-phenylpropyl isobutyrate (**4b**) as a colorless oil (96.0 mg, 93%). $\mathbf{R_f}$ = 0.55 (petroleum ether/ethyl acetate = 20/1, v/v). **^{1}H NMR** (400 MHz, $CDCl_3$) δ 7.33–7.24 (m, 2H), 7.23–7.15 (comp, 3H), 4.09 (t, J = 6.5 Hz, 2H), 2.69 (t, J = 7.7 Hz, 2H), 2.55 (hept, J = 7.0 Hz, 1H), 1.96 (tt, J = 14.0, 6.5 Hz, 2H), 1.18 (d, J = 7.0 Hz, 6H). **^{13}C NMR** (101 MHz, $CDCl_3$) δ 177.2, 141.3, 128.45 (2C), 128.41 (2C), 126.0, 63.5, 34.1, 32.2, 30.3, 19.0 (2C). **HRMS—ESI** (m/z) for $C_{13}H_{18}O_2$ $[M + Na]^+$: calcd 229.1199, found 229.1201.

Benzhydryl isobutyrate (**4c**): Compound **4c** was prepared according to the general procedure using **1a** (86.0 mg, 0.50 mmol, 1.00 equiv) and diphenylmethanol (101.3 mg, 0.55 mmol, 1.10 equiv) at 60 °C for 12 h. Purification by flash column chromatography (petroleum ether/ethyl acetate = 20/1, v/v) afforded benzhydryl isobutyrate (**4c**) as a colorless oil (114.4 mg, 90%). $\mathbf{R_f}$ = 0.55 (petroleum ether/ethyl acetate = 20/1, v/v). **^{1}H NMR** (400 MHz, $CDCl_3$) δ 7.39–7.27 (comp, 10H), 6.86 (s, 1H), 2.67 (hept, J = 7.0 Hz, 1H), 1.21 (d, J = 6.9 Hz, 6H). **^{13}C NMR** (101 MHz, $CDCl_3$) δ 176.0, 140.5 (2C), 128.5 (4C), 127.8 (2C), 127.0 (4C), 76.6, 34.2, 18.9 (2C). **HRMS—ESI** (m/z) for $C_{17}H_{18}O_2$ $[M + Na]^+$: calcd 277.1199, found 277.1198.

Cyclohexyl isobutyrate (**4d**): Compound **4d** was prepared according to the general procedure using **1a** (86.0 mg, 0.50 mmol, 1.00 equiv) and cyclohexanol (55.1 mg, 0.55 mmol, 1.10 equiv) at 80 °C for 12 h. Purification by flash column chromatography (petroleum ether/ethyl acetate = 20/1, v/v) afforded cyclohexyl isobutyrate (**4d**) as a colorless oil (69.8 mg, 82%). $\mathbf{R_f}$ = 0.55 (petroleum ether/ethyl acetate = 20/1, v/v). The NMR data of **4d** were in agreement with the literature data [111]. **HRMS—ESI** (m/z) for $C_{10}H_{18}O_2$ $[M + Na]^+$: calcd 193.1199, found 193.1205.

S-(4-Fluorophenyl) 2-methylpropanethioate (**4e**): Compound **4e** was prepared according to the general procedure using **1a** (86.0 mg, 0.50 mmol, 1.00 equiv) and 4-fluorothiophenol (74.5 mg, 0.55 mmol, 1.10 equiv) at rt for 12 h. Purification by flash column chromatography (petroleum ether/ethyl acetate = 10/1, v/v) afforded S-(4-fluorophenyl) 2-methylpropanethioate (**4e**) as a colorless oil (81.2 mg, 82%). $\mathbf{R_f}$ = 0.65 (petroleum ether/ethyl acetate = 10/1, v/v). **^{1}H NMR** (400 MHz, $CDCl_3$) δ 7.41–7.33 (m, 2H), 7.14–7.05 (m, 2H), 2.86 (hept, J = 6.9 Hz, 1H), 1.26 (d, J = 6.8 Hz, 6H). **^{19}F NMR** (377 MHz, $CDCl_3$) δ –111.6. **^{13}C NMR** (101 MHz, $CDCl_3$) δ 202.0, 163.5 (d, J = 249.6 Hz), 136.8 (d, J = 8.6 Hz, 2C), 123.3, 116.5 (d, J = 22.2 Hz, 2C), 43.1, 19.5 (2C). **HRMS—ESI** (m/z) for $C_{10}H_{11}FOS$ $[M + H]^+$: calcd 199.0587, found 199.0584.

S-Dodecyl 2-methylpropanethioate (**4f**): Compound **4f** was prepared according to the general procedure using **1a** (86.0 mg, 0.50 mmol, 1.00 equiv) and dodecane-1-thiol (111.3 mg, 0.55 mmol, 1.10 equiv) at rt for 12 h. Purification by flash column chromatography (petroleum ether/ethyl acetate = 3/1, *v*/*v*) afforded S-dodecyl 2-methylpropanethioate (**4f**) as a colorless oil (51.1 mg, 90%). **R$_f$** = 0.60 (petroleum ether/ethyl acetate = 10/1, *v*/*v*). **^{1}H NMR** (400 MHz, $CDCl_3$) δ 2.84 (t, *J* = 7.4 Hz, 2H), 2.72 (hept, *J* = 6.9 Hz, 1H), 1.65–1.49 (m, 2H), 1.42–1.21 (comp, 18H), 1.18 (d, *J* = 7.0 Hz, 6H), 0.88 (t, *J* = 6.7 Hz, 3H). **^{13}C NMR** (101 MHz, $CDCl_3$) δ 204.5, 43.3, 32.1, 29.8 (3C), 29.7, 29.6, 29.5, 29.3, 29.0, 28.7, 22.8, 19.6 (2C), 14.2. **HRMS−ESI** (*m*/*z*) for $C_{16}H_{32}OS$ [M + H]$^+$: calcd 273.2247, found 273.2247.

N-(4-Bromobenzyl)isobutyramide (**4g**): Compound **4g** was prepared according to the general procedure using **1a** (86.0 mg, 0.50 mmol, 1.00 equiv) and (4-bromophenyl)methanamine (102.3 mg, 0.55 mmol, 1.10 equiv) at 100 °C for 12 h. Purification by flash column chromatography (petroleum ether/ethyl acetate = 10/1, *v*/*v*) afforded *N*-(4-bromobenzyl)isobutyramide (**4g**) as a yellow solid (117.4 mg, 92%). **R$_f$** = 0.30 (petroleum ether/ethyl acetate = 10/1, *v*/*v*). **mp** 114–115 °C (petroleum ether). **^{1}H NMR** (400 MHz, $CDCl_3$) δ 7.44 (d, *J* = 8.4 Hz, 2H), 7.13 (d, *J* = 8.4 Hz, 2H), 5.83 (s, 1H), 4.37 (d, *J* = 5.9 Hz, 2H), 2.38 (hept, *J* = 6.9 Hz, 1H), 1.17 (d, *J* = 6.9 Hz, 6H). **^{13}C NMR** (101 MHz, $CDCl_3$) δ 177.0, 137.8, 131.9 (2C), 129.5 (2C), 121.4, 42.9, 35.8, 19.7 (2C). **HRMS−ESI** (*m*/*z*) for $C_{11}H_{14}BrNO$ [M + H]$^+$: calcd 256.0332 (^{79}Br), 258.0312 (^{81}Br), found 256.0032 (^{79}Br), 258.0312 (^{81}Br).

N-(3-Phenylpropyl)isobutyramide (**4h**): Compound **4h** was prepared according to the general procedure using **1a** (86.0 mg, 0.50 mmol, 1.00 equiv) and 3-phenylpropan-1-amine (74.4 mg, 0.55 mmol, 1.10 equiv) at 100 °C for 12 h. Purification by flash column chromatography (petroleum ether/ethyl acetate = 20/1, *v*/*v*) afforded *N*-(3-phenylpropyl)isobutyramide (**4h**) as a yellow oil (93.4 mg, 91%). **R$_f$** = 0.20 (petroleum ether/ethyl acetate = 20/1, *v*/*v*). **^{1}H NMR** (400 MHz, $CDCl_3$) δ 7.39–7.24 (m, 2H), 7.23–7.12 (comp, 3H), 5.43 (br, 1H), 3.29 (q, *J* = 6.5 Hz, 2H), 2.65 (t, *J* = 7.6 Hz, 2H), 2.28 (hept, *J* = 6.9 Hz, 1H), 1.91–1.77 (m, 2H), 1.12 (d, *J* = 6.9 Hz, 6H). **^{13}C NMR** (101 MHz, $CDCl_3$) δ 177.0, 141.7, 128.6 (2C), 128.5 (2C), 126.2, 39.2, 35.8, 33.5, 31.4, 19.7 (2C). **HRMS−ESI** (*m*/*z*) for $C_{13}H_{19}NO$ [M + H]$^+$: calcd 206.1540, found 206.1540.

N-(Heptadecan-9-yl)isobutyramide (**4i**): Compound **4i** was prepared according to the general procedure using **1a** (86.0 mg, 0.50 mmol, 1.00 equiv) and heptadecan-9-amine (140.5 mg, 0.55 mmol, 1.10 equiv) at 100 °C for 12 h. Purification by flash column chromatography (petroleum ether/ethyl acetate = 20/1, *v*/*v*) afforded *N-(heptadecan-9-yl)isobutyramide* (**4i**) as a white solid (146.5 mg, 90%). **R$_f$** = 0.50 (petroleum ether/ethyl acetate = 10/1, *v*/*v*). **mp** 85–86 °C (petroleum ether). **^{1}H NMR** (400 MHz, $CDCl_3$) δ 5.05 (d, *J* = 9.2 Hz, 1H), 3.88 (m, 1H), 2.31 (hept, *J* = 6.9 Hz, 1H), 1.47 (m, 2H), 1.27 (comp, 26H), 1.15 (d, *J* = 6.9 Hz, 6H), 0.87 (t, *J* = 6.7 Hz, 6H). **^{13}C NMR** (101 MHz, $CDCl_3$) δ 176.5, 49.0, 36.1, 35.5 (2C), 32.0 (2C), 29.75 (2C), 29.67 (2C), 29.4 (2C), 26.0 (2C), 22.8 (2C), 19.9 (2C), 14.2 (2C). **HRMS−ESI** (*m*/*z*) for $C_{21}H_{43}NO$ [M + H]$^+$: calcd 326.3418, found 326.3418.

N-Cyclohexylisobutyramide (**4j**): Compound **4j** was prepared according to the general procedure using **1a** (86.0 mg, 0.50 mmol, 1.00 equiv) and cyclohexanamine (54.5 mg, 0.55 mmol, 1.10 equiv) at 100 °C for 12 h. Purification by flash column chromatography (petroleum ether/ethyl acetate = 10/1, *v*/*v*) afforded *N*-cyclohexylisobutyramide (**4j**) as a white solid (71.9 mg, 85%). **R$_f$** = 0.50 (petroleum ether/ethyl acetate = 10/1, *v*/*v*). **mp** 116–117 °C (petroleum ether). **^{1}H NMR** (400 MHz, $CDCl_3$) δ 5.36 (s, 1H), 3.79–3.64 (m, 1H), 2.28 (hept, *J* = 6.8 Hz, 1H), 1.88 (m, 2H), 1.75–1.64 (m, 2H), 1.64–1.50 (m, 1H), 1.36 (m, 2H), 1.12 (comp, 9H). **^{13}C NMR** (101 MHz, $CDCl_3$) δ 176.1, 47.9, 35.9, 33.3 (2C), 25.7, 25.0 (2C), 19.8 (2C). **HRMS−ESI** (*m*/*z*) for $C_{10}H_{19}NO$ [M + H]$^+$: calcd 170.1540, found 170.1540.

2-Methyl-1-morpholinopropan-1-one (**4k**): Compound **4k** was prepared according to the general procedure using **1a** (86.0 mg, 0.50 mmol, 1.00 equiv) and morpholine (47.9 mg,

0.55 mmol, 1.10 equiv) at 100 °C for 12 h. Purification by flash column chromatography (petroleum ether/ethyl acetate = 3/1, *v*/*v*) afforded 2-methyl-1-morpholinopropan-1-one (**4k**) as a colorless oil (51.1 mg, 62%). $\mathbf{R_f}$ = 0.45 (petroleum ether/ethyl acetate = 3/1, *v*/*v*). **^{1}H NMR** (400 MHz, $CDCl_3$) δ 3.74–3.63 (comp, 4H), 3.63–3.56 (m, 2H), 3.50 (m, 2H), 2.74 (hept, *J* = 6.8 Hz, 1H), 1.11 (d, *J* = 6.8 Hz, 6H). **^{13}C NMR** (101 MHz, $CDCl_3$) δ 175.7, 67.1, 66.9, 46.1, 42.2, 30.0, 19.4 (2C). **HRMS—ESI** (*m*/*z*) for $C_8H_{15}NO_2$ $[M + H]^+$: calcd 158.1176, found 158.1176.

3.2.4. Gram-Scale Preparation of 4-Acetamidophenyl Isobutyrate (3z)

To a 50-mL round-bottom flask, 5,5-dimethyl-Meldrum's acid **1a** (1.72 g, 10.0 mmol, 1.00 equiv), BTMG (34.2 mg, 0.20 mmol, 0.02 equiv) were dissolved in anhydrous NMP (25.0 mL). Then, acetaminophen (1.66 g, 11.0 mmol, 1.10 equiv) was added and stirred at 60 °C for 12 h. After the reaction was completed, the mixture was diluted with EA (100 mL) and washed with 2 × 2 M aqueous HCl solution (50 mL). The organic layer was separated, washed with saturated brine (100 mL), dried over anhydrous sodium sulfate, filtered, and concentrated in vacuo. The crude product was then purified by silica gel column chromatography (petroleum ether/ethyl acetate = 3/1, *v*/*v*), which afforded 4-acetamidophenyl isobutyrate (**3z**) as a white solid (2.12 g, 96%). $\mathbf{R_f}$ = 0.35 (petroleum ether/ethyl acetate = 3/1, *v*/*v*). **mp** 111–112 °C (petroleum ether). **^{1}H NMR** (400 MHz, $CDCl_3$) δ 7.51 (d, *J* = 8.4 Hz, 2H), 7.23 (s, 1H), 7.04 (d, *J* = 8.4 Hz, 2H), 2.81 (hept, *J* = 7.0 Hz, 1H), 2.19 (s, 3H), 1.33 (d, *J* = 7.0 Hz, 6H). **^{13}C NMR** (101 MHz, $CDCl_3$) δ 176.1, 168.5, 147.0, 135.6, 121.8 (2C), 120.9 (2C), 34.1, 24.4, 18.9 (2C). **HRMS—ESI** (*m*/*z*) for $C_{12}H_{15}NO_3$ $[M + H]^+$: calcd 222.1125, found 222.1126.

3.2.5. Synthesis of 4-Acetamidophenyl 2-(((benzyloxy)carbonyl)amino)-2-Methylpropanoate (6)

Step 1: To a 25-mL round-bottom flask, 2,2,5,5-tetramethyl-1,3-dioxane-4,6-dione (**1a**) (688.3 mg, 4.0 mmol, 1.00 equiv) and BTMG (753.6 mg, 0.55 mmol, 1.10 equiv) were dissolved in anhydrous DCM (10.0 mL). Then, acetaminophen (665.1 mg, 4.4 mmol, 1.10 equiv) was added, and the mixture was stirred at rt for 4 h. After the reaction was completed, the mixture was diluted with DCM (20 mL) and washed with 2 M aqueous HCl solution (15 mL). The organic layer was separated, washed with saturated brine (20 mL), dried over anhydrous sodium sulfate, filtered, and concentrated in vacuo. The crude product was then purified by silica gel column chromatography (ethyl acetate), which afforded 3-(4-acetamidophenoxy)-2,2-dimethyl-3-oxopropanoic acid (**5**) as a white solid (912.5 mg, 86%). $\mathbf{R_f}$ = 0.20 (dichloromethane /methanol = 40/1, *v*/*v*). **mp** 166–168 °C (petroleum ether). **^{1}H NMR** (400 MHz, DMSO-d_6) δ 13.04 (br, s, 1H), 9.98 (s, 1H), 7.61 (d, *J* = 9.0 Hz, 2H), 7.00 (d, *J* = 8.9 Hz, 2H), 2.04 (s, 3H), 1.46 (s, 6H). **^{13}C NMR** (101 MHz, DMSO-d_6) δ 173.4, 171.6, 168.2, 145.5, 137.1, 121.4 (2C), 119.9 (2C), 49.4, 23.9, 22.4 (2C). **HRMS—ESI** (*m*/*z*) for $C_{13}H_{16}NO_5$ $[M + H]^+$: calcd 266.1023, found 266.1030.

Step 2: To a 4.0-mL vial, the malonate half-ester **5** (132.5 mg, 0.50 mmol, 1.00 equiv), DPPA (165.1 mg, 0.60 mmol, 1.20 equiv), and TEA (75.9 mg, 0.75 mmol, 1.50 equiv) were dissolved in anhydrous toluene (2.5 mL). The mixture was stirred at 100 °C for 12 h. After it was cooled to rt, benzyl alcohol (108.1 mg, 1.00 mmol, 2.00 equiv) was added and stirred at 100 °C for 12 h. After the reaction was completed, the mixture was diluted with EA (20 mL) and washed with 2 M aqueous HCl solution (15 mL). The organic layer was separated, washed with saturated brine (20 mL), dried over anhydrous sodium sulfate, filtered, and concentrated in vacuo. The crude product was then purified by silica gel column chromatography (petroleum ether/ethyl acetate = 1/1, *v*/*v*), which afforded 4-acetamidophenyl 2-(((benzyloxy)carbonyl)amino)-2-methylpropanoate (**6**) as a white solid (140.6 mg, 76%). $\mathbf{R_f}$ = 0.35 (petroleum ether/ethyl acetate = 1/1, *v*/*v*). **mp** 189–190 °C (petroleum ether). **^{1}H NMR** (400 MHz, DMSO-d_6) δ 9.97 (s, 1H), 7.98 (s, 1H), 7.57 (d, *J* = 8.4 Hz, 2H), 7.41–7.26 (comp, 5H), 6.90 (d, *J* = 8.5 Hz, 2H), 5.08 (s, 2H), 2.05 (s, 3H), 1.49 (s, 6H). **^{13}C NMR** (101 MHz, DMSO-d_6) δ 173.3, 168.2, 155.3, 145.9, 136.9, 136.8, 128.3 (2C), 127.8 (3C), 121.6 (2C), 119.8 (2C), 65.4, 55.6, 24.9 (2C), 23.9. **HRMS—ESI** (*m*/*z*) for $C_{20}H_{22}N_2O_5$ $[M + H]^+$: calcd 371.1602, found 371.1610.

3.2.6. One-Pot Preparation of 4-Acetamidophenyl 3-((4-bromobenzyl)amino)-2,2-dimethyl-3-oxopropanoate (7)

In a 4.0-mL vial, 2,2,5,5-tetramethyl-1,3-dioxane-4,6-dione (1a) (86.0 mg, 0.50 mmol, 1.00 equiv) and BTMG (94.2 mg, 0.55 mmol, 1.10 equiv) were dissolved in anhydrous DCM (1.25 mL). Then, acetaminophen (83.1 mg, 0.55 mmol, 1.10 equiv) was added, and the mixture was stirred at rt for 4 h. Then, *p*-BrBnNH$_2$ (102.3 mg, 0.55 mmol, 1.10 equiv), EDC·HCl (143.8 mg, 0.75 mmol, 1.50 equiv), and HOBt (101.3 mg, 0.75 mmol, 1.50 equiv) were added, and the mixture was stirred at rt for 6 h. After the reaction was completed, the mixture was diluted with EA (20 mL) and washed with 2 M aqueous HCl solution (15 mL). The organic layer was separated, washed with saturated brine (20 mL), dried over anhydrous sodium sulfate, filtered, and concentrated in vacuo. The crude product was then purified by silica gel column chromatography (petroleum ether/ethyl acetate = 3/1, *v*/*v*), which afforded 4-acetamidophenyl 3-((4-bromobenzyl)amino)-2,2-dimethyl-3-oxopropanoate (7) as a white solid (140.4 mg, 65%). **R_f** = 0.35 (petroleum ether/ethyl acetate = 3/1, *v*/*v*). **mp** 179–180 °C (petroleum ether). **^{1}H NMR** (400 MHz, DMSO-d_6) δ 9.97 (s, 1H), 8.50 (t, *J* = 6.0 Hz, 1H), 7.59 (d, *J* = 8.9 Hz, 2H), 7.48 (d, *J* = 8.3 Hz, 2H), 7.23 (d, *J* = 8.4 Hz, 2H), 6.95 (d, *J* = 8.9 Hz, 2H), 4.29 (d, *J* = 5.9 Hz, 1H), 2.04 (s, 3H), 1.49 (s, 6H). **^{13}C NMR** (101 MHz, DMSO-d_6) δ 172.2, 171.5, 168.2, 145.6, 139.0, 137.0, 131.0 (2C), 129.2 (2C), 121.5 (2C), 119.8 (2C), 119.7, 50.0, 41.9, 23.9, 22.7 (2C). **HRMS—ESI** (*m*/*z*) for $C_{20}H_{21}BrN_2O_4$ $[M + H]^+$: calcd 433.0758 (^{79}Br), 435.0737 (^{81}Br), found 433.0766 (^{79}Br), 435.0745 (^{81}Br).

4. Conclusions

We have identified disubstituted Meldrum's acid as a novel carbon-based scaffold with SuFEx-like reactivity. As exemplified in other SuFEx reactions, phenols are the optimal nucleophilic exchange partners. Notably, thiols and thiophenols, typically prone to oxidation by S(VI) electrophiles in classical SuFEx reactions, exhibit comparable reactivity to phenols in our method. In contrast, alcohols and amines require elevated temperatures to achieve full conversion. Sterically hindered nucleophiles, such as tertiary alcohols or bulky primary and secondary amines, remain challenging and will require the development of new catalytic systems. Alternative activation strategies for disubstituted Meldrum's acids are currently under investigation in our laboratory and will be reported in due course.

5. Patents

Sun Yat-sen University has filed a patent application.

Supplementary Materials: The following supporting information can be downloaded at: https://www.mdpi.com/article/10.3390/molecules30173534/s1. General Information, Synthesis of Starting Materials, Reaction Optimizations, Synthesis and Characterization Data, Preparation-scale Derivatization of Acetaminophen, Preliminary Mechanistic Experiments, and NMR spectra [112–114].

Author Contributions: Methodology, B.C. and Z.W.; validation, B.C., Z.W., X.P., J.X., Z.S.; investigation, B.C., Z.W., X.P., J.X., Z.S., L.L.; resources, L.L.; writing—original draft preparation, L.L.; writing—review and editing, B.C., Z.W., X.P., J.X., Z.S., L.L.; supervision, L.L., B.C. and Z.W. contributed to the work equally. All authors have read and agreed to the published version of the manuscript.

Funding: This research was funded by the National Natural Science Foundation of China (No. 22471292 and No. 21502241).

Institutional Review Board Statement: Not applicable.

Informed Consent Statement: Not applicable.

Data Availability Statement: Data is contained within the article or Supplementary Material.

Acknowledgments: L.L. thanks Suhua Li and Pengfei Ma (Sun Yat-sen University) and Pyh Li for helpful discussions and support.

Conflicts of Interest: The authors declare no conflict of interest.

References

1. Staudinger, H.; Meyer, J. Über neue organische Phosphorverbindungen III. Phosphinmethylenderivate und Phosphinimine. *Helv. Chim. Acta* **1919**, *2*, 635–646. [CrossRef]
2. Dong, J.J.; Krasnova, L.; Finn, M.G.; Sharpless, K.B. Sulfur(VI) Fluoride Exchange (SuFEx): Another Good Reaction for Click Chemistry. *Angew. Chem. Int. Ed.* **2014**, *53*, 9430–9448. [CrossRef]
3. Barrow, A.S.; Smedley, C.J.; Zheng, Q.; Li, S.; Dong, J.; Moses, J.E. The growing applications of SuFEx click chemistry. *Chem. Soc. Rev.* **2019**, *48*, 4731–4758. [CrossRef]
4. Lou, T.S.-B.; Willis, M.C. Sulfonyl fluorides as targets and substrates in the development of new synthetic methods. *Nat. Rev. Chem.* **2022**, *6*, 146–162. [CrossRef]
5. Homer, J.A.; Xu, L.; Kayambu, N.; Zheng, Q.H.; Choi, E.J.; Kim, B.M.; Sharpless, K.B.; Zuilhof, H.; Dong, J.J.; Moses, J.E. Sulfur fluoride exchange. *Nat. Rev. Methods Primers* **2023**, *3*, 58. [CrossRef]
6. Rojas, J.J.; Bull, J.A. Sulfonyl fluorides as novel click reagents: Unconventional reactivity of sulfonyl fluorides. *Trends Chem.* **2025**, *7*, 124–133. [CrossRef]
7. Zheng, Q.H.; Dong, J.J.; Sharpless, K.B. Ethenesulfonyl Fluoride (ESF): An On-Water Procedure for the Kilogram-Scale Preparation. *J. Org. Chem.* **2016**, *81*, 11360–11362. [CrossRef] [PubMed]
8. Lu, J.; Zhou, T.; Zhang, E. A Method for Sulfur(VI) Fluoride Exchange (SuFEx) Reaction. CN 107266392 A, 20 October 2017.
9. Zheng, Q.H.; Woehl, J.L.; Kitamura, S.; Santos-Martins, D.; Smedley, C.J.; Li, G.C.; Forli, S.; Moses, J.E.; Wolan, D.W.; Sharpless, K.B. SuFEx-enabled chemoproteomics platform. *Proc. Natl. Acad. Sci. USA* **2019**, *116*, 18808–18814. [CrossRef]
10. Meng, G.Y.; Guo, T.J.; Ma, T.C.; Zhang, J.; Shen, Y.C.; Sharpless, K.B.; Dong, J.J. A Modular click chemistry libraries for functional screens using a diazotizing reagent. *Nature* **2019**, *574*, 86–89. [CrossRef]
11. Zheng, M.-M.; Cai, L.; Ma, T.C.; Tan, H.-D.; Lai, X.Y.; Dong, J.J.; Xue, X.-S. Computational analysis of modular diazotransfer reactions for the development of predictive reactivity models and diazotransfer reagents. *Nat. Synth.* **2024**, *3*, 1507–1517. [CrossRef]
12. Cao, L.; Yu, B.C.; Klauser, P.C.; Zhang, P.; Li, S.S.; Wang, L. SuFEx Click Chemistry in Peptide Synthesis. *Angew. Chem. Int. Ed.* **2024**, *63*, e202412843. [CrossRef] [PubMed]
13. Mukherjee, P.; Woroch, C.P.; Cleary, L.; Rusznak, M.; Franzese, R.W.; Reese, M.R.; Tucker, J.W.; Humphrey, J.M.; Etuk, S.M.; Kwan, S.C.; et al. Sulfonamide Synthesis via Calcium Triflimide Activation of Sulfonyl Fluorides. *Org. Lett.* **2018**, *20*, 3943–3947. [CrossRef]
14. Mahapatra, S.; Woroch, C.P.; Butler, T.W.; Carneiro, S.N.; Kwan, S.C.; Khasnavis, S.R.; Gu, J.; Dutra, J.K.; Vetelino, B.C.; Bellenger, J.; et al. Unified Strategy to Access Sulfamides, Sulfamates and Sulfonamides from Sulfur(VI) Fluorides. *Org. Lett.* **2020**, *22*, 4389–4394. [CrossRef] [PubMed]
15. Gao, B.; Zhang, L.; Zheng, Q.H.; Zhou, F.; Klivansky, L.M.; Lu, J.M.; Liu, Y.; Dong, J.J.; Wu, P.; Sharpless, K.B. Bifluoride-catalysed sulfur(VI) fluoride exchange reaction for the synthesis of polysulfates and polysulfonates. *Nat. Chem.* **2017**, *9*, 1083–1088. [CrossRef]
16. Wei, M.J.; Liang, D.C.; Cao, X.H.; Luo, W.J.; Ma, G.J.; Liu, Z.Y.; Li, L. A Broad-Spectrum Catalytic Amidation of Sulfonyl Fluorides and Fluorosulfates. *Angew. Chem. Int. Ed.* **2021**, *60*, 7397–7404. [CrossRef]
17. Smedley, C.J.; Homer, J.A.; Gialelis, T.L.; Barrow, A.S.; Koelln, R.A.; Moses, J.E. Accelerated SuFEx Click Chemistry For Modular Synthesis. *Angew. Chem. Int. Ed.* **2022**, *61*, e202112375. [CrossRef]
18. Lin, M.Z.; Luo, J.Y.; Xie, Y.; Du, G.F.; Cai, Z.H.; Dai, B.; He, L. SuFEx Reactions of Sulfonyl Fluorides, Fluorosulfates, and Sulfamoyl Fluorides Catalyzed by N-Heterocyclic Carbenes. *ACS Catal.* **2023**, *13*, 14503–14512. [CrossRef]
19. Yassa, T.D.; Fang, Y.X.; Ravelo, L.K.; Anand, S.; Arora, S.; Ball, N.D. Lewis Acid-Catalyzed Sulfur Fluoride Exchange. *Org. Lett.* **2024**, *26*, 9897–9902. [CrossRef]

20. Homer, J.A.; Koelln, R.A.; Barrow, A.S.; Gialelis, T.L.; Boiarska, Z.; Steinohrt, N.S.; Lee, E.F.; Yang, W.H.; Johnson, R.M.; Chung, T.M.; et al. Modular synthesis of functional libraries by accelerated SuFEx click chemistry. *Chem. Sci.* **2024**, *15*, 3879–3892. [CrossRef]
21. Narayanan, A.; Jones, L.H. Sulfonyl fluorides as privileged warheads in chemical biology. *Chem. Sci.* **2015**, *6*, 2650–2659. [CrossRef] [PubMed]
22. Baranczak, A.; Liu, Y.; Connelly, S.; Du, W.G.H.; Greiner, E.R.; Genereux, J.C.; Wiseman, R.L.; Eisele, Y.S.; Bradbury, N.C.; Dong, J.J.; et al. A Fluorogenic Aryl Fluorosulfate for Intraorganellar Transthyretin Imaging in Living Cells and in Caenorhabditis elegans. *J. Am. Chem. Soc.* **2015**, *137*, 7404–7414. [CrossRef]
23. Chen, W.T.; Dong, J.J.; Plate, L.; Mortenson, D.E.; Brighty, G.J.; Li, S.H.; Liu, Y.; Galmozzi, A.; Lee, P.S.; Hulce, J.J.; et al. Arylfluorosulfates Inactivate Intracellular Lipid Binding Protein(s) through Chemoselective SuFEx Reaction with a Binding Site Tyr Residue. *J. Am. Chem. Soc.* **2016**, *138*, 7353–7364. [CrossRef]
24. Chen, W.; Dong, J.; Li, S.; Liu, Y.; Wang, Y.; Yoon, L.; Wu, P.; Sharpless, K.B.; Kelly, J.W. Synthesis of Sulfotyrosine-Containing Peptides by Incorporating Fluorosulfated Tyrosine Using an Fmoc-Based Solid-Phase Strategy. *Angew. Chem. Int. Ed.* **2016**, *55*, 1835–1838. [CrossRef] [PubMed]
25. Wang, N.X.; Yang, B.; Fu, C.Y.; Zhu, H.; Zheng, F.; Kobayashi, T.; Liu, J.; Li, S.S.; Ma, C.; Wang, P.G.; et al. Genetically Encoding Fluorosulfate-L-tyrosine To React with Lysine, Histidine, and Tyrosine via SuFEx in Proteins in Vivo. *J. Am. Chem. Soc.* **2018**, *140*, 4995–4999. [CrossRef] [PubMed]
26. Liu, F.; Wang, H.; Li, S.; Bare, G.A.L.; Chen, X.; Wang, C.; Moses, J.E.; Wu, P.; Sharpless, K.B. Biocompatible SuFEx Click Chemistry: Thionyl Tetrafluoride (SOF_4)-Derived Connective Hubs for Bioconjugation to DNA and Proteins. *Angew. Chem. Int. Ed.* **2019**, *58*, 8029–8033. [CrossRef]
27. Yang, L.Y.; Yuan, Z.N.; Li, Y.K.; Yang, S.Y.; Yu, B.C. Sulfur (VI) fluoride exchange (SuFEx): A versatile tool to profile protein-biomolecule interactions for therapeutic development. *Med. Chem. Res.* **2024**, *33*, 1315–1329. [CrossRef]
28. Mortenson, D.E.; Brighty, G.J.; Plate, L.; Bare, G.; Chen, W.; Li, S.; Wang, H.; Cravatt, B.F.; Forli, S.; Powers, E.T.; et al. "Inverse Drug Discovery" Strategy To Identify Proteins That Are Targeted by Latent Electrophiles As Exemplified by Aryl Fluorosulfates. *J. Am. Chem. Soc.* **2017**, *140*, 200–210. [CrossRef] [PubMed]
29. Liu, Z.L.; Li, J.; Li, S.H.; Li, G.C.; Sharpless, K.B.; Wu, P. SuFEx Click Chemistry Enabled Late-Stage Drug Functionalization. *J. Am. Chem. Soc.* **2018**, *140*, 2919–2925. [CrossRef]
30. Martín-Gago, P.; Olsen, C.A. Arylfluorosulfate-Based Electrophiles for Covalent Protein Labeling: A New Addition to the Arsenal. *Angew. Chem. Int. Ed.* **2019**, *58*, 957–966. [CrossRef]
31. Xu, H.T.; Ma, F.; Wang, N.; Hou, W.; Xiong, H.; Lu, F.P.; Li, J.; Wang, S.Y.; Ma, P.X.; Yang, G.; et al. DNA-Encoded Libraries: Aryl Fluorosulfonates as Versatile Electrophiles Enabling Facile On-DNA Suzuki, Sonogashira, and Buchwald Reactions. *Adv. Sci.* **2019**, *6*, 1901551. [CrossRef]
32. Smedley, C.J.; Li, G.C.; Barrow, A.S.; Gialelis, T.L.; Giel, M.C.; Ottonello, A.; Cheng, Y.F.; Kitamura, S.; Wolan, D.W.; Sharpless, K.B.; et al. Diversity Oriented Clicking (DOC): Divergent Synthesis of SuFExable Pharmacophores from 2-Substituted-Alkynyl-1-Sulfonyl Fluoride (SASF) Hubs. *Angew. Chem. Int. Ed.* **2020**, *59*, 12460–12469. [CrossRef]
33. Kitamura, S.; Zheng, Q.H.; Woehl, J.L.; Solania, A.; Chen, E.; Dillon, N.; Hull, M.V.; Kotaniguchi, M.; Cappiello, J.R.; Kitamura, S.; et al. Sulfur(VI) Fluoride Exchange (SuFEx)-Enabled High-Throughput Medicinal Chemistry. *J. Am. Chem. Soc.* **2020**, *142*, 10899–10904. [CrossRef]
34. Kline, G.M.; Nugroho, K.; Kelly, J.W. Inverse Drug Discovery identifies weak electrophiles affording protein conjugates. *Curr. Opin. Chem. Biol.* **2022**, *67*, 102113. [CrossRef]
35. Liu, Z.W.; Li, J.; Li, S.H.; Li, G.C.; Sharpless, K.B.; Wu, P. Sulfur-fluoride exchange (SuFEx)-enabled lead discovery of AChE inhibitors by fragment linking strategies. *Eur. J. Med. Chem.* **2023**, *257*, 115502. [CrossRef]
36. Huang, H.; Jones, L.H. Covalent drug discovery using sulfur(VI) fluoride exchange warheads. *Expert Opin. Drug Discov.* **2023**, *18*, 725–735. [CrossRef] [PubMed]
37. Wilson, L.S.; Qin, R.Z.; Rakesh, K.P.; Sharath, K.K.S.; Qin, H.L. Chemical and biology of sulfur fluoride exchange (SuFEx) click chemistry for drug discovery. *Bioorg. Chem.* **2023**, *130*, 106227. [CrossRef]
38. Du, S.Q.; Hu, X.P.; Lindsley, C.W.; Zhan, P. New Applications of Sulfonyl Fluorides: A Microcosm of the Deep Integration of Chemistry and Biology in Drug Design. *J. Med. Chem.* **2024**, *67*, 16925–16927. [CrossRef] [PubMed]
39. Dong, J.J.; Sharpless, K.B.; Kwisnek, L.; Oakdale, J.S.; Fokin, V.V. SuFEx-Based Synthesis of Polysulfates. *Angew. Chem. Int. Ed.* **2014**, *53*, 9466–9470. [CrossRef]
40. Yatvin, J.; Brooks, K.; Locklin, J. SuFEx on the Surface: A Flexible Platform for Postpolymerization Modification of Polymer Brushes. *Angew. Chem. Int. Ed.* **2015**, *54*, 13370–13373. [CrossRef]
41. Wang, H.; Zhou, F.; Ren, G.R.; Zheng, Q.H.; Chen, H.L.; Gao, B.; Klivansky, L.; Liu, Y.; Wu, B.; Xu, Q.F.; et al. SuFEx-Based Polysulfonate Formation from Ethenesulfonyl Fluoride–Amine Adducts. *Angew. Chem. Int. Ed.* **2017**, *56*, 11203–11208. [CrossRef]

42. Hmissa, T.; Zhang, X.F.; Dhumal, N.R.; McManus, G.J.; Zhou, X.; Nulwala, H.B.; Mirjafari, A. Autocatalytic Synthesis of Bifluoride Ionic Liquids by SuFEx Click Chemistry. *Angew. Chem. Int. Ed.* **2018**, *57*, 16005–16009. [CrossRef] [PubMed]
43. Gahtory, D.; Sen, R.; Pujari, S.; Li, S.H.; Zheng, Q.H.; Moses, J.E.; Sharpless, K.B.; Zuilhof, H. Quantitative and Orthogonal Formation and Reactivity of SuFEx Platforms. *Chem. Eur. J.* **2018**, *24*, 10550–10556. [CrossRef]
44. Yang, C.J.; Flynn, J.P.; Niu, J. Facile Synthesis of Sequence-Regulated Synthetic Polymers Using Orthogonal SuFEx and CuAAC Click Reactions. *Angew. Chem. Int. Ed.* **2018**, *57*, 16194–16199. [CrossRef] [PubMed]
45. Park, S.; Song, H.; Ko, N.; Kim, C.; Kim, K.; Lee, E. SuFEx in Metal−Organic Frameworks: Versatile Postsynthetic Modification Tool. *ACS Appl. Mater. Interfaces* **2018**, *10*, 33785–33789. [CrossRef]
46. Demay-Drouhard, P.; Du, K.; Samanta, K.; Wan, X.T.; Yang, W.W.; Srinivasan, R.; Sue, A.C.H.; Zuilhof, H. Functionalization at Will of Rim-Differentiated Pillar[5]arenes. *Org. Lett.* **2019**, *21*, 3976–3980. [CrossRef]
47. Kulow, W.; Wu, J.W.; Kim, C.; Michaudel, Q. Synthesis of unsymmetrical sulfamides and polysulfamides via SuFEx click chemistry. *Chem. Sci.* **2020**, *11*, 7807–7812. [CrossRef] [PubMed]
48. Sun, W.; Lu, K.Y.; Wang, L.; Hao, Q.; Liu, J.R.; Wang, Y.; Wu, Z.Q.; Chen, H. Introducing SuFEx click chemistry into aliphatic polycarbonates: A novel toolbox/platform for post-modification as biomaterials. *Mater. Chem. B* **2022**, *10*, 5203–5210. [CrossRef]
49. Wang, M.L.; Hou, J.M.; Do, H.; Wang, C.; Zhang, X.H.; Du, Y.; Dong, Q.X.; Wang, L.J.; Ni, K.; Ren, F.Z.; et al. Intramolecular chalcogen bonding activated SuFEx click chemistry for efficient organic-inorganic linking. *Nat. Commun.* **2024**, *15*, 6849. [CrossRef]
50. Li, S.H.; Li, G.C.; Gao, B.; Pujari, S.P.; Chen, X.Y.; Kim, H.; Zhou, F.; Klivansky, L.M.; Liu, Y.; Driss, H.; et al. SuFExable polymers with helical structures derived from thionyl tetrafluoride. *Nat. Chem.* **2021**, *13*, 858–867. [CrossRef]
51. Kim, H.; Zhao, J.Y.; Bae, J.; Klivansky, L.M.; Dailing, E.A.; Liu, Y.; Cappiello, J.R.; Sharpless, K.B.; Wu, P. Chain-Growth Sulfur(VI) Fluoride Exchange Polycondensation: Molecular Weight Control and Synthesis of Degradable Polysulfates. *ACS Cent. Sci.* **2021**, *7*, 1919–1928. [CrossRef]
52. Kim, M.P.; Sahoo, M.K.; Chun, J.-H.; Hong, S.Y. The First Decade of SuFEx Chemistry: Advancements in SuFEx Polymerization, Non-Canonical SuFEx Reactions, and SuFEx Radiochemistry. *Synthesis* **2025**, *57*, 1551–1568. [CrossRef]
53. Qin, H.L.; Zheng, Q.H.; Bare, G.A.L.; Wu, P.; Sharpless, K.B. A Heck–Matsuda Process for the Synthesis of β-Arylethenesulfonyl Fluorides: Selectively Addressable Bis-electrophiles for SuFEx Click Chemistry. *Angew. Chem. Int. Ed.* **2016**, *55*, 14155–14158. [CrossRef] [PubMed]
54. Li, S.H.; Wu, P.; Moses, J.E.; Sharpless, K.B. Multidimensional SuFEx Click Chemistry: Sequential Sulfur(VI) Fluoride Exchange Connections of Diverse Modules Launched From An SOF_4 Hub. *Angew. Chem. Int. Ed.* **2017**, *56*, 2903–2908. [CrossRef] [PubMed]
55. Gao, B.; Li, S.H.; Wu, P.; Moses, J.E.; Sharpless, K.B. SuFEx Chemistry of Thionyl Tetrafluoride (SOF4) with Organolithium Nucleophiles: Synthesis of Sulfonimidoyl Fluorides, Sulfoximines, Sulfonimidamides, and Sulfonimidates. *Angew. Chem. Int. Ed.* **2018**, *57*, 1939–1943. [CrossRef] [PubMed]
56. Guo, T.J.; Meng, G.Y.; Zhan, X.J.; Yang, Q.; Ma, T.C.; Xu, L.; Sharpless, K.B.; Dong, J.J. A New Portal to SuFEx Click Chemistry: A Stable Fluorosulfuryl Imidazolium Salt Emerging as an "F@SO2+" Donor of Unprecedented Reactivity, Selectivity, and Scope. *Angew. Chem. Int. Ed.* **2018**, *57*, 2605–2610. [CrossRef]
57. Meng, Y.P.; Wang, S.M.; Fang, W.Y.; Xie, Z.Z.; Leng, J.; Alsulami, H.; Qin, H.L. Ethenesulfonyl Fluoride (ESF) and Its Derivatives in SuFEx Click Chemistry and More. *Synthesis* **2020**, *52*, 673–687. [CrossRef]
58. Liang, D.D.; Streefkerk, D.E.; Jordaan, D.; Wagemakers, J.; Baggerman, J.; Zuilhof, H. Silicon-Free SuFEx Reactions of Sulfonimidoyl Fluorides: Scope, Enantioselectivity, and Mechanism. *Angew. Chem. Int. Ed.* **2020**, *59*, 7494–7500. [CrossRef]
59. Nie, X.L.; Xu, T.X.; Hong, Y.H.; Zhang, H.H.; Mao, C.X.; Liao, S.H. Introducing A New Class of Sulfonyl Fluoride Hubs via Radical Chloro-Fluorosulfonylation of Alkynes. *Angew. Chem. Int. Ed.* **2021**, *60*, 22035–22042. [CrossRef]
60. Zeng, D.M.; Ma, Y.H.; Deng, W.P.; Wang, M.; Jiang, X.F. The Linkage of Sulfonimidoyl Fluorides and Unactivated Alkenes via Hydrosulfonimidoylation. *Angew. Chem. Int. Ed.* **2022**, *61*, e202207100. [CrossRef]
61. Zeng, D.M.; Deng, W.P.; Jiang, X.F. Advances in the construction of diverse SuFEx linkers. *Natl. Sci. Rev.* **2023**, *10*, nwad123. [CrossRef]
62. Erchinger, J.E.; Hoogesteger, R.; Laskar, R.; Dutta, S.; Huempel, C.; Rana, D.; Daniliuc, C.G.; Glorius, F. EnT-Mediated N−S Bond Homolysis of a Bifunctional Reagent Leading to Aliphatic Sulfonyl Fluorides. *J. Am. Chem. Soc.* **2023**, *145*, 2364–2374. [CrossRef]
63. Aleksandrenko, S.; Dobrydnev, A.V.; Zhersh, S.; Grygorenko, O.O. Saturated Heterocyclic Sulfamoyl Fluorides: Building Blocks for the SuFEx Chemistry. *Eur. J. Org. Chem.* **2024**, *27*, e202400611. [CrossRef]
64. Li, H.Y.; Wang, Y. Recent Advances in SuFEx Chemistry. *Synthesis* **2025**, *57*, 1690–1706.
65. Serbetci, D.; Marraffa, L.; Natho, P.; Andresini, M.; Luisi, R. A Practical Guide to SuFEx Chemistry: An Overview of S(VI)-SuFEx Linkers and Their Reactivity. *Synthesis* **2025**, *57*, 1569–1582. [CrossRef]
66. Chao, Y.; Krishna, A.; Subramaniam, M.; Liang, D.D.; Pujari, S.P.; Sue, A.C.H.G.; Li, G.N.; Miloserdov, F.M.; Zuilhof, H. Sulfur–Phenolate Exchange: SuFEx-Derived Dynamic Covalent Reactions and Degradation of SuFEx Polymers. *Angew. Chem. Int. Ed.* **2022**, *61*, e202207456. [CrossRef] [PubMed]

67. Boom, A.F.J.; Subramaniam, M.; Zuilhof, H. Sulfur-Phenolate Exchange As a Fluorine-Free Approach to S(VI) Exchange Chemistry on Sulfonyl Moieties. *Org. Lett.* **2022**, *24*, 8621–8626. [CrossRef] [PubMed]
68. Boom, A.F.J.; Zuilhof, H. Sulfur-Phenolate Exchange as a Mild, Fast, and High-Yielding Method toward the Synthesis of Sulfonamides. *Org. Lett.* **2023**, *25*, 788–793. [CrossRef] [PubMed]
69. Chao, Y.; Subramaniam, M.; Namitharan, K.; Zhu, Y.M.; Koolma, V.; Hao, Z.T.; Li, S.K.; Wang, Y.X.; Hudoynazarov, I.; Miloserdov, F.M.; et al. Synthesis of Large Macrocycles with Chiral Sulfur Centers via Enantiospecific SuFEx and SuPhenEx Click Reactions. *J. Org. Chem.* **2023**, *88*, 15658–15665. [CrossRef]
70. Sun, S.J.; Homer, J.A.; Smedley, C.J.; Cheng, Q.-Q.; Sharpless, K.B.; Moses, J.E. Phosphorus fluoride exchange: Multidimensional catalytic click chemistry from phosphorus connective hubs. *Chem* **2023**, *9*, 2128–2143. [CrossRef]
71. Cao, L.; Yu, B.C.; Li, S.S.; Zhang, P.; Li, Q.K.; Wang, L. Genetically enabling phosphorus fluoride exchange click chemistry in proteins. *Chem* **2024**, *10*, 1868–1884. [CrossRef]
72. Homer, J.A.; Sun, S.J.; Koelln, R.A.; Moses, J.E. Protocol for producing phosphoramidate using phosphorus fluoride exchange click chemistry. *STAR Protoc.* **2024**, *5*, 102824. [CrossRef]
73. Wang, Z.F.; Vishwakarma, D.S.; Sun, S.J.; Huang, Q.Y.; Pati, S.; Johnson, R.M.; Rufrano, R.M.; Gembicky, M.J.; Homer, J.A.; Moses, J.E. Phosphorus Fluoride Exchange (PFEx) Click Chemistry: 2-Substituted-Alkynyl-1-Cyclotriphosphazene (SACP) Hubs for Diversity Oriented Clicking. *Adv. Synth. Catal.* **2025**, *367*, e202401573. [CrossRef]
74. Arnett, E.M.; Harrelson, J.A., Jr. A Spectacular Example of the Importance of Rotational Barriers: The Ionization of Meldrum's Acid. *J. Am. Chem. Soc.* **1987**, *109*, 809–812. [CrossRef]
75. Zhang, X.M.; Bordwell, F.G. Acidities and Homolytic Bond Dissociation Enthalpies (BDEs) of the Acidic H-A Bonds in Acyclic and Cyclic Alkoxycarbonyl Compounds (Esters and Carbamates). *J. Org. Chem.* **1994**, *59*, 6456–6458. [CrossRef]
76. Byun, K.; Mo, Y.; Gao, J. New Insight on the Origin of the Unusual Acidity of Meldrum's Acid from ab Initio and Combined QM/MM Simulation Study. *J. Am. Chem. Soc.* **2001**, *123*, 3974–3979. [CrossRef]
77. Nakamura, S.; Hirao, H.; Ohwada, T. Rationale for the Acidity of Meldrum's Acid. Consistent Relation of C-H Acidities to the Properties of Localized Reactive Orbital. *J. Org. Chem.* **2004**, *69*, 4309–4316. [CrossRef]
78. Dumas, A.M.; Fillion, E. Meldrum's Acids and 5-Alkylidene Meldrum's Acids in Catalytic Carbon-Carbon Bond-Forming Processes. *Acc. Chem. Res.* **2010**, *43*, 440–454. [CrossRef]
79. Chen, B.-C. Meldrum's Acid in Orgnaic Synthesis. *Heterocycles* **1991**, *32*, 529–597. [CrossRef]
80. Brosge, F.; Singh, P.; Almqvist, F.; Bolm, C. Selected applications of Meldrum's acid – a tutorial. *Org. Biomol. Chem.* **2021**, *19*, 5014–5027. [CrossRef]
81. Hiratake, J.; Shibata, K.; Baba, N.; Oda, J. Enantiotopic-Group Differentiation. Asymmetric Monoesterification of Malonic Acids Using Cinchona Alkaloid Derivatives. *Synthesis* **1988**, *4*, 278–280. [CrossRef]
82. Korotkov, V.S.; Larionov, O.V.; Hofmeister, A.; Magull, J.; Meijere, A.D. $GaCl_3$-Catalyzed Insertion of Diazene Derivatives into the Cyclopropane Ring. *J. Org. Chem.* **2007**, *72*, 7504–7510. [CrossRef]
83. Lau, K.-N.; Chow, H.-F.; Chan, M.-C.; Wong, K.-W. Dendronized Polymer Organogels from Click Chemistry: A Remarkable Gelation Property Owing to Synergistic Functional-Group Binding and Dendritic Size Effects. *Angew. Chem. Int. Ed.* **2008**, *47*, 6912–6916. [CrossRef]
84. Chang, T.T.; More, S.V.; Lu, I.-H.; Hsu, J.-C.; Chen, T.-J.; Jen, Y.C.; Lu, C.-K.; Li, W.-S. Isomalyngamide A, A-1 and their analogs suppress cancer cell migration in vitro. *Eur. J. Med. Chem.* **2011**, *46*, 3810–3819. [CrossRef]
85. Choi, L.-S.; Chow, H.-F. Vetteerrsatile Synthesis of Amphiphilic Oligo(Aliphatic-Glycerol) Layer-Block Dendrons with Different Hydrophilic-Lipophilic Balance Values. *Synlett* **2013**, *24*, 201–206. [CrossRef]
86. Ariyarathna, Y.; Tunge, J.A. Decarboxylative allylations of ester enolate equivalents. *Org. Biomol. Chem.* **2014**, *12*, 8386–8389. [CrossRef] [PubMed]
87. Ambrogio, I.; Cacchi, S.; Fabrizi, G.; Goggiamani, A.; Iazzetti, A. Palladium-Catalyzed Nucleophilic Substitution of Propargylic Carbonates and Meldrum's Acid Derivatives. *Eur. J. Org. Chem.* **2015**, *14*, 3147–3151. [CrossRef]
88. Sui, X.L.; Gutekunst, W.R. Cascade Alternating Metathesis Cyclopolymerization of Diynes and Dihydrofuran. *ACS Macro Lett.* **2022**, *11*, 630–635. [CrossRef] [PubMed]
89. Ronzon, Q.; Zhang, W.; Charote, T.; Casaretto, N.; Frison, G.; Nay, B. Total Synthesis of (+)-Cinereain and (-)-Janoxepin through a Fragment Coupling/Retro-Claisen Rearrangement Cascade. *Angew. Chem. Int. Ed.* **2022**, *61*, e202212855. [CrossRef]
90. Ariyarathna, Y.; Tunge, J.A. Multicomponent decarboxylative allylations. *Chem. Commun.* **2014**, *50*, 14049–14052. [CrossRef] [PubMed]
91. Legros, F.; Martzel, T.; Brière, J.-F.; Oudeyer, S.; Levacher, V. Organocatalytic Enantioselective Decarboxylative Protonation Reaction of Meldrum's Acid Derivatives under PTC Conditions. *Eur. J. Org. Chem.* **2018**, *17*, 1975–1983. [CrossRef]
92. Martzel, T.; Annibaletto, J.; Levacher, V.; Brière, J.F.; Oudeyer, S. C5-Disubstituted Meldrum's Acid Derivatives as Platform for the Organocatalytic Synthesis of C3-Alkylated Dihydrocoumarins. *Adv. Synth. Catal.* **2019**, *361*, 995–1000. [CrossRef]

93. Oikawa, Y.; Hirasawa, H.; Yonemitsu, O. Meldrum's acid in organic synthesis. 1. A convenient one-pot synthesis of ethyl indolepropionates. *Tetrahedron Lett.* **1978**, *20*, 1759–1762. [CrossRef]
94. Cheawchan, S.; Koyama, Y.; Uchida, S.; Takata, T. Catalyst-free click cascade functionalization of unsaturated-bondcontaining polymers using masked-ketene-tethering nitrile N-oxide. *Polymer* **2013**, *54*, 4501–4510. [CrossRef]
95. Nakatani, K.; Natsuhara, N.; Mori, Y.; Mukherjee, S.; Das, B.; Murata, A. Synthesis of Naphthyridine Dimers with Conformational Restriction and Binding to DNA and RNA. *Chem. Asian J.* **2017**, *12*, 3077–3087. [CrossRef] [PubMed]
96. Adamson, N.J.; Wilbur, K.C.E.; Malcolmson, S.J. Enantioselective Intermolecular Pd-Catalyzed Hydroalkylation of Acyclic 1,3-Dienes with Activated Pronucleophiles. *J. Am. Chem. Soc.* **2018**, *140*, 2761–2764. [CrossRef]
97. Liu, M.; Zhao, H.Y.; Li, C.K. Rh(I)-catalyzed regio- and enantioselective allylic alkylation of Meldrum's acid. *Chin. Chem. Lett.* **2021**, *32*, 385–388. [CrossRef]
98. Tabti, R.; Lamoureux, F.; Charrier, C.; Ory, B.; Heymann, D.; Bentouhami, E.; Desaubry, L. Development of prohibitin ligands against osteoporosis. *Eur. J. Med. Chem.* **2021**, *210*, 112961. [CrossRef]
99. Das, B.; Nagano, K.; Kawai, G.; Murata, A.; Nakatani, K. 2-Amino-1,8-naphthyridine Dimer (ANP77), a High-Affinity Binder to the Internal Loops of C/CC and T/CC Sites in Double-Stranded DNA. *J. Org. Chem.* **2022**, *87*, 340–350. [CrossRef] [PubMed]
100. Lin, X.-W.; Han, M.; Shen, M.-H.; Zhu, C.-F.; Xu, H.-D. Synthesis of functionalized γ-lactams by a lewis acid catalyzed ketene formation/cyclization/claisen rearrangement sequence of 5,5-disubstituted Meldrum's acids. *Tetrahedron Lett.* **2022**, *99*, 153816. [CrossRef]
101. Avula, S.K.; Ullah, S.; Ebrahimi, A.; Rostami, A.; Halim, S.A.; Khan, A.; Anwar, M.U.; Gibbons, S.; Csuk, R.; Al-Harrasi, A. Dihydrofolate reductase inhibitory potential of 1H-indole-based-meldrum linked 1H-1,2,3-triazoles as new anticancer derivatives: *In-vitro* and in-silico studies. *Eur. J. Med. Chem.* **2025**, *283*, 117174. [CrossRef]
102. Tite, T.; Sabbah, M.; Levacher, V.; Brière, J.-F. Organocatalysed decarboxylative protonation process from Meldrum's acid: Enantioselective synthesis of isoxazolidinones. *Chem. Commun.* **2013**, *49*, 11569–11571. [CrossRef]
103. Engl, O.D.; Saadi, J.; Cosimi, E.; Wennemers, H. Synthesis of Monothiomalonates – Versatile Thioester Enolate Equivalents for C–C Bond Formations. *Helv. Chim. Acta* **2017**, *100*, e1700196. [CrossRef]
104. Brown, R.F.C.; Eastwood, F.W.; Harrington, K.J. Methyleneketenes and Methylenecarbenes. I Formation of Arylmethyleneketenes and Alkylideneketenes by Pyrolysis of Substituted 2,2-Dimethyl-1,3-dioxan-4,6-diones. *Aust. J. Chem.* **1974**, *27*, 2373–2384. [CrossRef]
105. Baxter, G.J.; Brown, R.F.C.; Eastwood, F.W.; Harrington, K.J. Pyrolytic generation of carbonylcyclopropane (dimethylene ketene) and its dimerization to dispiro-[2,1,2,1]-octane-4,8-dione. *Tetrahedron Lett.* **1975**, *16*, 4283–4284. [CrossRef]
106. Leibfarth, F.A.; Kang, M.; Ham, M.; Kim, J.; Campos, L.M.; Gupta, N.; Moon, B.; Hawker, C.J. A facile route to ketene-functionalized polymers for general materials applications. *Nat. Chem.* **2010**, *2*, 207–212. [CrossRef]
107. Leibfarth, F.A.; Wolffs, M.; Campos, L.M.; Delany, K.; Treat, N.; Kade, M.J.; Moon, B.; Hawker, C.J. Low-temperature ketene formation in materials chemistry through molecular engineering. *Chem. Sci.* **2012**, *3*, 766–771. [CrossRef]
108. Armarego, W.L.F.; Perrin, D.D. *Purification of Laboratory Chemicals*, 4th ed.; Butterworth-Heinemann: Oxford, UK, 1997.
109. Sakakura, A.; Kawajiri, K.; Ohkubo, T.; Kosugi, Y.; Ishihara, K. Widely Useful DMAP-Catalyzed Esterification under Auxiliary Base- and Solvent-Free Conditions. *J. Am. Chem. Soc.* **2007**, *129*, 14775–14779. [CrossRef]
110. Mensah, E.; Earl, L. Mild and Highly Efficient Copper(I) Inspired Acylation of Alcohols and Polyols. *Catalysts* **2017**, *7*, 33. [CrossRef]
111. Yang, C.-H.; Fan, W.-W.; Liu, G.-Q.; Duan, L.; Li, L.; Li, Y.-M. On the Understanding of $BF_3 \cdot Et_2O$-Promoted Intra- and Intermolecular Amination and Oxygenation of Unfunctionalized Olefins. *RSC Adv.* **2015**, *5*, 61081–61093. [CrossRef]
112. More, S.-V.; Chang, T.-T.; Chiao, Y.-P.; Jao, S.-C.; Lu, C.-K.; Li., W.-S. Glycosylation enhances the anti-migratory activities of isomalyngamide A analogs. *Eur. J. Med. Chem.* **2013**, *64*, 169–178. [CrossRef]
113. Kawamoto, K.; Zhong, M.; Wang, R.; Olsen, B.D.; Johnson, J.A. Loops versus Branch Functionality in Model Click Hydrogels. *Macromolecules* **2015**, *48*, 8980–8988. [CrossRef]
114. Li, J.-S.; Da, Y.-D.; Chen, G.-Q.; Yang, Q.; Li, Z.-W.; Yang, F.; Huang, P.-M. Solvent-, and Catalyst-Free Acylation of Anilines with Meldrum's Acids: A Neat Access to Anilides. *ChemistrySelect* **2017**, *2*, 1770–1773. [CrossRef]

molecules

MDPI

Article

Ni-Catalyzed [2 + 2 + 2] Cycloaddition via the Capture of Azametallacyclopentadienes with Allyl Boronate: Facile Access to Fused Pyridine Derivatives

Kesi Du [1,†], Tao Zhu [2,†], Guangyu Li [2], Taohong Shi [2], Chunsheng Li [3,*], Siting Hu [3], Ruiran Gao [1], Zhao-Yang Wang [4,*] and Jiuzhong Huang [2,*]

1 Guizhou Provincial Engineering Technology Research Center for Chemical Drug R&D, School of Pharmacy, Guizhou Medical University, Guiyang 550004, China
2 Jiangxi Province Key Laboratory of Pharmacology of Traditional Chinese Medicine, School of Pharmacy, Gannan Medical University, Ganzhou 341000, China
3 School of Environmental and Chemical Engineering, Zhaoqing University, Zhaoqing 526061, China
4 School of Chemistry, South China Normal University, Guangzhou 510006, China
* Correspondence: lichunsheng@zqu.edu.cn (C.L.); wangzy@scnu.edu.cn (Z.-Y.W.); huangjz@gmu.edu.cn (J.H.)
† These authors contributed equally to this work.

Abstract

An unprecedented nickel-catalyzed [2 + 2 + 2] cycloaddition that enables efficient construction of fused pyridine frameworks with allyl boronate was reported. This transformation is proposed to occur through a mechanism involving aza-nickelacyclopentadiene intermediates, wherein the boryl group of the allyl boronate plays a critical role in enabling the following cyclization via the control experiments. This work not only expands the structural diversity accessible via transition-metal-catalyzed [2 + 2 + 2] cycloadditions but also showcases the untapped potential of unsaturated substrates in cycloaddition reactions.

Keywords: [2 + 2 + 2] cycloaddition; nickel catalysis; azanickelcyclopentadiene; allyl boronate; fused pyridine derivatives

1. Introduction

Fused pyridine skeleton represents a privileged scaffold prevalent in numerous heterocyclic compounds and natural products (Figure 1), serving as fundamental structural units in pharmaceuticals, functional materials, and as versatile ligands or catalysts [1–7]. Although significant progress has been made in developing synthetic strategies for pyridine derivatives [8–13], the catalytic construction of densely substituted pyridines remains a formidable challenge in synthetic chemistry.

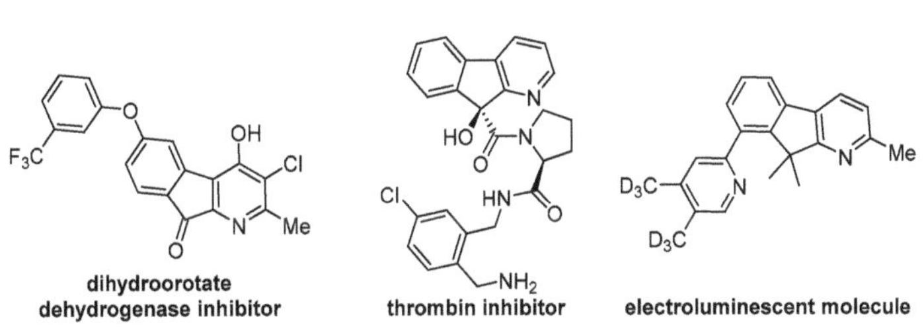

Figure 1. Pyridine-based functional molecules.

De novo synthetic approaches offer distinct advantages for assembling pyridyl cores with diverse substitution patterns from readily accessible building blocks. In this context, transition-metal-catalyzed [2 + 2 + 2] cycloaddition of two alkyne units with a nitrile component has emerged as an atom-economical and versatile strategy for synthesizing six-membered cyclic and aromatic compounds [14–16].

A key intermediate in these transformations is the azametallacyclopentadiene, featuring one M-C(sp^2) and one M-N(sp^2) bond, which forms via metal-mediated oxidative cyclometalation of two triple-bond units [17–19]. Typically, azametallacyclopentadienes subsequently undergo alkyne insertion to afford the final cyclic/aromatic products (Scheme 1I) [20–23]. Considerable efforts have explored diverse catalytic systems based on (aza)metallacyclopentadienes, with successful implementations reported using ruthenium [24], rhodium [25], iridium [26], cobalt [27], iron [28], nickel [29,30], and niobium [31] catalysts [14,15]. For instance, the Liu group reported a Ni/BPh_3 co-catalyzed [2 + 2 + 2] cycloaddition of alkyne-nitriles with internal alkynes, providing an efficient route to fused pyridines (Scheme 1(IIa)) [32]. Recently, Liu and coauthors developed a palladium/copper dual-catalyzed [2 + 2 + 2] cycloaddition of alkyne-tethered malononitriles and alkynes (Scheme 1(IIb)) [33].

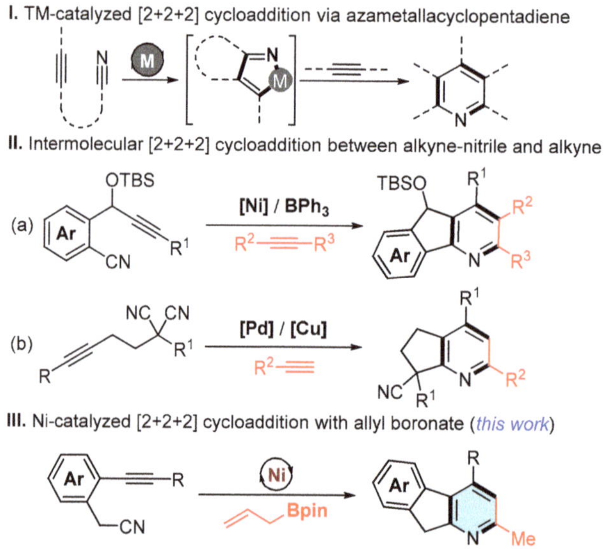

Scheme 1. Background and project synopsis.

Notably, despite the diverse transformations of azametallacyclopentadienes in pyridine synthesis, alkene derivatives remained insurmountable substrates in this process due to subtle electrical property differences with the triple bond. Motivated by our interest in transition-metal-catalyzed transformations of unsaturated hydrocarbons for heterocycle assembly [34–36], we herein report a nickel-catalyzed [2 + 2 + 2] cycloaddition for constructing pyridine scaffolds using allyl boronate as cycloaddition partner (Scheme 1III).

2. Results and Discussion

The [2 + 2 + 2] cycloaddition of an alkyne-nitrile substrate with allyl boronate was investigated using a nickel catalytic system, affording **3a** in 80% isolated yield under optimal conditions (Table 1, entry 1). Firstly, control experiments established that the nickel catalyst, diphosphine ligand, and base were all essential for the conversion (entries

2–4). Replacing $Ni(Ph_3P)_2Cl_2$ with $Ni(acac)_2$ as the catalyst significantly decreased reaction efficiency (entry 5), while other ligands, such as DPEphos, dppp, dppf, and Cy_3P, failed to produce the desired cycloaddition product (entries 6–9). Additionally, performing the transformation with Na_3PO_4 as a base, a very low yield is obtained (entry 10). Reactions in other solvents, particularly polar solvents, resulted in a complex mixture (entries 11–12). On the other hand, performing the reaction under air did not improve the outcome (entry 13), and lower reaction temperatures were detrimental to the [2 + 2 + 2] cycloaddition (entry 14). Therefore, the optimal reaction conditions were identified employing $Ni(PPh_3)_2Cl_2$ as the catalyst, XantPhos as the ligand, and K_3PO_4 as the base in trifluorotoluene.

Table 1. Optimization of the reaction conditions.

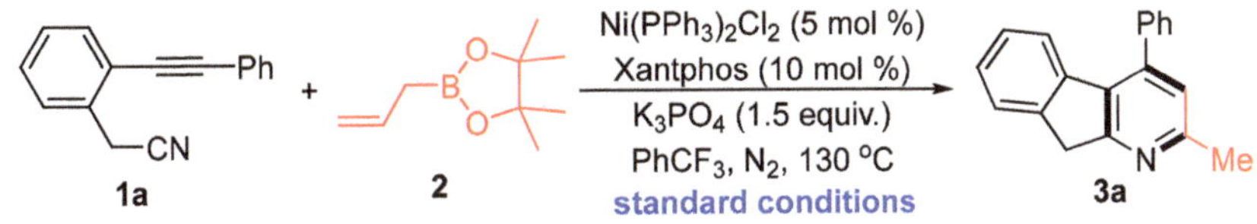

Entry [a]	Variation from Standard Conditions	Yield of 3a [b]
1	none	84% (80%)
2	w/o $Ni(PPh_3)_2Cl_2$	N.R.
3	w/o XantPhos	N.R.
4	w/o K_3PO_4	N.R.
5	$Ni(acac)_2$ instead of $Ni(PPh_3)_2Cl_2$	55%
6	DPEphos instead of XantPhos	30%
7	dppp instead of XantPhos	35%
8	dppf instead of XantPhos	<5%
9	Cy_3P instead of XantPhos	32%
10	Na_3PO_4 instead of K_3PO_4	15%
11	Toluene instead of $PhCF_3$	70%
12	CH_3CN instead of $PhCF_3$	25%
13	under air atmosphere	72%
14	reaction temperature 120 °C	70%

[a] Conditions: **1a** (0.2 mmol), **2** (1.5 equiv), catalyst (5 mol %), ligand (10 mol %), base (1.5 equiv), solvent (2.0 mL) under N_2 atmosphere at 130 °C for 24 h in seal tube; [b] Yields were determined by ^1H NMR with CH_2Br_2 as internal standard, isolated yield is in the parentheses; N.R. = no reaction.

After establishing optimal conditions, the scope of the nickel-catalyzed [2 + 2 + 2] cycloaddition was explored (Scheme 2). Generally, *para*-substituted internal alkynes bearing both electron-donating (Me, OMe, Ph, ^{t}Bu) and electron-withdrawing groups (F, Cl, CF_3, CO_2Me) proved compatible, affording tricyclic derivatives in moderate yields (**3b**–**3i**). The constitution of product **3h** was confirmed by X-ray crystallographic analysis (CCDC: 2474292). *meta*-Substituted substrates (^{t}Bu, OMe, F) also exhibited good reactivity under standard conditions (**3j**–**3l**). Notably, *ortho*-substituted substrates afforded the desired products in lower yields (**3m**–**3o**), indicating steric hindrance influenced reaction efficiency. Significantly, fused pyridine tricyclic derivatives were synthesized from biaryl alkynes bearing diverse substituents (silyl ether, 2-naphthyl, triphenylenyl, thienyl, benzothienyl, etc.), yielding products **3p**–**3v** in moderate yields. Finally, variations in substituents on the acetonitrile-derived phenyl ring were well-tolerated with negligible impact on yields (**3w**–**3y**).

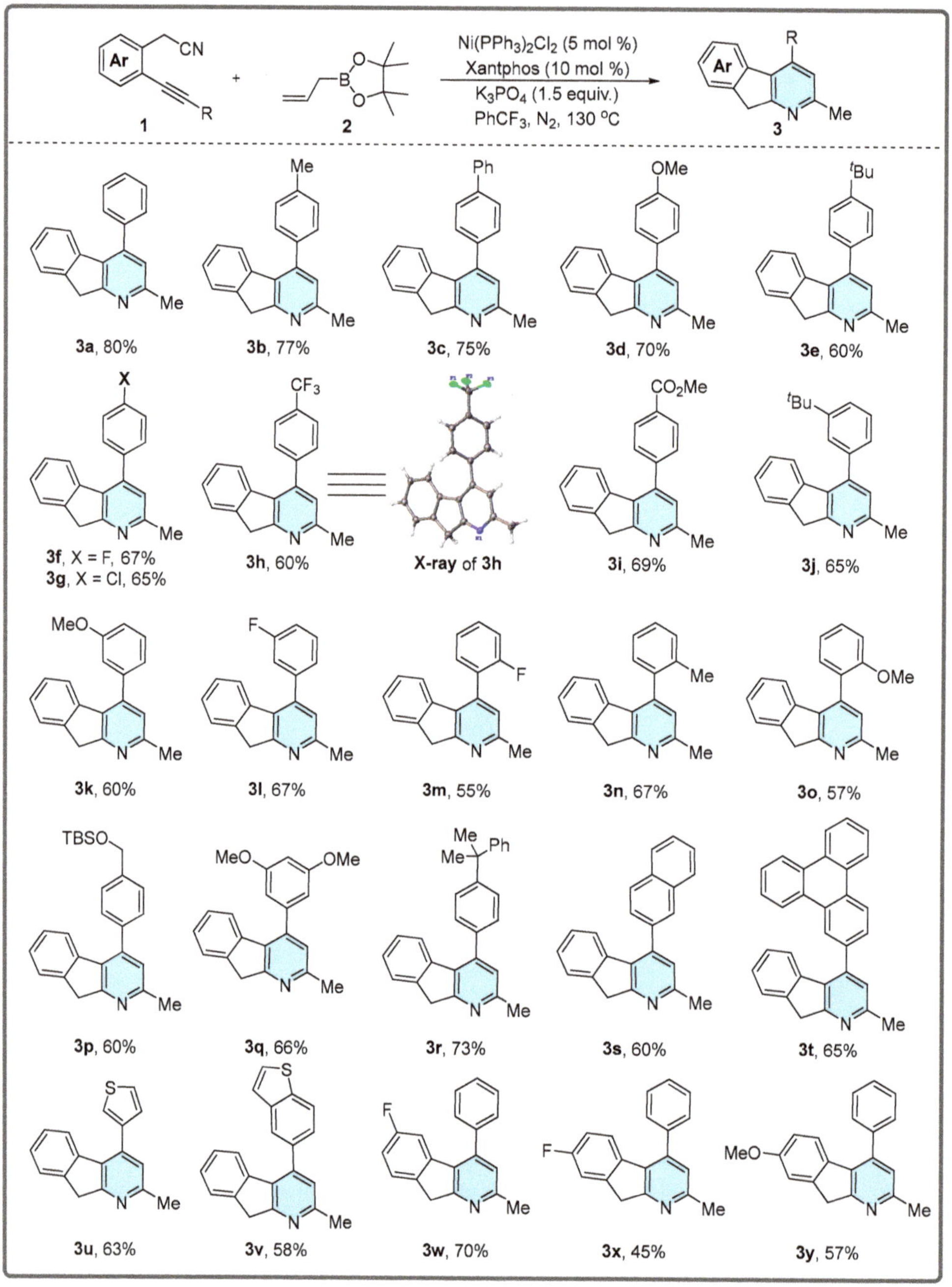

Scheme 2. Substrate scope of the Ni-catalyzed [2 + 2 + 2] cycloaddition. The synthetic utility of this reaction was demonstrated through a gram-scale synthesis and product derivatizations. Compound **3a** was successfully synthesized on a gram scale under the optimized conditions, affording the product in good yield (Scheme 3I). Subsequently, compounds **3a** and **3i** were subjected to a copper-mediated oxidation system, yielding the corresponding oxidative products **4a** and **4i** in moderate to good yields (Scheme 3II).

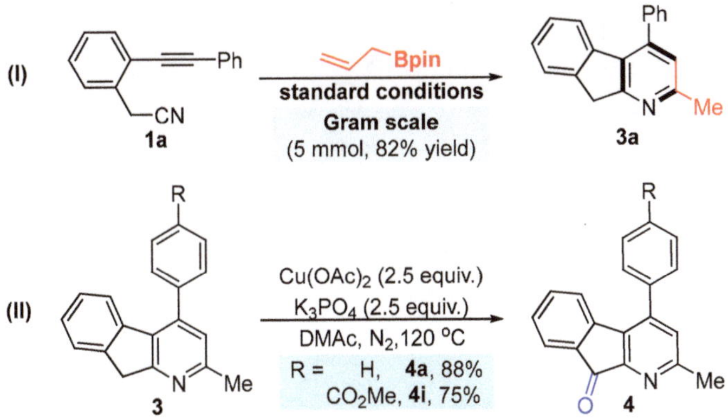

Scheme 3. The gram-scale experiment and synthetic utility.

To gain insight into the reaction mechanism, several control experiments were conducted (Scheme 4). First, various allyl derivatives, such as trifluoroborate, trimethylsilyl, halide, and acetate groups, were used in place of allyl boronate under the standard conditions (Scheme 4I). However, these failed to afford the desired product due to the low conversion of **1a**. Furthermore, crotyl boronate also failed to produce the fused pyridine products **3z** or **3aa** under the optimal conditions (Scheme 4II). These results indicate that both the boronate group and a terminal double bond are essential for the [2 + 2 + 2] cycloaddition.

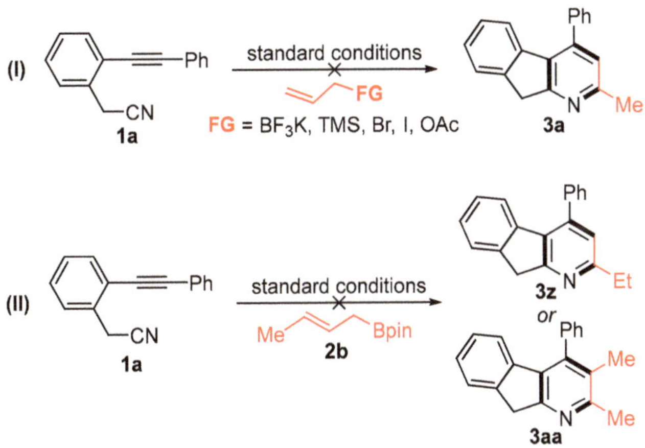

Scheme 4. Control experiments.

Based on experimental results and the previous literature [32,33,37,38], a plausible mechanism is proposed in Scheme 5. Initially, coordination of the substrate's alkyne group to the nickel(0) catalyst forms intermediate **Int-1**. Subsequent oxidative heterocyclometallation then generates azanickelcyclopentadiene intermediate **Int-2**. This species undergoes migration insertion of allyl boronate's double bond, yielding seven-membered aza-nickelacycle **Int-3**. Reductive elimination of **Int-3** releases both the active nickel(0) species and the six-membered framework complex **Int-4**. Finally, Int-4 undergoes base-facilitated olefin isomerization to afford the target product **3a**.

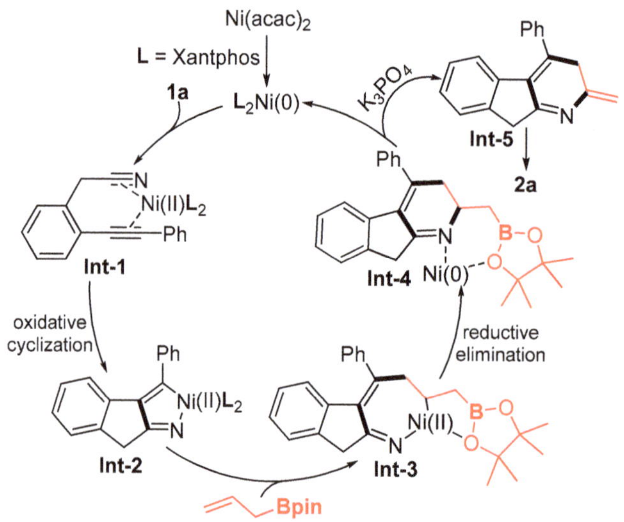

Scheme 5. Plausible mechanistic pathways.

3. Materials and Methods

3.1. Materials

All the reagents were obtained from commercial sources and used directly without further purification, unless otherwise noted. Synthetic methods and spectral data for the start substrates were consistent with the methods and data reported in the studies. ^{1}H NMR, ^{19}F NMR, and ^{13}C NMR spectra were recorded on a Bruker AVANCE III 400 MHz. ^{1}H NMR, ^{19}F NMR, and ^{13}C NMR chemical shifts were determined relative to the internal standard TMS at δ 0.0. Chemical shifts (δ) are reported in ppm, and coupling constants (J) are reported in Hertz (Hz).

3.2. General Methods for the Preparation of Fused Pyridine Derivatives

To a 25 mL oven-dried Schlenk-tube with magnetic stirrer bar, substrate (**1**, 0.2 mmol), $Ni(PPh_3)Cl_2$ (5 mol%), Xantphos (10 mol%), K_3PO_4 (1.5 equiv), allyl boronate (**2**, 1.5 equiv, 0.3 mmol), and $PhCF_3$ (2.0 mL) were successively added and vigorously stirred together in 130 °C oil bath under N_2 atmosphere for 12 h. After the reaction was finished, the mixture was cooled to room temperature. The reaction was quenched with saturated NH_4Cl aq. and extracted with EtOAc (3 × 25 mL). The combined ethyl acetate layer was washed with brine (25 mL) and dried over anhydrous Na_2SO_4. The solvent was removed under vacuum. The crude product was purified by flash column chromatography (eluting with petroleum ether/ethyl acetate) on silica gel to afford the product **3**.

2-methyl-4-phenyl-9H-indeno [2,1-b]pyridine (**3a**): Compound **3a** was prepared according to the general procedure using **1a** with allyl borate **2**. Purification by flash column chromatography (petroleum ether/ethyl acetate = 8/1, *v*/*v*) afforded **3a** as a brown solid, m.p. = 127.4—129.6 °C, 41.1 mg, 80% yield. ^{1}H NMR (400 MHz, $CDCl_3$) δ 7.56—7.46 (m, 6H), 7.26—7.22 (m, 1H), 7.12—7.07 (m, 2H), 7.01 (s, 1H), 4.02 (s, 2H), 2.65 (s, 3H). ^{13}C NMR (101 MHz, $CDCl_3$) δ 164.77, 155.93, 144.92, 141.38, 139.44, 138.83, 129.56, 128.71, 128.43, 128.41, 126.92, 126.55, 125.04, 122.84, 122.69, 38.85, 24.24. HRMS-ESI (*m*/*z*): calcd for $C_{19}H_{15}N$, $[M+H]^+$: 258.1283, found, 258.1302.

2-methyl-4-(p-tolyl)-9H-indeno [2,1-b]pyridine (**3b**): Compound **3b** was prepared according to the general procedure using **1b** with allyl borate **2**. Purification by flash column chromatography (petroleum ether/ethyl acetate = 8/1, *v*/*v*) afforded **3b** as a brown solid, m.p. = 99.2—103.3 °C, 41.7 mg, 77% yield. ^{1}H NMR (400 MHz, CDCl$_3$) δ 7.54 (d, *J* = 7.5 Hz, 1H), 7.38 (d, *J* = 7.9 Hz, 2H), 7.32 (d, *J* = 7.8 Hz, 2H), 7.26—7.23 (m, 1H), 7.17 (d, *J* = 7.6 Hz, 1H), 7.11 (t, *J* = 7.5 Hz, 1H), 6.99 (s, 1H), 4.02 (s, 2H), 2.65 (s, 3H), 2.48 (s, 3H). ^{13}C NMR (101 MHz, CDCl$_3$) δ 164.70, 155.83, 145.09, 141.35, 139.55, 138.27, 135.85, 129.64, 129.38, 128.32, 126.86, 126.51, 125.01, 122.90, 122.83, 38.82, 24.19, 21.40. HRMS-ESI (*m*/*z*): calcd for $C_{20}H_{17}N$, [M+H]$^+$: 272.1439, found, 272.1432.

4-([1,1'-biphenyl]-4-yl)-2-methyl-9H-indeno [2,1-b]pyridine (**3c**): Compound **3c** was prepared according to the general procedure using **1c** with allyl borate **2**. Purification by flash column chromatography (petroleum ether/ethyl acetate = 6/1, *v*/*v*) afforded **3c** as a brown solid, m.p. = 180.1—185.4 °C, 50 mg, 75% yield. ^{1}H NMR (400 MHz, CDCl$_3$) δ 7.79—7.70 (m, 4H), 7.60—7.55 (m, 3H), 7.50 (dd, *J* = 8.4, 6.9 Hz, 2H), 7.43—7.38 (m, 1H), 7.28 (dd, *J* = 7.5, 1.2 Hz, 1H), 7.25—7.22 (m, 1H), 7.15—7.10 (m, 1H), 7.06 (s, 1H), 4.04 (s, 2H), 2.67 (s, 3H). ^{13}C NMR (101 MHz, CDCl$_3$) δ 164.81, 155.92, 144.64, 141.40, 141.25, 140.44, 139.41, 137.70, 129.61, 128.97, 128.95, 127.70, 127.37, 127.16, 127.02, 126.61, 125.10, 122.93, 122.77, 38.84, 24.23. HRMS-ESI (*m*/*z*): calcd for $C_{25}H_{19}N$, [M+H]$^+$: 334.1596, found, 334.1609.

4-(4-methoxyphenyl)-2-methyl-9H-indeno [2,1-b]pyridine (**3d**): Compound **3d** was prepared according to the general procedure using **1d** with allyl borate **2**. Purification by flash column chromatography (petroleum ether/ethyl acetate = 3/1, *v*/*v*) afforded **3d** as brown solid, m.p. = 133.2—135.4 °C, 40.2 mg, 70% yield. ^{1}H NMR (400 MHz, CDCl$_3$) δ 7.57—7.52 (m, 1H), 7.45—7.39 (m, 2H), 7.27 (d, *J* = 1.2 Hz, 1H), 7.24—7.18 (m, 1H), 7.12 (t, *J* = 7.6 Hz, 1H), 7.07—7.03 (m, 2H), 6.99 (s, 1H), 4.02 (s, 2H), 3.92 (s, 3H), 2.65 (s, 3H). ^{3}C NMR (101 MHz, CDCl$_3$) δ 164.72, 159.81, 155.82, 144.81, 141.35, 139.57, 131.07, 129.73, 129.71, 126.86, 126.52, 125.03, 122.90, 122.84, 114.10, 55.40, 38.83, 24.17. HRMS-ESI (*m*/*z*): calcd for $C_{25}H_{19}N$, [M+H]$^+$: 288.1388, found, 288.1388.

4-(4-(tert-butyl)phenyl)-2-methyl-9H-indeno [2,1-b]pyridine (**3e**): Compound **3e** was prepared according to the general procedure using **1e** with allyl borate **2**. Purification by flash column chromatography (petroleum ether/ethyl acetate = 9/1, *v*/*v*) afforded **3e** as a brown solid, m.p. = 120.2-125.4 °C, 37.6 mg, 60% yield. ^{1}H NMR (400 MHz, CDCl$_3$) δ 7.57—7.50 (m, 3H), 7.46—7.40 (m, 2H), 7.26—7.23 (m, 1H), 7.20 (dt, *J* = 7.8, 1.0 Hz, 1H), 7.14—7.10 (m, 1H), 7.01 (s, 1H), 4.02 (s, 2H), 2.64 (s, 3H), 1.42 (s, 9H). ^{13}C NMR (101 MHz, CDCl$_3$) δ 164.72, 155.81, 151.58, 145.05, 141.35, 139.57, 135.77, 129.61, 128.12, 126.86, 126.52, 125.57, 125.00, 122.93, 122.91, 38.84, 34.80, 31.43, 24.17. HRMS-ESI (*m*/*z*): calcd for $C_{23}H_{23}N$, [M+H]$^+$: 314.1909, found, 314.1928.

4-(4-fluorophenyl)-2-methyl-9H-indeno [2,1-b]pyridine (**3f**): Compound **3f** was prepared according to the general procedure using **1f** with allyl borate **2**. Purification by flash column chromatography (petroleum ether/ethyl acetate = 7/1, *v*/*v*) afforded **3f** as a brown solid, m.p. = 159.4—162.2 °C, 36.8 mg, 67% yield. ^{1}H NMR (400 MHz, CDCl$_3$) δ 7.56 (d, *J* = 7.5 Hz, 1H), 7.49—7.44 (m, 2H), 7.29—7.19 (m, 4H), 7.15—7.06 (m, 2H), 6.98 (s, 1H), 4.02 (s, 2H), 2.66 (s, 3H).^{13}C NMR (101 MHz, CDCl$_3$) δ 164.85, 162.88 (d, *J* = 247.8 Hz), 156.01, 143.85, 141.41, 139.25, 134.78, 130.24 (d, *J* = 8.3 Hz), 129.64, 126.84 (d, *J* = 45.5 Hz), 125.16, 122.74, 122.67, 115.90, 115.69, 38.83, 24.22. ^{19}F NMR (377 MHz, CDCl$_3$) δ -113.29. HRMS-ESI (*m*/*z*): calcd for $C_{19}H_{14}FN$, [M+H]$^+$: 276.1189, found, 276.1188.

4-(4-chlorophenyl)-2-methyl-9H-indeno [2,1-b]pyridine (**3g**): Compound **3g** was prepared according to the general procedure using **1g** with allyl borate **2**. Purification by flash column chromatography (petroleum ether/ethyl acetate = 7/1, *v*/*v*) afforded **3g** as a brown solid, m.p. = 133.2—135.4 °C, 37.8 mg, 65% yield. ^{1}H NMR (400 MHz, CDCl$_3$) δ 7.58—7.49 (m, 3H), 7.46—7.42 (m, 2H), 7.29 (dd, *J* = 7.3, 1.5 Hz, 1H), 7.16—7.09 (m, 2H), 6.98 (s, 1H), 4.03 (s, 2H), 2.66 (s, 3H). ^{13}C NMR (101 MHz, CDCl$_3$) δ 164.87, 156.02, 141.41, 139.11, 137.21, 129.88, 129.52, 129.02, 127.16, 126.67, 125.19, 122.72, 122.57, 38.81, 24.21.HRMS-ESI (*m*/*z*): calcd for $C_{19}H_{14}ClN$, [M+H]$^+$: 292.0893, found, 292.0893.

2-methyl-4-(4-(trifluoromethyl)phenyl)-9H-indeno [2,1-b]pyridine (**3h**): Compound **3h** was prepared according to the general procedure using **1h** with allyl borate **2**. Purification by flash column chromatography (petroleum ether/ethyl acetate = 7/1, *v*/*v*) afforded **3h** as a brown solid, m.p. = 139—142 °C, 39 mg, 60% yield. ^{1}H NMR (400 MHz, $CDCl_3$) δ 7.80 (d, *J* = 8.0 Hz, 2H), 7.60 (dd, *J* = 20.3, 7.8 Hz, 3H), 7.31—7.27 (m, 1H), 7.13 (t, *J* = 7.6 Hz, 1H), 7.05—6.97 (m, 2H), 4.05 (s, 2H), 2.68 (s, 3H). ^{13}C NMR (101 MHz, $CDCl_3$) δ 164.99, 156.14, 143.24, 142.50, 141.46, 138.90, 130.81, 129.39, 128.95, 127.31, 126.74, 125.77 (q, *J* = 3.7 Hz), 125.26, 122.62, 122.41, 38.82, 24.22. ^{19}F NMR (377 MHz, $CDCl_3$) δ -62.45. HRMS-ESI (*m*/*z*): calcd for $C_{20}H_{14}F_3N$, $[M+H]^+$: 326.1157, found, 326.1154.

methyl 4-(2-methyl-9H-indeno [2,1-b]pyridin-4-yl)benzoate (**3i**): Compound **3i** was prepared according to the general procedure using **1i** with allyl borate **2**. Purification by flash column chromatography (petroleum ether/ethyl acetate = 2/1, *v*/*v*) afforded **3i** as a brown solid, m.p. = 164.8—168.8 °C, 43.5 mg, 69% yield. ^{1}H NMR (400 MHz, $CDCl_3$) δ 8.23—8.18 (m, 2H), 7.59—7.55 (m, 3H), 7.27 (td, *J* = 7.4, 1.2 Hz, 2H), 7.10 (td, *J* = 7.6, 1.1 Hz, 1H), 7.05—6.99 (m, 2H), 4.04 (s, 2H), 3.99 (s, 3H), 2.67 (s, 3H). ^{13}C NMR (101 MHz, $CDCl_3$) δ 166.84, 164.89, 156.03, 143.76, 143.45, 141.43, 138.99, 130.17, 130.05, 129.39, 128.63, 127.22, 126.69, 125.19, 122.74, 122.30, 52.39, 38.81, 24.21. HRMS-ESI (*m*/*z*): calcd for $C_{21}H_{17}NO_2$, $[M+H]^+$: 316.1338, found, 316.1317.

4-(3-(tert-butyl)phenyl)-2-methyl-9H-indeno [2,1-b]pyridine (**3j**): Compound **3i** was prepared according to the general procedure using **1j** with allyl borate **2**. Purification by flash column chromatography (petroleum ether/ethyl acetate = 8/1, *v*/*v*) afforded **3j** as a brown solid, m.p. = 115.3—118.4 °C, 40.7 mg, 65% yield. ^{1}H NMR (400 MHz, $CDCl_3$) δ 7.57—7.44 (m, 4H), 7.32—7.27 (m, 1H), 7.25 (dd, *J* = 7.3, 1.5 Hz, 1H), 7.15—7.07 (m, 2H), 7.04 (s, 1H), 4.03 (s, 2H), 2.67 (s, 3H), 1.37 (s, 9H). ^{13}C NMR (101 MHz, $CDCl_3$) δ 164.71, 155.85, 151.46, 145.56, 141.37, 139.50, 138.31, 129.63, 128.56, 126.91, 126.45, 125.83, 125.44, 125.27, 125.03, 122.96, 122.78, 38.82, 34.92, 31.36, 24.21. HRMS-ESI (*m*/*z*): calcd for $C_{23}H_{23}N$, $[M+H]^+$: 314.1909, found, 314.1891.

4-(3-methoxyphenyl)-2-methyl-9H-indeno [2,1-b]pyridine (**3k**): Compound **3k** was prepared according to the general procedure using **1k** with allyl borate **2**. Purification by flash column chromatography (petroleum ether/ethyl acetate = 3/1, *v*/*v*) afforded **3k** as a brown solid, m.p. = 119.4—120.2 °C, 34.4 mg, 60% yield. ^{1}H NMR (400 MHz, $CDCl_3$) δ 7.56 (d, *J* = 7.6 Hz, 1H), 7.44 (td, *J* = 7.9, 2.2 Hz, 1H), 7.31—7.24 (m, 2H), 7.17—7.11 (m, 2H), 7.09—7.00 (m, 4H), 4.04 (s, 2H), 3.85 (d, *J* = 2.2 Hz, 3H), 2.67 (d, *J* = 2.2 Hz, 3H). ^{13}C NMR (101 MHz, $CDCl_3$) δ 164.60, 159.76, 155.74, 144.93, 141.34, 140.06, 139.28, 129.86, 129.65, 127.02, 126.62, 125.05, 122.99, 122.65, 120.73, 114.28, 113.61, 55.40, 38.76, 24.12. HRMS-ESI (*m*/*z*): calcd for $C_{20}H_{17}NO$, $[M+H]^+$: 288.1388, found, 288.1388.

4-(3-fluorophenyl)-2-methyl-9H-indeno [2,1-b]pyridine (**3l**): Compound **3l** was prepared according to the general procedure using **1l** with allyl borate **2**. Purification by flash column chromatography (petroleum ether/ethyl acetate = 7/1, *v*/*v*) afforded **3l** as a brown solid, m.p. = 130.2—135.2 °C, 36.9 mg, 67% yield. ^{1}H NMR (400 MHz, $CDCl_3$) δ 7.57 (dt, *J* = 7.5, 1.0 Hz, 1H), 7.53—7.47 (m, 1H), 7.31—7.27 (m, 2H), 7.24—7.18 (m, 2H), 7.16—7.07 (m, 2H), 7.00 (s, 1H), 4.04 (s, 2H), 2.67 (s, 3H). ^{13}C NMR (101 MHz, $CDCl_3$) δ 164.80, 162.85 (d, *J* = 248.0 Hz), 155.94, 143.55, 141.40, 140.84, 138.99, 130.42 (d, *J* = 8.2 Hz), 129.53, 126.95 (d, *J* = 50.2 Hz), 125.17, 124.26 (d, *J* = 2.9 Hz), 122.75, 122.50, 115.68, 115.49 (d, *J* = 5.2 Hz), 115.31, 38.77, 24.14. ^{19}F NMR (377 MHz, $CDCl_3$) δ -112.17. HRMS-ESI (*m*/*z*): calcd for $C_{19}H_{14}FN$, $[M+H]^+$: 276.1189, found, 276.1188.

4-(2-fluorophenyl)-2-methyl-9H-indeno [2,1-b]pyridine (**3m**): Compound **3m** was prepared according to the general procedure using **1m** with allyl borate **2**. Purification by flash column chromatography (petroleum ether/ethyl acetate = 7/1, *v*/*v*) afforded **3m** as a brown solid, m.p. = 158.9—162.4 °C, 30.2 mg, 55% yield. ^{1}H NMR (400 MHz, $CDCl_3$) δ

7.58—7.47 (m, 2H), 7.40 (td, J = 7.4, 1.9 Hz, 1H), 7.34—7.26 (m, 2H), 7.24 (dd, J = 6.0, 1.1 Hz, 1H), 7.13 (td, J = 7.6, 1.1 Hz, 1H), 7.04 (s, 1H), 6.95 (d, J = 7.8 Hz, 1H), 4.04 (d, J = 3.5 Hz, 2H), 2.67 (s, 3H). ^{13}C NMR (101 MHz, $CDCl_3$) δ 164.62, 159.47 (d, J = 247.9 Hz), 155.89, 141.35, 139.27, 138.13, 130.82 (d, J = 3.3 Hz), 130.58, 130.50, 130.47, 126.99 (d, J = 33.3 Hz), 126.25 (d, J = 16.3 Hz), 125.06, 124.57 (d, J = 3.7 Hz), 123.01, 122.28, 116.10 (d, J = 21.5 Hz), 38.79, 24.23. ^{19}F NMR (377 MHz, $CDCl_3$) δ -114.66. HRMS-ESI (m/z): calcd for $C_{19}H_{14}FN$, $[M+H]^+$: 276.1189, found, 276.1188.

2-methyl-4-(o-tolyl)-9H-indeno [2,1-b]pyridine (**3n**): Compound **3n** was prepared according to the general procedure using **1n** with allyl borate **2**. Purification by flash column chromatography (petroleum ether/ethyl acetate = 7/1, v/v) afforded **3n** as a brown solid, m.p. = 138.9—142.4 °C, 36.3 mg, 67% yield. ^{1}H NMR (400 MHz, $CDCl_3$) δ 7.55 (dt, J = 7.5, 1.0 Hz, 1H), 7.44—7.31 (m, 3H), 7.22 (ddd, J = 10.7, 7.5, 1.3 Hz, 3H), 7.08 (td, J = 7.6, 1.1 Hz, 1H), 6.97 (s, 1H), 6.63 (dt, J = 7.8, 0.9 Hz, 1H), 4.04 (d, J = 3.3 Hz, 2H), 2.67 (s, 3H), 2.09 (s, 3H). ^{13}C NMR (101 MHz, $CDCl_3$) δ 164.31, 155.98, 144.41, 141.20, 139.58, 138.23, 135.54, 130.28, 130.22, 128.45, 128.43, 126.94, 126.25, 124.94, 122.42, 122.23, 38.80, 24.27, 19.78. HRMS-ESI (m/z): calcd for $C_{20}H_{17}N$, $[M+H]^+$: 272.1439, found, 272.1432.

4-(2-methoxyphenyl)-2-methyl-9H-indeno [2,1-b]pyridine (**3o**): Compound **3o** was prepared according to the general procedure using **1o** with allyl borate **2**. Purification by flash column chromatography (petroleum ether/ethyl acetate = 3/1, v/v) afforded **3o** as a brown solid, m.p. = 152.1—153.3 °C, 32.8 mg, 57% yield. ^{1}H NMR (400 MHz, $CDCl_3$) δ 7.55—7.46 (m, 2H), 7.29—7.26 (m, 1H), 7.23 (dd, J = 7.5, 1.2 Hz, 1H), 7.13—7.05 (m, 3H), 7.02 (s, 1H), 6.86 (d, J = 7.8 Hz, 1H), 4.03 (d, J = 6.9 Hz, 2H), 3.69 (s, 3H), 2.66 (s, 3H). ^{13}C NMR (101 MHz, $CDCl_3$) δ 164.02, 156.53, 141.20, 139.88, 130.26, 130.04, 127.49, 126.77, 126.62, 124.82, 123.23, 122.43, 120.97, 110.94, 55.56, 38.72, 24.17. HRMS-ESI (m/z): calcd for $C_{20}H_{17}NO$, $[M+H]^+$: 288.1388, found, 288.1388.

4-(4-(((tert-butyldimethylsilyl)oxy)methyl)phenyl)-2-methyl-9H-indeno.[2,1-b]pyridine (**3p**): Compound **3p** was prepared according to the general procedure using **1p** with allyl borate **2**. Purification by flash column chromatography (petroleum ether/ethyl acetate = 10/1, v/v) afforded **3p** as Brown oil, 48.1 mg, 60% yield. ^{1}H NMR (400 MHz, $CDCl_3$) δ 7.38 (dt, J = 7.5, 1.0 Hz, 1H), 7.33—7.27 (m, 4H), 7.11—7.06 (m, 2H), 6.99—6.89 (m, 2H), 6.84 (s, 1H), 4.71 (s, 2H), 3.86 (s, 2H), 2.49 (s, 3H), 0.82 (s, 9H). ^{13}C NMR (101 MHz, $CDCl_3$) δ 164.69, 155.82, 144.99, 141.82, 141.35, 139.45, 137.36, 129.67, 128.32, 126.91, 126.52, 126.32, 125.01, 122.93, 122.79, 64.82, 38.80, 26.00, 24.17, 18.49, -5.16. HRMS-ESI (m/z): calcd for $C_{26}H_{31}NOSi$, $[M+H]^+$: 402.2253, found, 402.2273.

4-(3,5-dimethoxyphenyl)-2-methyl-9H-indeno [2,1-b]pyridine (**3q**): Compound **3q** was prepared according to the general procedure using **1q** with allyl borate **2**. Purification by flash column chromatography (petroleum ether/ethyl acetate = 2/1, v/v) afforded **3q** as a brown solid, m.p. = 133.4—135.5 °C, 41.9 mg, 66% yield. ^{1}H NMR (400 MHz, $CDCl_3$) δ 7.56 (d, J = 7.5 Hz, 1H), 7.30—7.27 (m, 1H), 7.26—7.21 (m, 1H), 7.15 (t, J = 7.5 Hz, 1H), 7.03 (s, 1H), 6.63—6.58 (m, 3H), 4.03 (s, 2H), 3.83 (s, 6H), 2.66 (s, 3H). ^{13}C NMR (101 MHz, $CDCl_3$) δ 164.68, 160.98, 155.84, 144.86, 141.34, 140.71, 139.28, 129.49, 126.98, 126.66, 125.03, 123.12, 122.40, 106.24, 100.62, 55.54, 38.80, 24.20. HRMS-ESI (m/z): calcd for $C_{21}H_{19}NO_2$, $[M+H]^+$: 318.1494, found, 318.1496.

2-methyl-4-(4-(2-phenylpropan-2-yl)phenyl)-9H-indeno [2,1-b]pyridine (**3r**): Compound **3r** was prepared according to the general procedure using **1r** with allyl borate **2**. Purification by flash column chromatography (petroleum ether/ethyl acetate = 5/1, v/v) afforded **3r** as a brown solid, m.p. = 130.8—131.8 °C, 54.7 mg, 73% yield. ^{1}H NMR (400 MHz, $CDCl_3$) δ 7.55 (d, J = 7.5 Hz, 1H), 7.44—7.35 (m, 4H), 7.33 (d, J = 5.2 Hz, 4H), 7.24—7.20 (m, 1H), 7.19—7.09 (m, 2H), 7.02 (s, 1H), 4.02 (s, 2H), 2.65 (s, 3H), 1.78 (s, 6H). ^{13}C NMR (101 MHz, $CDCl_3$) δ 164.68, 155.79, 151.16, 150.46, 144.98, 141.36, 139.50, 135.98, 129.65, 128.14, 128.11,

127.15, 126.91, 126.86, 126.52, 125.84, 125.04, 122.88, 43.06, 38.82, 30.81, 24.18. HRMS-ESI (*m/z*): calcd for $C_{28}H_{25}N$, $[M+H]^+$: 376.2065, found, 376.2085.

2-methyl-4-(naphthalen-2-yl)-9H-indeno [2,1-b]pyridine (**3s**): Compound **3s** was prepared according to the general procedure using **1s** with allyl borate **2**. Purification by flash column chromatography (petroleum ether/ethyl acetate = 10/1, *v/v*) afforded **3s** as a brown solid, m.p. = 138.0—142.8 °C, 36.8 mg, 60% yield. ^{1}H NMR (400 MHz, $CDCl_3$) δ 8.02—7.95 (m, 3H), 7.93—7.89 (m, 1H), 7.63—7.56 (m, 4H), 7.26 (dd, *J* = 14.7, 1.4 Hz, 2H), 7.14—7.02 (m, 3H), 4.09 (s, 2H), 2.70 (s, 3H). ^{13}C NMR (101 MHz, $CDCl_3$) δ 164.74, 155.86, 141.39, 139.35, 136.24, 133.37, 133.10, 128.40, 128.28, 127.92, 127.43, 127.04, 126.66, 126.64, 126.51, 125.08, 123.02, 122.96, 38.84, 24.20. HRMS-ESI (*m/z*): calcd for $C_{25}H_{17}N$, $[M+H]^+$: 308.1439, found, 308.1460.

2-methyl-4-(triphenylen-2-yl)-9H-indeno [2,1-b]pyridine (**3t**): Compound **3t** was prepared according to the general procedure using **1t** with allyl borate **2**. Purification by flash column chromatography (petroleum ether/ethyl acetate = 5/1, *v/v*) afforded **3t** as a brown solid, m.p. = 143—147 °C, 52.9 mg, 65% yield. ^{1}H NMR (400 MHz, $CDCl_3$) δ 8.90—8.53 (m, 7H), 7.83—7.55 (m, 7H), 7.27—7.15 (m, 4H), 7.02 (t, *J* = 7.7 Hz, 1H), 4.11 (s, 2H), 2.76—2.70 (m, 3H). ^{13}C NMR (101 MHz, $CDCl_3$) δ 164.94, 156.06, 144.90, 141.45, 139.44, 137.48, 130.08, 130.05, 130.03, 129.81, 129.78, 129.55, 129.45, 127.68, 127.66, 127.50, 127.46, 127.43, 127.06, 126.74, 125.14, 123.88, 123.51, 123.48, 123.45, 123.36, 122.88, 122.85, 38.91, 24.30. HRMS-ESI (*m/z*): calcd for $C_{31}H_{21}N$, $[M+H]^+$: 408.1751, found, 408.1765.

2-methyl-4-(thiophen-3-yl)-9H-indeno [2,1-b]pyridine (**3u**): Compound **3u** was prepared according to the general procedure using **1u** with allyl borate **2**. Purification by flash column chromatography (petroleum ether/ethyl acetate = 4/1, *v/v*) afforded **3u** as a brown solid, m.p. = 138.9—142.2 °C, 33.2 mg, 63% yield. ^{1}H NMR (400 MHz, $CDCl_3$) δ 7.58—7.54 (m, 1H), 7.51 (dd, *J* = 4.9, 3.0 Hz, 1H), 7.45 (dd, *J* = 3.0, 1.3 Hz, 1H), 7.30—7.27 (m, 2H), 7.20—7.15 (m, 1H), 7.05 (s, 1H), 4.02 (s, 2H), 2.65 (s, 3H). ^{13}C NMR (101 MHz, $CDCl_3$) δ 141.29, 139.32, 139.10, 128.17, 127.11, 126.73, 126.38, 125.09, 123.81, 122.91, 122.76, 38.74, 24.01. HRMS-ESI (*m/z*): calcd for $C_{17}H_{13}NS$, $[M+H]^+$: 264.0847, found, 264.0823.

4-(benzo[b]thiophen-5-yl)-2-methyl-9H-indeno [2,1-b]pyridine (**3v**): Compound **3v** was prepared according to the general procedure using **1v** with allyl borate **2**. Purification by flash column chromatography (petroleum ether/ethyl acetate = 5/1, *v/v*) afforded **3v** as a brown solid, m.p. = 147.9—150.2 °C, 36.3 mg, 58% yield. ^{1}H NMR (400 MHz, $CDCl_3$) δ 8.02 (d, *J* = 8.1 Hz, 1H), 7.94 (d, *J* = 1.7 Hz, 1H), 7.58—7.54 (m, 2H), 7.47 (dt, *J* = 8.4, 1.6 Hz, 1H), 7.41 (d, *J* = 5.4 Hz, 1H), 7.25 (dd, *J* = 7.4, 1.8 Hz, 1H), 7.08 (dt, *J* = 7.9, 5.4 Hz, 3H), 4.05 (s, 2H), 2.68 (d, *J* = 1.2 Hz, 3H). ^{13}C NMR (101 MHz, $CDCl_3$) δ 164.77, 155.89, 145.02, 141.39, 139.91, 139.77, 139.43, 134.96, 129.80, 127.53, 126.99, 126.59, 125.08, 124.79, 124.09, 123.36, 123.11, 122.90, 122.78, 38.85, 24.24. HRMS-ESI (*m/z*): calcd for $C_{21}H_{15}NS$, $[M+H]^+$: 314.1003, found, 314.1021.

6-fluoro-2-methyl-4-phenyl-9H-indeno [2,1-b]pyridine (**3w**): Compound **3w** was prepared according to the general procedure using **1w** with allyl borate **2**. Purification by flash column chromatography (petroleum ether/ethyl acetate = 7/1, *v/v*) afforded **3w** as a brown solid, m.p. = 120.3—124.5 °C, 38.5 mg, 70% yield. ^{1}H NMR (400 MHz, $CDCl_3$) δ 7.53 (pd, *J* = 4.7, 1.7 Hz, 3H), 7.50—7.44 (m, 3H), 7.03 (s, 1H), 6.97—6.91 (m, 1H), 6.76 (dd, *J* = 9.9, 2.5 Hz, 1H), 3.98 (s, 2H), 2.66 (s, 3H). ^{13}C NMR (101 MHz, $CDCl_3$) δ 165.45, 161.79 (d, *J* = 242.5 Hz), 156.58, 145.29, 141.09 (d, *J* = 9.4 Hz), 138.17, 136.65, 136.62, 129.03, 129.00, 128.88, 128.73, 128.29, 125.92 (d, *J* = 8.9 Hz), 122.80, 113.83 (d, *J* = 23.0 Hz), 109.90 (d, *J* = 24.3 Hz), 38.24, 24.28. ^{19}F NMR (377 MHz, $CDCl_3$) δ -115.19. HRMS-ESI (*m/z*): calcd for $C_{19}H_{14}FN$, $[M+H]^+$: 276.1189, found, 276.1188.

7-fluoro-2-methyl-4-phenyl-9H-indeno [2,1-b]pyridine (**3x**): Compound **3x** was prepared according to the general procedure using **1x** with allyl borate **2**. Purification by flash column chromatography (petroleum ether/ethyl acetate = 6/1, *v*/*v*) afforded **3x** as a brown solid, m.p. = 123.4—125.5 °C, 24.7 mg, 45% yield. ^{1}H NMR (400 MHz, $CDCl_3$) δ 7.58—7.45 (m, 6H), 7.04 (s, 1H), 6.95 (td, *J* = 8.7, 2.5 Hz, 1H), 6.76 (dd, *J* = 9.9, 2.5 Hz, 1H), 3.99 (s, 2H), 2.67 (s, 3H). ^{13}C NMR (101 MHz, $CDCl_3$) δ 165.39, 161.79 (d, *J* = 242.4 Hz), 156.52, 145.36, 141.06 (d, *J* = 9.2 Hz), 138.14, 136.61, 128.89, 128.75, 128.28, 125.93 (d, *J* = 9.1 Hz), 122.86, 113.86 (d, *J* = 22.9 Hz), 109.91 (d, *J* = 24.4 Hz), 38.20, 24.23.^{19}F NMR (377 MHz, $CDCl_3$) δ -115.19. HRMS-ESI (*m*/*z*): calcd for $C_{19}H_{14}FN$, $[M+H]^+$: 276.1189, found, 276.1188.

7-methoxy-2-methyl-4-phenyl-9H-indeno [2,1-b]pyridine (**3y**): Compound **3y** was prepared according to the general procedure using **1y** with allyl borate **2**. Purification by flash column chromatography (petroleum ether/ethyl acetate = 3/1, *v*/*v*) afforded **3y** as a brown solid, m.p. = 117.3—120.5 °C, 32.7 mg, 57% yield. ^{1}H NMR (400 MHz, $CDCl_3$) δ 7.57—7.48 (m, 2H), 7.40 (td, *J* = 7.4, 1.9 Hz, 1H), 7.33—7.27 (m, 2H), 7.26—7.23 (m, 1H), 7.13 (td, *J* = 7.6, 1.1 Hz, 1H), 7.04 (s, 1H), 6.95 (d, *J* = 7.8 Hz, 1H), 4.04 (d, *J* = 3.5 Hz, 2H), 2.67 (s, 3H). ^{13}C NMR (101 MHz, $CDCl_3$) δ 192.69, 164.06, 159.19, 143.31, 138.81, 132.15, 129.83, 128.73, 128.42, 128.40, 123.64, 122.68, 112.81, 110.44, 55.46, 38.88, 23.94. HRMS-ESI (*m*/*z*): calcd for $C_{20}H_{17}NO$, $[M+H]^+$: 288.1388, found, 288.1388.

3.3. General Procedure for the Derivatization of Pyridine Products

To a 25 mL Schlenk tube with a magnetic stirrer bar, substrates (**3**, 0.2 mmol), $Cu(OAc)_2$ (1.5 equiv, 0.3 mmol), K_3PO_4 (2.5 equiv), and DMAc (2.0 mL) were successively added and vigorously stirred together in a 120 °C oil bath under N_2 atmosphere for 8 h. After the reaction was finished, the mixture was cooled to room temperature. The reaction was quenched with saturated NH_4Cl aq. and extracted with EtOAc (3 × 20 mL). The combined ethyl acetate layer was washed with brine (15 mL) and dried over anhydrous Na_2SO_4. The solvent was removed under vacuum. The crude product was purified by flash column chromatography (eluting with petroleum ether/ethyl acetate) on silica gel to afford the product **4**.

2-methyl-4-phenyl-9H-indeno [2,1-b]pyridin-9-one (**4a**): Compound **4a** was prepared according to the general procedure using **3a**. Purification by flash column chromatography (petroleum ether/ethyl acetate = 3/1, *v*/*v*) afforded **4a** as a light yellow solid, m.p. = 116.5—119.5 °C, 47.7 mg, 88% yield. ^{1}H NMR (400 MHz, Chloroform-*d*) δ 7.71 (dd, *J* = 5.7, 3.0 Hz, 1H), 7.57—7.46 (m, 5H), 7.26—7.23 (m, 2H), 7.07 (s, 1H), 6.90 (dd, *J* = 6.4, 2.6 Hz, 1H), 2.66 (s, 3H). ^{13}C NMR (101 MHz, Chloroform-*d*) δ 193.02, 159.49, 153.24, 145.59, 142.21, 137.26, 135.11, 134.70, 132.45, 129.20, 129.11, 128.99, 128.17, 128.05, 124.69, 123.14, 24.12. HRMS-ESI (*m*/*z*): calcd for $C_{19}H_{13}NO$, $[M+H]^+$: 272.1070, found, 272.1061.

methyl 4-(2-methyl-9-oxo-9H-indeno [2,1-b]pyridin-4-yl)benzoate (**4i**): Compound **4i** was prepared according to the general procedure using **3i**. Purification by flash column chromatography (petroleum ether/ethyl acetate = 1/1, *v*/*v*) afforded **4i** as a light yellow solid, m.p. = 112.5—114.5 °C, 49.3 mg, 75% yield. ^{1}H NMR (400 MHz, Chloroform-*d*) δ 8.28—8.17 (m, 2H), 7.73 (d, *J* = 6.6 Hz, 1H), 7.61—7.54 (m, 2H), 7.28 (d, *J* = 9.0 Hz, 2H), 7.08 (s, 1H), 6.84 (d, *J* = 6.8 Hz, 1H), 4.00 (d, *J* = 1.5 Hz, 3H), 2.68 (s, 3H). ^{13}C NMR (101 MHz, Chloroform-*d*) δ 192.69, 166.54, 159.72, 153.34, 144.38, 141.82, 141.80, 135.21, 134.48, 132.44, 130.84, 130.26, 129.47, 128.40, 127.54, 124.87, 123.04, 52.48, 24.15. HRMS-ESI (*m*/*z*): calcd for $C_{21}H_{15}NO_3$, $[M+H]^+$: 330.1125, found, 330 1112.

4. Conclusions

In summary, we have developed a nickel-catalyzed [2 + 2 + 2] cycloaddition of alkynes, nitriles, and allyl boronates using a concise and stable catalytic system. This protocol employs readily available starting materials, enabling the efficient synthesis of fused pyridine derivatives with good functional group compatibility and excellent regioselectivity. Mechanistic studies revealed the essential roles of the terminal double bond and the Bpin group. Collectively, these findings provide fundamental insights into the [2 + 2 + 2] cycloaddition mechanism and the reactivity of azametallacyclopentadienes, thereby opening new avenues for metal-catalyzed cycloadditions of unsaturated compounds.

Supplementary Materials: The following supporting information can be downloaded at: https://www.mdpi.com/article/10.3390/molecules30173629/s1, the X-ray of **3h**, NMR data and spectra of the catalytic products. References [36,37,39–43] are cited in the Supplementary Materials.

Author Contributions: Conceptualization, K.D. and J.H.; methodology, K.D., T.Z. and G.L.; investigation, K.D., T.Z., T.S., S.H. and R.G.; writing—original draft preparation, J.H. and C.L.; writing—review and editing, Z.-Y.W. and C.L.; supervision, Z.-Y.W. and J.H.; project administration, J.H.; funding acquisition, Z.-Y.W., C.L. and J.H. All authors have read and agreed to the published version of the manuscript.

Funding: This research was funded by the National Natural Science Foundation of China (22361003), Guizhou Province Science and Technology Support Program (QKHZC-[2025]YB133), the Jiangxi Provincial Natural Science Foundation (20242BAB25591), Zhaoqing University Innovative Research Team Funding Program (TD202413).

Institutional Review Board Statement: Not applicable.

Informed Consent Statement: Not applicable.

Data Availability Statement: Data are contained within the article and Supplementary Materials.

Conflicts of Interest: The authors declare no conflicts of interest.

References

1. Marshall, C.M.; Federice, J.G.; Bell, C.N.; Cox, P.B.; Njardarson, J.T. An Update on the Nitrogen Heterocycle Compositions and Properties of U.S. FDA Approved Pharmaceuticals (2013–2023). *J. Med. Chem.* **2024**, *67*, 11622–11655. [CrossRef]
2. Guan, A.-Y.; Liu, C.-L.; Sun, X.-F.; Xie, Y.; Wang, M.-A. Discovery of Pyridine-based Agrochemicals by Using Intermediate Derivatization Methods. *Bioorg. Med. Chem.* **2016**, *24*, 342–353. [CrossRef]
3. Desimoni, G.; Faita, G.; Quadrelli, P. Pyridine-2,6-bis-(oxazolines), Helpful Ligands for Asymmetric Catalysts. *Chem. Rev.* **2003**, *103*, 3119–3154. [CrossRef]
4. Gibson, V.C.; Redshaw, C.; Solan, G.A. Bis(imino)pyridines: Surprisingly Reactive Ligands and a Gateway to New Families of Catalysts. *Chem. Rev.* **2007**, *107*, 1745–1776. [CrossRef] [PubMed]
5. Wurz, R.P. Chiral Dialkylaminopyridine Catalysts in Asymmetric Synthesis. *Chem. Rev.* **2007**, *107*, 5570–5595. [CrossRef] [PubMed]
6. Kwong, H.-L.; Yeung, H.-L.; Yeung, C.-T.; Lee, W.-S.; Lee, C.-S.; Wong, W.-L. Chiral Pyridine-containing Ligands in Asymmetric Catalysis. *Coord. Chem. Rev.* **2007**, *251*, 2188–2222. [CrossRef]
7. Yang, G.; Zhang, W. Renaissance of Pyridine-oxazolines as Chiral Ligands for Asymmetric Catalysis. *Chem. Soc. Rev.* **2018**, *47*, 1783–1810. [CrossRef] [PubMed]
8. Hill, M.D. Recent Strategies for the Synthesis of Pyridine Derivatives. *Chem. Eur. J.* **2010**, *16*, 12052–12062. [CrossRef]
9. Gulevich, A.V.; Dudnik, A.S.; Chernyak, N.; Gevorgyan, V. Transition Metal-mediated Synthesis of Monocyclic Aromatic Heterocycles. *Chem. Rev.* **2013**, *113*, 3084–3213. [CrossRef]
10. Allais, C.; Grassot, J.-M.; Rodriguez, J.; Constantieux, T. Metal-free Multicomponent Syntheses of Pyridines. *Chem. Rev.* **2014**, *114*, 10829–10868. [CrossRef]
11. Cao, X.-Y.; Li, Z.-H.; Cao, Z.-H.; Li, Z.; Pang, C.-M.; Zhang, Z.-Q.; Wang, Z.-Y. Multifunctional 3-Cyanopyridine Compounds: Synthesis Based on A Tandem Reaction with 100% Atom Economy and Their Applications. *Green Chem.* **2025**, *27*, 7300–7306. [CrossRef]
12. Zeng, J.; Zhou, T.; Liu, J.; Wan, J.-P. Photocatalytic Pyridine Synthesis with Enaminones and TMEDA under Metal-Free Conditions. *J. Org. Chem.* **2024**, *89*, 11060–11066. [CrossRef]
13. Zhan, J.-L.; Wu, M.-W.; Wei, D.; Wei, B.-Y.; Jiang, Y.; Yu, W.; Han, B. 4-HO-TEMPO-Catalyzed Redox Annulation of Cyclopropanols with Oxime Acetates toward Pyridine Derivatives. *ACS Catal.* **2019**, *9*, 4179–4188. [CrossRef]
14. Roglans, A.; Pla-Quintana, A.; Solà, M. Mechanistic Studies of Transition-Metal-Catalyzed [2 + 2 + 2] Cycloaddition Reactions. *Chem. Rev.* **2021**, *121*, 1894–1979. [CrossRef] [PubMed]

15. Cai, J.; Cen, K.; Shen, W.; Bai, L.-G.; Liu, W.-B. [2 + 2 + 2] Cycloaddition of Nitriles to Enantioenriched and Highly Substituted Pyridines. *Chem. Catal.* **2022**, *2*, 2889–2897. [CrossRef]
16. Domínguez, G.; Pérez-Castells, J. Alkenes in [2 + 2 + 2] Cycloadditions. *Chem. Eur. J.* **2016**, *22*, 6720–6739. [CrossRef]
17. Lv, Z.-J.; Liu, W.; Zhang, W.-X. Progress of Azametallacyclopentadienes in the New Century. *Chem. Eur. J.* **2023**, *29*, e202204079. [CrossRef]
18. Whitehurst, W.G.; Kim, J.; Koenig, S.G.; Chirik, P.J. Three-Component Coupling of Arenes, Ethylene, and Alkynes Catalyzed by a Cationic Bis(phosphine) Cobalt Complex: Intercepting Metallacyclopentenes for C-H Functionalization. *J. Am. Chem. Soc.* **2022**, *144*, 4530–4540. [CrossRef]
19. Ning, C.; Rui, K.-H.; Wei, Y.; Shi, M. Rh(I)-Catalyzed Dimerization of Ene-Vinylidenecyclopropanes for the Construction of Spiro[4,5]decanes and Mechanistic Studies. *Chem. Sci.* **2022**, *13*, 7310–7317. [CrossRef]
20. Peng, J.-H.; Zheng, Y.-Q.; Bai, L.-G.; Liu, W.-B. Chiral Discrimination of Small Substituents in Biaryl Atropisomer Construction: Enantioselective Synthesis of Axially Chiral 1-Azafluorene via Ni-catalyzed [2 + 2 + 2] Cycloaddition. *Sci. China Chem.* **2023**, *66*, 3148–3153. [CrossRef]
21. Huh, D.N.; Cheng, Y.; Frye, C.W.; Egger, D.T.; Tonks, I.A. Multicomponent Syntheses of 5- and 6-Membered Aromatic Heterocycles using Group 4-8 Transition Metal Catalysts. *Chem. Sci.* **2021**, *12*, 9574–9590. [CrossRef]
22. Sheng, J.; Wang, Y.; Su, X.; He, R.; Chen, C. Copper-catalyzed [2 + 2 + 2] Modular Synthesis of Multisubstituted Pyridines: Alkenylation of Nitriles with Vinyliodonium Salts. *Angew. Chem. Int. Ed.* **2017**, *56*, 4824–4828. [CrossRef]
23. Kumar, P.; Prescher, S.; Louie, J. A Serendipitous Discovery: Nickel Catalyst for the Cycloaddition of Diynes with Unactivated Nitriles. *Angew. Chem. Int. Ed.* **2011**, *50*, 10694–10698. [CrossRef] [PubMed]
24. Yamamoto, Y.; Ogawa, R.; Itoh, K. Significant Chemo- and Regioselectivies in the Ru(II)-Catalyzed [2 + 2 + 2] Cycloaddition of 1,6-Diynes with Dicyanides. *J. Am. Chem. Soc.* **2001**, *123*, 6189–6190. [CrossRef] [PubMed]
25. Cioni, P.; Diversi, P.; Ingrosso, G.; Lucherini, A.; Ronca, P. Rhodium-catalyzed Synthesis of Pyridines from Alkynes and Nitriles. *J. Mol. Catal.* **1987**, *40*, 337–357. [CrossRef]
26. Onodera, G.; Shimizu, Y.; Kimura, J.; Kobayashi, J.; Ebihara, Y.; Kondo, K.; Sakata, K.; Takeuchi, R. Iridium-Catalyzed [2 + 2 + 2] Cycloaddition of α,ω-Diynes with Nitriles. *J. Am. Chem. Soc.* **2012**, *134*, 10515–10531. [CrossRef]
27. Wakatsuki, Y.; Yamazaki, H. Cobalt-catalyzed Synthesis of Pyridines from Acetylenes and Nitriles. *Tetrahedron Lett.* **1973**, *14*, 3383–3384. [CrossRef]
28. Schmidt, U.; Zenneck, U. Katalytische Cocyclisierungen von Ethin Mit Nitrilen an Bis(η^2-ethen)(η^6-toluol)eisen als Katalysator. *J. Organomet. Chem.* **1992**, *440*, 187–190. [CrossRef]
29. McCormick, M.M.; Duong, H.A.; Zuo, G.; Louie, J. A Nickel Catalyzed Route to Pyridines. *J. Am. Chem. Soc.* **2005**, *127*, 5030–5031. [CrossRef]
30. Stolley, R.M.; Duong, H.A.; Thomas, D.R.; Louie, J. The Discovery of $[Ni(NHC)RCN]_2$ Species and Their Role as Cycloaddition Catalysts for the Formation of Pyridines. *J. Am. Chem. Soc.* **2012**, *134*, 15154–15162. [CrossRef]
31. Satoh, Y.; Obora, Y. Low-Valent Niobium-Catalyzed Intermolecular [2 + 2 + 2] Cycloaddition of *tert*-Butylacetylene and Arylnitriles to Form 2,3,6-Trisubstituted Pyridine Derivatives. *J. Org. Chem.* **2013**, *78*, 7771–7776. [CrossRef]
32. Mulcahy, S.P.; Varelas, J.G. Three-step Synthesis of an Annulated β-Carboline via Palladium Catalysis. *Tetrahedron Lett.* **2013**, *54*, 6599–6601. [CrossRef] [PubMed]
33. Saliba, B.M.; Khanal, S.; O'Donnell, M.A.; Queenan, K.E.; Song, J.; Gentile, M.R.; Mulcahy, S.P. Parallel Strategies for the Synthesis of Annulated Pyrido[3,4-b]indoles via Rh(I)-and Pd(0)-Catalyzed Cyclotrimerization. *Tetrahedron Lett.* **2018**, *59*, 4311–4314. [CrossRef] [PubMed]
34. Chen, Z.; Nie, B.; Li, X.; Liu, T.; Li, C.; Huang, J. Ligand-controlled Regiodivergent Ni-Catalyzed trans-Hydroboration/Carboboration of Internal Alkynes with B_2pin_2. *Chem. Sci.* **2024**, *15*, 2236–2242. [CrossRef] [PubMed]
35. Chen, W.; Liu, T.; Li, S.; Li, G.; Wu, G.; Gao, Y.; Xu, Z.; Wu, Y.; Peng, X.; Huang, J. Redox-Neutral Nickel-Catalyzed Selective Hydroalkynylation of Internal Alkyne and Its Application in Anticancer Agent Discovery. *Chin. J. Chem.* **2024**, *42*, 3317–3323. [CrossRef]
36. Huang, J.; Yan, W.; Tan, C.; Wu, W.; Jiang, H. Palladium(II)-catalyzed Hydroboration of Alkene with B_2pin_2. *Chem. Comm.* **2018**, *54*, 1770–1773. [CrossRef]
37. Ma, W.; Yu, C.; Chen, T.; Xu, L.; Zhang, W.-X.; Xi, Z. Metallacyclopentadienes: Synthesis, Structure and Reactivity. *Chem. Soc. Rev.* **2017**, *46*, 1160–1192. [CrossRef]
38. Li, M.; Wu, W.; Jiang, H. Recent Advances in Silver-Catalyzed Transformations of Electronically Unbiased Alkenes and Alkyne. *Chem. Cat. Chem.* **2020**, *12*, 5034–5050. [CrossRef]
39. Zhang, N.; Zhang, C.; Hu, X.; Xie, X.; Liu, Y. Nickel-Catalyzed C(sp^3)-H Functionalization of Benzyl Nitriles: Direct Michael Addition to Terminal Vinyl Ketones. *Org. Lett.* **2021**, *23*, 6004–6009. [CrossRef]
40. Chen, X.; He, Q.; Xie, Y.; Yang, C. Palladium(II)-Catalyzed Synthesis of Functionalized Indenones via Oxidation and Cyclization of 2-(2-Arylethynylphenyl)acetonitriles. *Org. Biomol. Chem.* **2013**, *11*, 2582–2585. [CrossRef]

41. Chen, L.L.; Zhang, J.W.; Yang, W.W.; Fu, J.Y.; Zhu, J.Y.; Wang, Y.B. Synthesis of 1-Cyano-3-acylnaphthalenes via Formal [4+2] Benzannulation of 2-(2-Alkynylphenyl)acetonitriles and Alkynones. *J. Org. Chem.* **2019**, *84*, 8090–8099. [CrossRef]
42. Lin, H.S.; Pan, Y.Z.; Tian, Y.H.; Pan, Y.M.; Wang, X. Palladium-Catalyzed Tandem Cyclization of 2-(2 Ethynylphenyl)acetonitriles and Isocyanides: Access to Indeno[2,1-b]pyrroles. *Adv. Synth. Catal.* **2022**, *364*, 1117–1121. [CrossRef]
43. Sedelmeier, J.; Ley, S.V.; Lange, H.; Baxendale, I.R. Pd-EnCat^{TM} TPP30 as a Catalyst for the Generation of Highly Functionalized Aryl- and Alkenyl-Substituted Acetylenes via Microwave-Assisted Sonogashira Type Reactions. *Eur. J. Org. Chem.* **2009**, *26*, 4412–4420. [CrossRef]

MDPI AG
Grosspeteranlage 5
4052 Basel
Switzerland
Tel.: +41 61 683 77 34

Molecules Editorial Office
E-mail: molecules@mdpi.com
www.mdpi.com/journal/molecules

www.ingramcontent.com/pod-product-compliance
Lightning Source LLC
Chambersburg PA
CBHW062059220926
51850CB00010B/2826
* 9 7 8 3 7 2 5 8 5 8 6 1 3 *